Student Workbook to Accompany

Delmar's Comprehensive Medical Assisting
Administrative and Clinical Competencies

WILBURTA (BILLIE) Q. LINDH, CMA
Current Instructor and Former Coordinator,
Medical Assisting Program
Highline Community College
Des Moines, Washington

MARILYN S. POOLER, RN, CMA-C, Med
Professor, Medical Assisting Department
Springfield Technical Community College
Springfield, Massachusetts

CAROL D. TAMPARO, CMA-A, PhD
Coordinator, Medical Assistant and Paralegal
Programs, Highline Community College
Des Moines, Washington

JOANNE U. CERRATO, BS, MT (ASCP), MA
Professor, Department Chairperson, and Program
Director, Clinical Laboratory Science Department
Springfield Technical Community College
Springfield, Massachusetts

Contributors

Lee Ann Chearney
Mary Kay Linge
Anne Pierce
Candace Levy, Ph.D.
Jenny Bolster, RN, CIC
Alison Molumby
Marianne LeVert
Melissa Johnson
Donna Baker, RN
Mary Fahsbender, DO.

Delmar Publishers

I(T)P® an International Thomson Publishing company

Albany • Bonn • Boston • Cincinnati • Detroit • London • Madrid
Melbourne • Mexico City • New York • Pacific Grove • Paris • San Francisco
Singapore • Tokyo • Toronto • Washington

Produced by PublisherStudio

Printed in the United States of America
For more information, contact:

Delmar Publishers
3 Columbia Circle, Box 15015
Albany, New York 12212-5015

International Thomson Publishing Europe
Berkshire House 168-173
High Holborn
London, WC1V 7AA
England

Thomas Nelson Australia
102 Dodds Street
South Melbourne, 3205
Victoria, Australia

Nelson Canada
1120 Birchmount Road
Scarborough, Ontario
Canada, M1K 5G4

International Thomson Editores
Campos Eliseos 385, Piso 7
Col Polanco
11560 Mexico D F Mexico

International Thomson Publishing GmbH
Konigswinterer Strasse 418
53227 Bonn
Germany

International Thomson Publishing Asia
221 Henderson Road
#05-10 Henderson Building
Singapore 0315

International Thomson Publishing—Japan
Hirakawacho Kyowa Building, 3F
2-2-1 Hirakawacho
Chiyoda-ku, Tokyo 102
Japan

3 4 5 6 7 8 9 10 XXX 03 02 01 00 99 98

Library of Congress Card No. 96-45520
ISBN: 0-8273-6765—1

Table of Contents

SECTION I: GENERAL PROCEDURES

Unit 1: Introduction to Medical Assisting and Health Professions

Unit 2: Federal Regulations and Emergency Procedures

Unit 3: The Therapeutic Approach

Unit 4: Responsible Medical Practice

SECTION II ADMINISTRATIVE PROCEDURES

Unit 5:Integrated Administrative Procedures

Unit 6: Managing Facility Finances

SECTION III: CLINICAL PROCEDURES

Unit 7: Integrated Clinical Procedures

Unit 8: Diagnostic Procedures

Unit 9: Laboratory Procedures

SECTION IV: PROFESSIONAL PROCEDURES

Unit 10: Office and Human Resource Management

Unit 11: Entry Into the Profession

To the Learner

This workbook is designed to accompany *Delmar's Comprehensive Medical Assisting: Administrative and Clinical Competencies.* Using the textbook, study guide software, videos, CD-ROM and this workbook will provide you with the most creative and dynamic learning system available. This complete learning package will help reinforce all the essential competencies you will need to enter the field of medical assisting and become a highly skilled professional in today's multiskilled health care environment. In addition the workbook will challenge you to apply basic skills, use critical thinking abilities, and integrate your knowledge effectively.

WORKBOOK ORGANIZATION

Workbook chapters are divided into the following sections: Vocabulary Builder, Learning Review, Investigation Activity, Case Study, Skills Competency Assessments, and Evaluations of Chapter Knowledge.

Vocabulary Builder

Includes exercises designed to put vocabulary into situational or applied contexts and/or to build spelling skills. Exercises range from word scrambles, crossword puzzles, and word searches to matching and fill in the blank. Very often, vocabulary builder exercises will utilize simulation characters to create applied scenarios that put the key term in a situational workplace context that makes the meaning real and requires you to truly understand the term in usage—going beyond just supplying rote definitions.

Learning Review

These exercises cover the basic chapter content, reinforcing and applying your understanding of chapter content. Simulation characters are often used here to bring the information and place it in a working context for you to consider.

Investigation Activity

These activities take the you beyond the classroom walls. The activities include games, role-playing, research activities, self-tests that probe your response to issues related to chapter content (such as reactions to bioethical issues in chapter 10) or ability of certain skills (such as the "how observant are you self-test in chapter 32: Introduction to the Medical Laboratory), therapeutic communication building exercises, (such as the nonverbal skills exercise in chapter 6; the family medical history genogram exercise in chapter 22; the living will form in chapter 10, etc.). These exercises help you develop a set of personal and professional viewpoints and ethical values that will help you build asuccessful career as a medical assistant, recognize health and medical issues faced by patients and in the community.

Case Study

These use simulation characters to apply chapter knowledge in a situational context requiring you to exhibit the proper clinical or administrative knowledge necessary to handle the situation and/or to examine the role of the medical assistant in a variety of situations and contexts.

In general, the workbook has been conceived to give you a creative and interpretive forum to apply your knowledge learned, not simply to repeat it to answer workbook questions. Realistic simulations appear throughout the workbook referencing characters referred to in the textbook, software, CD-ROM and videos. This gives the material a "real world" feel that comes as close as possible to your future experiences in an ambulatory setting. Clinical principles, such as those of infection control, are repeatedly reinforced through simulation exercises that require the ability to use your knowledge effectively and readily.

CHECKLIST SHEETS

By enrolling in a medical assisting program, you have chosen a special goal for yourself. Each step you master takes you closer to your ultimate goal. Remember that the longest journey begins with a single step, the steps you take are the lessons you study and the skills you practice!

This workbook provides two types of worksheets: Evaluation of Chapter Knowledge sheets and Skills Competency Assessment Checklists sheets. These sheets are designed to correlate with specific information and procedures discussed in *Delmar's Comprehensive Medical Assisting: Administrative and Clinical Competencies* textbook.

The Evaluation of Chapter Knowledge sheets are incorporated at the end of each chapter to review theoretical understanding and define competency, while at the same time incorporating essential interpersonal communication and professional skills. The evaluation and grading of these sheets can be done by self-evaluation, by another individual, or by instructor, and are based on a good, average, or poor checklist. If you perform poorly, the instructor may require re-evaluation at a future time.

The Skills Competency Assessment Checklist sheets are designed to set criteria or standards that should be observed while a specific procedure is being performed. They follow the same procedural steps as listed in the textbook. As you perform each procedure, the Evaluation Section of this sheet can be used to judge your performance. The instructor will use this sheet to evaluate your competency in performing this skill. A Skill Tracking sheet is also provided for you on page ix to use as an overview for all competency assessment checklists included in the workbook. This tracking sheet can serve as a table of contents for all checklists, as well as a guide to easily view your performance on the assessment checklists.

The format of the Skills Competency Assessment Checklist sheet is designed to provide specific conditions, standards, skill steps, and evaluation and documentation sections for essential skills necessary for an entry level medical assistant. The Competency Assessment Checklist sheet is organized as follows:

Conditions

These provide clues defining how and when to perform a task. Conditions should be stated in actual terms used in current medical practice. For example, when performing venipuncture, the tourniquet must be removed before removing the needle from the patient's vein.

Standards

Time and accuracy are very good measures of execution and performance. Where appropriate, the time standard pertains to how much time you will be allowed to complete a set of tasks. Accuracy entails how many times the task must be performed and the degree of correctness with which the task must be executed based on the conditions given for each skill. For some laboratory procedures, the exact time required for you to complete the procedure competently will vary according to your preparation and skill, the instructor's requirements, and the equipment and supplies available in the laboratory.

Skill Step Checklist

There are three columns provided for each step of a procedure. The first column includes a checkbox to indicate whether the task step was performed accurately, the second column indicates the point values assigned to each specific task, and the third column defines the specific task. A score for each procedure can easily be determined by dividing the total points earned by the total points possible and multiplying the results by 100). For example, if you earn 110 points out of 125 points possible, your score for that procedure would be:

$110 \div 125 = .88 \qquad .88 \times 100 = 88\%$

Evaluation Summary

This summary includes the actual time you need to complete the specific procedure and will be graded by your evaluator based on your performance of procedural steps and whether standards were met. Your instructor may also provide suggestions for improving your skills which can also be noted in this section.

Documentation

Charting is an extremely valuable part of a performing any medical procedure. This section will assist with hands-on charting exercises based on actual procedures performed. Including charting as a part of every Skill Competency Assessment will help you associate performing a procedure, then immediately charting it—which closely simulates the actual workplace environment.

GENERAL STUDY TIPS

Here are some tips to help you learn more effectively:

- Feel certain that each procedure and concept you master is an important step toward preparing your skills and knowledge for the workplace. The textbook, study guide software, student workbook, and instructor materials have all been coordinated to meet the core objectives. Review the textbook Objectives before you begin to study; they are a road map that will take you to your goal.
- Remember that you are the learner, so you can take credit for your success. The instructor is an important guide on this journey, and the text, workbook, software and clinical experiences are tools, but whether or not you use the tools wisely is ultimately up to you.
- Evaluate yourself and your study habits. Take positive steps toward improving ourself, and avoid habits that could limit your success. For example, do you let family responsibilities or social opportunities interfere with your study? If so, sit down with your family and plan a schedule for study that they will support and to which you will adhere. Find a special place to study that is free from distraction.

Because regulations vary from state to state regarding which procedures can be performed by a medical assistant, it will be important to check specific regulations in your state. A medical assistant should never perform any procedure without being aware of legal responsibilities, correct procedure, and proper authorization.

Enjoy your career in medical assisting!

SKILLS COMPETENCY ASSESSMENT TRACKING SHEET

Procededure No. and Title	Workbook Page No.	Date Assessment Completed & Competency Achieved			
		School Program Date/Initials	Externship Site 1 Date/Initials	Externship Site 2 Date/Initials	Externship Site 3 Date/Initials
EXAMPLE: 21–1 Medical Asepsis Handwash	###	2/23/97 MP	3/15/97 BG	4/20/97	
12–1 Selecting Appropriate Software	124				
12–2 Basic Computer Operations	125				
13–1 Answering Incoming Calls	140				
13–2 Handling Problem Calls	142				
13–3 Placing Outgoing Calls	144				
14–1 Establishing the Appointment Matrix	161				
14–2 Checking In Patients	162				
14–3 Cancellation Procedures	164				
15–1 Steps for Manual Filing with Numeric System	175				
15–2 Steps for Manual Filing with a Subject Filing System	176				
16–1 Preparing and Composing Business Corrrspondence Using All Components	185				
16–2 Addressing Envelopes According to United States Postal Regulations	187				
16–3 Folding Letters for Standard Envelopes	188				
16–4 Preparing Outgoing Mail According to United States Postal Regulations	190				
16–5 Preparing, Sending, and Receiving a Fax	191				
17–1 Preparation for Posting a Day Sheet	203				
17–2 Recording Charges and Payments Requiring a Charge Slip (Patient Visits)	204				
17–3 Receiving a Payment on Account Requiring a Receipt	206				
17–4 Recording Payments Received Through the Mail	207				
17–5 Balancing Day Sheets	208				
17–6 Preparing a Deposit	210				
17–7 Reconciling a Bank Statement	211				
17–8 Balancing Petty Cash	213				
21–1 Medical Aseptic Handwash	247				
21–2 Instrument Sanitzation	249				
21–3 Removing Contaminated Gloves	251				
21–4 Instrument/Equipment Chemical Disinfection or Chemical Sterilization	252				
21–5 Wrapping Instruments for Sterilization in Autoclave	255				
21–6 Steam Sterilization of Instruments (Autoclave)	258				
22–1 Taking a Medical History	267				
23–1 Taking an Oral Temperature Using a Mercury Thermometer	280				

SKILLS COMPETENCY ASSESSMENT TRACKING SHEET (cont'd)

Procededure No. and Title	Workbook Page No.	Date Assessment Completed & Competency Achieved			
		School Program Date/Initials	Externship Site 1 Date/Initials	Externship Site 2 Date/Initials	Externship Site 3 Date/Initials
23–2 Taking an Oral Temperature Using a Disposable Oral Strip	281				
23–3 Taking an Oral Temperature Using a Digital Thermometer	284				
23–4 Obtaining an Aural Temperature Using a Tympanic Thermometer	286				
23–5 Taking a Rectal Temperature Using a Mercury Thermometer	288				
23–6 Taking a Rectal Temperature Using a Digital Thermometer	290				
23–7 Taking an Axillary Temperature	292				
23–8 Taking a Radial Pulse	294				
23–9 Taking an Apical Pulse	296				
23–10 Measuring the Respiration Rate	298				
23–11 Measuring a Blood Pressure	300				
23–12 Measuring Height	302				
23–13 Measuring Adult Weight	304				
24–1 Positioning Patient in the Supine Position	313				
24–2 Positioning Patient in the Dorsal Recumbent Position	314				
24–3 Positioning Patient in the Lithotomy Position	315				
24–4 Positioning Patient in the Fowler's Position	317				
24–5 Positioning Patient in the Knee-Chest Position	318				
24–6 Positioning Patient in Prone Position	320				
24–7 Positioning Patient in the Sims' Position	322				
24–8 Positioning Patient in the Trendelenburg Position	324				
24–9 Assisting with a Complete Physical Examination	326				
25–1 Chemical "Cold" Sterilization	335				
25–2 Applying Sterile Gloves	337				
25–3 Setting Up and Covering a Sterile Field	339				
25–4 Opening Sterile Packages of Instruments and Applying Them to a Sterile Field	341				
25–5 Pouring a Sterile Solution into a Cup on a Sterile Field	343				
25–6 Preparation of Patient Skin for Minor Surgery	345				
25–7 Assisting with Minor Surgery	347				
25–8 Suturing of Laceration or Incision Repair	350				
25–9 Dressing Change	352				
25–10 Suture Removal	354				
25–11 Application of Sterile Adhesive Skin Closure Strips	356				
25–12 Sebaceous Cyst Excision	358				

SKILLS COMPETENCY ASSESSMENT TRACKING SHEET (cont'd)

Procededure No. and Title	Workbook Page No.	Date Assessment Completed & Competency Achieved			
		School Program Date/Initials	Externship Site 1 Date/Initials	Externship Site 2 Date/Initials	Externship Site 3 Date/Initials
25–13 Incision and Drainage of Localized Infections	360				
25–14 Aspiration of Joint Fluid	362				
25–15 Hemorrhoid Thrombectomy	364				
26–1 Transferring Patient from Wheelchair to Examination Table	376				
26–2 Transferring Patient from Examination Table to Wheelchair	378				
26–3 Assisting the Patient to Stand and Walk	380				
26–4 Care of the Falling Patient	382				
26–5 Assisting a Patient to Ambulate with a Walker	384				
26–6 Teaching the Patient to Ambulate with Axillary Crutches	386				
26–7 Assisting a Patient to Ambulate with a Cane	388				
26–8 Range of Motion Exercises, Upper Body	390				
26–9 Range of Motion Exercises, Lower Body	393				
29–1 Administration of Oral Medications	426				
29–2 Administration of Subcutaneous, Intramuscular, and/or Intradermal Injections	428				
29–3 Withdrawing (Aspirating) Medicationfrom a Vial	431				
29–4 Withdrawing (Aspirating) Medication from an Ampule	433				
29–5 Administering a Subcutaneous Injection	435				
29–6 Administering an Intramuscular Injection	437				
29–7 Administering an Intradermal Injection	439				
29–8 Reconstituting a Powder Medication for Administration	441				
29–9 "Z"-Track Intramuscular Injection Technique	443				
30–1 Measuring the Infant: Weight, Height, Head, and Chest Circumference	450				
30–2 Taking an Infant's Rectal Temperature with a Mercury or Digital Thermometer	453				
30–3 Taking an Apical Pulse on an Infant	456				
30–4 Measuring Infant's Respiration Rate	458				
30–5 Obtaining a Urine Specimen from an Infant or Young Child	460				
30–6 Instructing Patient in Self–Breast Examination	462				
30–7 Assisting with Gynecologic or Pelvic Examination and a Papanicolaou (Pap) Test	464				
30–8 Instructing Patient in Testicular Self-Examination	489				

SKILLS COMPETENCY ASSESSMENT TRACKING SHEET (cont'd)

Procededure No. and Title	Workbook Page No.	Date Assessment Completed & Competency Achieved			
		School Program Date/Initials	Externship Site 1 Date/Initials	Externship Site 2 Date/Initials	Externship Site 3 Date/Initials
30–9 Performing a Urinary Catheterization on a Female Patient	468				
30–10 Performing a Urine Drug Screening	471				
30–11 Assisting with Proctosigmoidoscopy	473				
30–12 Fecal Occult Blood Test	476				
30–13 Performing Visual Acuity Testing Using a Snellen Chart	478				
30–14 Measuring Near Visual Acuity	480				
30–15 Performing Color Vision Test Using the Ishihara Plates	482				
30–16 Performing Eye Instillation	484				
30–17 Performing Eye Patch Dressing Application	486				
30–18 Performing Eye Irrigation	488				
30–19 Assisting with Audiometry	490				
30–20 Performing Ear Irrigation	492				
30–21 Performing Ear Instillation	494				
30–22 Assisting with Nasal Examination	496				
30–23 Procedure for Obtaining a Throat Culture	497				
30–24 Performing Nasal Irrigation	499				
30–25 Performing Nasal Instillation	501				
30–26 Obtaining a Sputum Specimen	503				
30–27 Administer Oxygen by Nasal Cannula for Minor Respiratory Distress	505				
30–28 Instructing Patient in Use of Metered Dose Nebulizer	507				
30–29 Assisting with Spirometry	509				
30–30 Assisting with Plaster-of- Paris Cast Application	511				
30–31 Assisting with Cast Removal	513				
30–32 Assisting the Physician during a Lumbar Puncture	515				
30–33 Assistin\g the Physician with a Neurological Screening Examination	518				
31–1 Perform Twelve-Lead Electrocardiogram, Single Channel	527				
31–2 Perform Twelve-Lead Electrocardiogram, Three Channel	531				
31–3 Perform Holter Monitor Application	533				
32–1 Using the Microscope	549				
33–1 Finding a Vein in the Upper Arm	558				
33–2 Venipuncture by Syringe Procedure	560				
33–3 Venipuncture by Evacuated Tube System	563				
33–4 Venipuncture by Butterfly Needle System	566				
34–1 Hemoglobin Determination (Manual Method Using a Spectrophotometer)	575				

SKILLS COMPETENCY ASSESSMENT TRACKING SHEET (cont'd)

Procededure No. and Title	Workbook Page No.	Date Assessment Completed & Competency Achieved			
		School Program Date/Initials	Externship Site 1 Date/Initials	Externship Site 2 Date/Initials	Externship Site 3 Date/Initials
34–2 Hemoglobin Determination (Hemoglobin Analyzer)	578				
34–3 Microhematocrit	580				
34–4 White Blood Cell Count (Unopette Method)	582				
34–5 Red Blood Cell Count (Unopette Method)	585				
34–6 Preparation of a Differential Blood Smear Slide	588				
34–7 Staining a Differential Blood Smear Slide	590				
34–8 Differential Leukocyte Count	592				
34–9 Erythrocyte Sedimentation Rate	594				
35–1 Assessing Urine Volume	607				
35–2 Observing Urine Color	609				
35–3 Observing Urine Clarity	611				
35–4 Using the Refractometer to Measure Specific Gravity	613				
35–5 Performing a Urinalysis Chemical Examination	615				
35–6 Testing for Reducing Sugars	617				
35–7 Microscopic Examination of Urine Sediment	619				
35–8 Performing a Urinalysis	621				
36–1 Preparing a Bacteriological Smear	631				
36–2 Gram Stain	632				
36–3 Ziehl-Neelsen Stain	634				
36–4 Wet Slide and Hanging Drop Slide Preparations	636				
36–5 Specimen Inoculation and Dilution Streaking	638				
36–6 Broth Tube Inoculation	640				
36–7 Deep Inoculation/Slant	642				
37–1 Pregnancy Tests	651				
37–2 Slide Test for Infectious Mononucleosis	654				
37–3 Analyzing Semen	656				
37–4 Obtaining Blood Sample for Phenylketonuria (PKU) Test	658				
37–5 Obtaining Urine Sample for Phenylketonuria (PKU) Test	660				
37–6 Mantoux Test	662				
37–7 Measurement of Blood Glucose Using an Automated Analyzer	664				
37–8 Cholesterol Testing	666				
38–1 Supervise Student Practicum	674				
38–2 Developing and Maintaining a Procedures Manual	676				
39–1 Develop and Maintain a Policy Manual	683				
39–2 Preparing a Job Description	684				
39–3 Interviewing	685				
39–4 Orient and Train Personnel	687				

CHAPTER 1

Medical Assisting as a Profession

PERFORMANCE OBJECTIVES

The medical assistant is a member of a highly skilled team of health care providers, working on a daily basis with physicians, nurses, allied health care professionals, and patients. It is important to display the professionalism that the medical assisting profession requires. Students entering a program of medical assisting education can use this workbook chapter to consider the scope of the medical assistant's duties and strive to cultivate the qualities of a professional medical assistant.

EXERCISES AND ACTIVITIES

Vocabulary Builder

Replace the **highlighted** *words in the following paragraph with the proper key vocabulary terms from the list below.*

accredits
ambulatory care settings
attributes
baccalaureate
certify
competency
compliance
credential
disposition
empathy
facilitates
improvising
integrate
licensed
licensure
litigious
practicums
versatile

The medical assistant is a **multiskilled** ____________________ health care professional who performs many clinical and administrative duties in physicians' offices and **outpatient facilities** ____________________. In today's **lawsuit-prone** ____________________ society, health care consumers are demanding educated, skilled health care professionals. The American Association of Medical Assistants is a national organization that **recognizes qualifying standards for** ____________________ medical assisting education programs and

practical applications of theory ______________________; provides national **proficiency** ______________________ exams that **guarantee** ______________________ the skills of medical assistants at entry job level, earning them the **official credit** ______________________ of CMA; and encourages continuing education. Medical assistants are educated at community, junior and technical colleges, and proprietary schools in programs that are in **agreement** ______________________ with essential guidelines and standards, and they sometimes earn **4-year undergraduate** ______________________ college degrees. The medical assistant must **combine** ______________________ several **characteristics** ______________________ that will enhance a professional appearance and attitude. Several of these include a warm and friendly **temperament** ______________________ that **allows for easy** ______________________ communication, **an insight into another's feelings or emotions** ______________________, and a talent for **performing without previous preparation** ______________________ good solutions to unexpected situations. Medical assistants work with **legally authorized to practice** ______________________ medical and nursing professionals, who have gone through a process of **granting of licenses to practice** ______________________.

Learning Review

1. Name the nine personal attributes of a professional medical assistant. Then, for each attribute, write a sentence that describes how possessing it contributes to better patient care and good relationships with co-workers and employers.

(1) ____

____

____

(2) ____

____

____

(3) ____

____

____

(4) ____

____

____

(5) ____

____

____

(6) ____

____

____

(7) ______________________________

____

____

(8) ______________________________

____

____

(9) ______________________________

____

____

2. Name four reasons why the medical assisting profession has grown to require more formal, skilled education and credentialing for medical assistants.

(1) ______________________________

____

(2) ______________________________

____

(3) ______________________________

____

(4) ______________________________

____

3. To show both health care consumers and other health care professionals that medical assistants are properly educated to handle a wide range of clinical procedures, the AAMA, starting with the June 1998 national certification exam, requires that only graduates of CAAHEP-accredited medical assisting programs are eligible to take the exam. Name the three anticipated benefits of this new requirement.

(1) ______________________________

____

(2) ______________________________

____

(3) ______________________________

____

4. *Circle the two correct responses.* Medical assistants must recertify their credential every five years. The two ways to recertify for the CMA credential are

A. Accumulate approved continuing education hours.
B. Obtain a good recommendation from a physician employer.
C. Become licensed.
D. Retake the certification examination.

5. The U. S. Department of Labor, Bureau of Statistics, lists medical assisting as the fastest growing allied health profession. Name eight settings where medical assistants are usually employed.

(1) ______________________ (5) ______________________

(2) ______________________ (6) ______________________

(3) ______________________ (7) ______________________

(4) ______________________ (8) ______________________

6. *Circle the two correct responses.* The DACUM (Developing *A* Curricul*um*) is a list of competencies compiled by practicing medical assistants. These guidelines are used by medical assisting program directors to develop curricula that ensures

A. Certification.
B. Employment preparedness.
C. Continuing education.
D. High-quality medical assisting education.

7. Medical assistants study a variety of clinical, administrative, and general education courses. Place a "C" next to each clinical course, an "A" next to each administrative course, and a "G" next to each general course listed below.

____ Maintaining medical records	____ Medical law and ethics
____ Coding/insurance claims	____ Scheduling appointments
____ Basic laboratory procedures	____ Anatomy and physiology
____ Patient education	____ Cardiopulmonary resuscitation
____ Assisting with minor surgery	____ Pharmacology

Investigation Activity

Write or call the American Association of Medical Assistants (AAMA) and the American Medical Technologists Association (AMT) to get information about the standards and requirements to become a Certified Medical Assistant (CMA) through AAMA or a Registered Medical Assistant (RMA) through AMT.

1. Fill in the addresses and phone numbers of the organizations below:

American Association of Medical Assistants	American Medical Technologists Association
______________________	______________________
______________________	______________________
______________________	______________________
______________________	______________________
______________________	______________________

2. What is needed to become a member of these organizations? What are the advantages of membership in these organizations?

American Association of Medical Assistants ______________________________

____

____

____

____

American Medical Technologists Association ______________________________

____

____

____

____

CASE STUDIES

Case 1

During your course of studies to become a medical assistant, you volunteer to help out at a multi-doctor urgent care center in the center of a large city to gain some firsthand experience in a professional setting.

Discuss the following issues:

1. What about this opportunity is interesting you to the extent that you want to volunteer in a professional setting?
2. Even though you are a volunteer, why is it important to look and behave like a professional? What does this entail?
3. You work with the CMA on staff who gives you administrative tasks to perform, such as updating patient information. What is important in order for you to perform this work professionally?
4. You ask the CMA if you can be allowed to watch the performance of some basic clinical procedures. The CMA must get permission from the center's office manager and physician and obtain the consent of the patient. Why are these necessary? How are patients' rights effected by your request?
5. After volunteering at the urgent care center for a period of time, you decide to try volunteering in another setting to get a new experience. How are your personal interests and goals important in choosing the right setting? Why are different personal qualities and ambitions needed in each setting; for example, how does a hospital setting differ from a medical laboratory?

Case 2

You are scheduled to go for your yearly complete physical examination. You decide to use this as an opportunity to study an ambulatory care setting.

Consider the following:

1. How is a patient's first impression of the physician's office and staff important in establishing a good relationship between the patient and the health care professionals who work there?

2. What, if anything, would you change about the experience to make it more successful from the patient's point of view?
3. Describe how the CMA at the physician's office interacted with patients. How did the CMA interact with the other health care professionals there? What kind of duties did the CMA perform?

SUPPLEMENTARY RESOURCES

Study Guide Disk: Additional practice exercises for this chapter are available on the Student Guide disk found in the back of the textbook.

Medical Assisting Videos: Appropriate content is available on Delmar's Medical Assisting Videos, 2nd ed., Tape 1, for the following topics:

Your Career as a Medical Assistant
Display Professionalism
Work as a Team Member
Career-Seeking Skills
Examinations and Certification through AAMA
RMA/AMT
Explanation of DACUM
Communication Skills

EVALUATION OF CHAPTER KNOWLEDGE

Evaluate your classroom professionalism. Compare this evaluation to the one provided by your instructor.

	Student Self-Evaluation			Instructor Evaluation		
Skill	*Good*	*Average*	*Poor*	*Good*	*Average*	*Poor*
Attendance/punctuality	_____	_____	_____	_____	_____	_____
Personal appearance	_____	_____	_____	_____	_____	_____
Applies effort	_____	_____	_____	_____	_____	_____
Is self-motivated	_____	_____	_____	_____	_____	_____
Is courteous	_____	_____	_____	_____	_____	_____
Has positive attitude	_____	_____	_____	_____	_____	_____
Completes assignments on time	_____	_____	_____	_____	_____	_____

Student's Initials:_____ Instructor's Initials:_____

Grade: ________

CHAPTER 2

Health Care Settings and the Health Care Team

PERFORMANCE OBJECTIVES

The medical assistant is one member of a dynamic, growing health care industry. As medical settings evolve to meet the challenges of technology and societal needs, the medical assistant represents a vital link in the health care team and is responsible for many duties, both clinical and administrative. Students beginning a course of study to become a medical assistant can use this workbook chapter to understand the medical settings where medical assistants are employed, learn about the shift of the health care industry toward managed care, and discover the wide range of health care professionals the medical assistant comes into contact with in various medical settings.

EXERCISES AND ACTIVITIES

Vocabulary Builder

Match each of the key vocabulary terms listed below to its proper definition.

A. Acupuncture
B. Allied health professionals
C. Ambulatory care settings
D. Fringe benefits
E. Health maintenance organizations (HMOs)
F. Holistic
G. Independent physician association (IPA)
H. Integrative medicine
I. Managed care
J. Managed care operations

1.___ Organizations designed to provide a full range of health care services under one roof, or, more recently, through a network of participating physicians within a defined geographic area.

2.___ Medical care in which physicians and hospitals compete for patients.

3.___ Advantages added to the terms of employment, such as health insurance and vacation time.

4.___ The type of medical practice management in which two or more physicians join together under a legal agreement to share in the total business operations of the practice.

5.___ An independent organization of physicians, whose members agree to treat patients for an agreed-upon fee.

K. Managed competition
L. Partnership
M. Preferred provider organizations (PPOs)
N. Sole proprietorship
O. Triage

6.___ An approach to patient care that considers the needs of the patient as a whole person, including physical, emotional, social, spiritual, and economic areas.
7.___ This kind of medical setting includes environments such as a medical office, an urgent or primary care center, and a managed care organization.
8.___ A solo practice in which one physician holds exclusive rights to all aspects of the medical practice.
9.___ A nontraditional medical approach proving to be effective in treating drug dependency and managing pain that requires insertion of needles at specified sites of the body.
10.___ Organizations in which physicians network to offer discounts to employers and other purchasers of health care.
11.___ Types of organizations that have been formed by demands on the health care industry to curtail costs while still maintaining high standards of patient care.
12.___ Members of the health care team, other than physicians and nurses, who have specific educational backgrounds and a broad array of skills and who perform supportive health care tasks.
13.___ Alternative forms of health care increasingly perceived as complements to traditional health care.
14.___ Determine priorities for medical action and assess patient needs.
15.___ A standard of patient care that seeks to provide quality care while containing costs.

Learning Review

1. How has managed care changed medical settings as the health care profession works to offer high-quality, cost-effective care to patients? What is the medical assistant's role in contributing to the efforts of the health care team in an era of managed care?

___

___

___

___

2. For each of the three forms of medical practice management, list appropriate medical settings. Then describe the patient's experience of care under each form of medical practice management. Note how patient experiences may differ and why this is possible.

Sole Proprietorships:

A. Medical Settings ___

___

___

___

B. Patient Experience ____

____

____

____

Partnerships:

A. Medical Settings ____

____

____

____

____

B. Patient Experience ____

____

____

____

____

Corporations:

A. Medical Settings ____

____

____

____

____

B. Patient Experience ____

____

____

____

____

3. Name three ways in which insurers, providers, and patients are working creatively to meet the challenge of managed care to keep costs down.

(1) ____

____

____

(2) ____

____

____

(3) ____

____

____

4. A. Name six administrative duties of the medical assistant as a member of the health care team.

(1) ____________________ (4) ____________________

(2) ____________________ (5) ____________________

(3) ____________________ (6) ____________________

B. Name five clinical duties of the medical assistant as a member of the health care team.

(1) ____________________

(2) ____________________

(3) ____________________

(4) ____________________

(5) ____________________

5. A. In the medical field, the abbreviation *Dr.* is used and the title *doctor* is addressed to the person qualified by education, training, and licensure to practice medicine. List the medical degree associated with each of the following credentials, and define each specialty.

MD ____________________

DPM ____________________

DC ____________________

ND ____________________

DO ____________________

OD ____________________

DDS ____________________

B. Using a medical dictionary or encyclopedia to help you, define the following six medical and surgical specialists. Study Table 2–1 of your textbook for a complete listing of medical and surgical specialties.

(1) Radiation oncologist ______________________________

____

____

(2) Obstetrician/gynecologist ______________________________

____

____

(3) Neurologist ______________________________

____

____

(4) Gerontologist ______________________________

____

____

(5) Ophthalmologist ______________________________

____

____

(6) Pediatrician ______________________________

____

____

6. Medical assistants are only one of many allied health and other health care professionals who form the health care team. While medical assistants may not work directly with each professional, they are likely to come into contact with many of them through telephone, written, or electronic communication. Work the crossword puzzle on the next page to see how many allied and other health care professionals you can identify.

Allied and Other Health Care Professionals

Clues

Across

1. Applies scientific knowledge and theory to practical clinical problems of respiratory care.
6. Prepares sections of body tissue for examination by a pathologist.
7. RN who, by advanced education and clinical experience, has acquired expert knowledge in a specific medical specialty.
12. Creates visual material designed to facilitate the recording and dissemination of medical, biological, and related knowledge through communication media.
13. Physically and chemically analyzes and cultures urine, blood, and other body fluids and tissues, working under supervision of the physician specialists such as oncologists, pathologists, and hematologists.

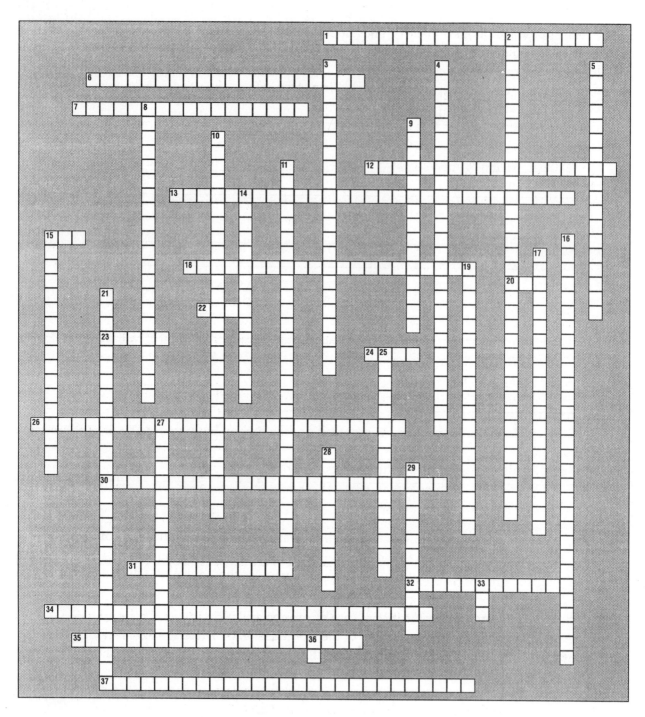

15. Trained to use and apply physical therapy procedures such as exercise and physical agents under the supervision of a physical therapist.
18. Performs nonclinical patient care tasks for the nursing unit of a hospital. Also called unit secretary, administrative specialist, ward clerk or ward secretary.
20. Works under direction of an OT.
22. Administers general respiratory care.
23. A person educated and licensed in the practice of nursing.
24. Recognizes, assesses, and manages medical emergencies of acutely ill or injured patients in prehospital settings, working under the direction of a physician.

26. Assists ophthalmologists to carry out diagnostic and therapeutic procedures.
30. Performs tasks such as airway management during surgery under the supervision of a licensed and qualified anesthesiologist.
31. Draws blood for diagnostic laboratory testing. Also called laboratory liaison technicians.
32. Operates extracorpeal circulation equipment.
34. Provides patient services using medical ultrasound under the supervision of a physician.
35. Educates and trains individuals in the application of purposeful, goal-oriented activity in the evaluation, diagnosis, and/or treatment of loss of the ability to cope with the tasks of living.
37. Assists the nuclear medicine physician to make diagnostic evaluations of the anatomic or physiologic conditions of the body and to provide therapy with unsealed radioactive sources.

Down

2. Possesses the knowledge, attributes, and skills to obtain interpretable recordings of a patient's nervous system functions.
3. Professional trained in basic nursing techniques and direct patient care.
4. Performs diagnostic exams under the direction of a physician in invasive cardiology, noninvasive cardiology, and noninvasive peripheral vascular study.
5. Administers radiation therapy services to patients under the supervision of radiation oncologists.
8. Participates in autopsies and examination, dissection, and processing of tissue specimens; functions as physician extenders.
9. Professionals who have completed a minimum of a two-year course of study at a state-approved school of nursing and passed the National Council Licensure Examination.
10. Develops data on the blood, tissues, and fluids of the human body, using a variety of precision instruments.
11. Processes, maintains, compiles, and reports patient data.
14. Provides services including injury prevention, recognition, immediate care, and treatment rehabilitation after athletic trauma.
15. Licensed professionals who assist in the examination, testing, and treatment of physically disabled or challenged people.
16. Manages health information systems consistent with medical, administrative, ethical, and legal requirements of the health care delivery system.
17. Designs and fits devices for patients.
19. Specialized training in the nutritional care of groups and individuals. This professional must successfully complete an examination of the Commission on Dietetic Registration.
21. Performs all routine tests in a medical laboratory under the direction of a pathologist, physician, medical technologist, or scientist.
25. Functions under the supervision of licensed medical professionals and is competent in both adminstrative/office and clinical/laboratory procedures.
27. Works with pathologists to detect changes in body cells, primarily through microscopic analysis.
28. Licensed by each state to prepare and dispense all types of medications as well as medical supplies related to medication administration.
29. Provides patient services using imaging modalities, as directed by physicians qualified to order and/or perform radiologic procedures.
33. Performs both routine and specialized tests in blood bank immunohematology in technical areas of the modern blood bank and performs transfusion services
36. Practices medicine under the direction and responsible supervision of a doctor of medicine or osteopathy.

7. In an effort to receive holistic, or whole person, care, many health care providers and patients are pursuing integrative medicine as a complement to traditional health care. Name seven alternative forms of health care that may be currently perceived to supplement traditional health care.

(1) ____________________

(2) ____________________

(3) ____________________

(4) ____________________

(5) ____________________

(6) ____________________

(7) ____________________

Investigation Activity

A. Identify a medical setting in your community that fits the definition of each of the three models of medical practice management: sole proprietorship, partnership, and corporation. List each practice, complete with the name, address, and phone number. What criteria must each setting meet in order to fit the definition of its appropriate medical practice management model?

Sole Proprietorship:

Name: ____________________

Address: ____________________

____

____

Phone: ____________________

____

____

____

Partnership:

Name: ____________________

Address: ____________________

____

____

Phone: ____________________

____

____

____

Corporation:

Name: ______________________________

Address: ______________________________

____

____

Phone: ______________________________

____

____

____

B. List five questions that could be used on a questionnaire to gather data about medical practices. For example, "Which services does your practice provide on site to patients?" and "Which kinds of insurance are accepted by your practice?"

(1) ______________________________

____

____

____

(2) ______________________________

____

____

____

(3) ______________________________

____

____

____

(4) ______________________________

____

____

____

(5) ______________________________

____

____

____

CASE STUDIES

In each of the following scenarios, consider the following: 1. How can the patients be encouraged to consider themselves as a part of the health care team? and 2. What is the role of the medical assistant?

Abigail Johnson is an older woman in her seventies with mature-onset diabetes. She is having trouble managing her diet; she lives alone but craves social contact and seems to enjoy her visits to the family physician's office.

Herb Fowler is an African-American man in his early fifties. Herb is a heavy smoker, is significantly overweight, and has a chronic cough. He feels the cough is due to bronchitis and stubbornly insists on being prescribed antibiotics.

Juanita Hansen is a single mother in her mid-twenties with one son, Henry. Juanita arrives at the urgent care clinic for the fourth time in a month. Henry has fallen twice, suffered a burn on the hand, and is now refusing to eat.

Lenore McDonell is a disabled woman in her early thirties who lives independently, with the aid of a motorized wheelchair. Lenore functions well in her home environment, but has grown fearful of venturing out—even to the physician's office for her routine follow-up examinations. She has canceled three appointments in a row.

SUPPLEMENTARY RESOURCES

Student Guide Disks: Additional practice exercises for this chapter are available on the Study Guide disk found in the back of the textbook.

Medical Assisting Videos: Appropriate content is available on Delmar's Medical Assisting Videos, 2nd ed., Tape 1, for the following topics:

Your Career as a Medical Assistant
Display Professionalism
Work as a Team Member
Career-Seeking Skills
Communication Skills

EVALUATION OF CHAPTER KNOWLEDGE

Skills achieved:

Skills	Instructor Evaluation *Good*	 *Average*	 *Poor*
Understanding of managed care	_____	_____	_____
Ability to distinguish medical management models	_____	_____	_____
Empathy with patient experience of medical settings	_____	_____	_____
Ability to identify members of health care team	_____	_____	_____
Respect for professionalism	_____	_____	_____
Understanding of medical assistant's role	_____	_____	_____

Student's Initials:____ Instructor's Initials:____

Grade: _______

CHAPTER 3

History of Medicine

PERFORMANCE OBJECTIVES

The medical assistant is a part of the constantly evolving history of medicine. Medicine developed from the contributions of individuals from various cultures throughout history who held many different theories and attitudes about medicine and the treatment of patients. So, too, today, the advances made in medicine continue to be shaped by more than one discipline or philosophy of care and treatment. Students of medical assisting can use this workbook chapter to discover the rich history of medicine and to think about the medical assistant's role in the future of medicine and health care.

EXERCISE AND ACTIVITIES

Vocabulary Builder

Fill in the blanks with the correct key vocabulary term.

acupuncture	malaria	septicemia
allopathic	moxibustion	typhus
asepsis	pharmacopoeias	yellow fever
bubonic plague	pluralistic	

1. In our ______________________________ society, we rely on several philosophies of medicine that serve an individual's needs by respecting ethnic, cultural, and religious traditions while providing the best standard of care to patients and their families.
2. ______________________________ is an ancient Chinese technique that requires the use of a powdered plant substance that is made into a small mound on the patient's skin and then burned, usually leaving a blister.

3. The piercing of the skin by long needles into any of 365 points along twelve meridians that transverse the body and transmit an active life force called *chi'i* is the practice of ______________________________, an ancient Chinese technique thought by many today to be effective in the treatment of chronic pain.
4. The fact that bacteria can enter the bloodstream to cause infection , ________________________, was observed in the nineteenth century by Hungarian physician and obstetrician Ignaz Phillipp Semmeweis. He proved that physicians who came from an autopsy directly to the care of postpartum women, without scrubbing their hands and washing instruments, carried infection with them that often caused puerperal fever and death to new mothers.
5. In the twentieth century, the discovery of antibiotics, the development of vaccines, and the institution of proper health and sanitation measures have largely contributed to the containment of many infectious diseases, including ____________________, ____________________, and ____________________. However, new, drug-resistant strains of tuberculosis, ____________________, and other diseases are not responding to known treatments, presenting medical researchers with new challenges for the twenty-first century.
6. Homeopathic physicians treat illness and disease by nonsurgical methods using small doses of medicine, based on the theory that "like cures like." ____________________ physicians treat illness and disease with medical and surgical interventions intended to alleviate the condition or effect a cure.
7. World cultures throughout history have compiled unique____________________________: books describing drugs and their preparation that detail plant, animal, and mineral substances as essential ingredients in effecting cures.
8. In the nineteenth century, ____________________, the process of sterilizing surgical environments to discourage the growth of bacteria, and anesthesia, the process of alleviating pain during surgery, revolutionized surgical practices throughout the world.

Learning Review

1. A. Religion, magic, and science all play a vital part in the history of medicine. Why?

Religion ____

____

____

Magic ____

____

____

Science ____

____

____

B. For each of the following, write an "R" if belief in religion, an "M" if belief in magic, or an "S" if belief in science underlies the treatment or practice.

____ 1. A recent research study involved two groups of AIDS patients: one group received daily prayers from an anonymous prayer group hundreds of miles away, the other received no prayers. The group receiving the prayers responded better to treatment.

____ 2. Trephination was used by prehistoric cultures to release evil spirits responsible for illness.

____ 3. Chinese acupuncture techniques are used to control pain or treat drug dependency.

____ 4. Botanicals are effective in treating certain conditions. The Chinese pharmacopoeia is rich in the use of herbs.

____ 5. Some Native Americans believe that someone recovering from a serious illness might hold extraordinary powers.

____ 6. Some physicians throughout history have held to the belief that healing involves not just medical treatment, but attention to the purity of the patient's soul and an attention to the faith of the individual.

2. Name the five methods of treatment important to the practice of medicine according to ancient Chinese tradition. How are these methods relevant for allopathic physicians today?

(1) ____

____

(2) ____

____

(3) ____

____

(4) ____

____

(5) ____

____

3. Individual cultures and peoples throughout history have conferred different, and often changing, status to women in medicine. For each of the five cultures, describe the status of women in medicine.

Primitive Societies ____________________

Chinese ____________________

Muslim ____________________

Italian ____________________

American ____________________

4. Trace the progression of medical education by listing the important advances, discoveries, or medical philosophies for each period or century listed. What do you expect for the twenty-first century?

Prehistoric Times ____________________

Ancient Times ____________________

Seventh Century ______________________________

Ninth Century ______________________________

Renaissance ______________________________

Nineteenth Century ______________________________

Twentieth Century ______________________________

Twenty-first Century ______________________________

5. Attitudes toward illness have changed throughout the history of medicine and also often differ between cultures. For each situation listed, give both historical and current attitudes toward the sick person; discuss how attitudes toward illness may, or may not, have changed through history.

A. Elderly and infirm people are encouraged to end their own lives or are outcast from society.

____

____

____

B. Individuals with a frightening illness, for which there is no cure, are shunned or quarantined.

____

____

____

C. Sickness is seen as a moral or spiritual failing of an individual.

____

____

____

D. Survivors of illness are viewed as heroic individuals.

____

____

____

E. People with disabilities are valued as individuals and receive care that allows them to function in mainstream society.

____

____

____

6. Name twelve infectious and/or epidemic diseases that have been controlled in the twentieth century through medical advances and discoveries like antibiotics, vaccines, asepsis, and insulin.

(1) ____________ (6) ____________ (11) ____________

(2) ____________ (7) ____________ (12) ____________

(3) ____________ (8) ____________

(4) ____________ (9) ____________

(5) ____________ (10) ____________

7. The Hippocratic Oath, originated in ancient Greece, embodied within it many ethical standards of treatment and care that physicians espouse even today. List, in contemporary layperson's language, the five basic standards contained in the oath:

(1) ____

(2) ____

(3) ____

(4) ______________________________

(5) ______________________________

8. *Match each individual to their contribution to the history of medicine. In the space following each name, fill in the century in which the individual lived.*

____ 1. Andreas Vesalius ______

____ 2. Sir Alexander Fleming ______

____ 3. W. T. G. Morton ______

____ 4. Moses ______

____ 5. Edward Jenner ______

____ 6. Clark Baron ______

____ 7. Louis Pasteur ______

____ 8. Elizabeth Blackwell ______

____ 9. Hippocrates ______

____ 10. René Laënnec ______

____ 11. Robert Koch ______

____ 12. Florence Nightingale ______

____ 13. Anton van Leeuwenhoek ______

____ 14. Wilhelm Roetgen ______

____ 15. John Hunter ______

____ 16. Elizabeth G. Anderson ______

____ 17. Leonardo da Vinci ______

____ 18. Joseph Lister ______

____ 19. Jonas Salk ______

____ 20. Frederick G. Banting ______

A. Developed a vaccine for poliomyelitis

B. Father of Medicine

C. Developed smallpox vaccine

D. Discovered penicillin

E. Father of Bacteriology

F. Advocate of health rules in Hebrew religion

G. Invented the stethoscope

H. First female physician in the United States

I. Rendered accurate anatomical drawings of body systems

J. Wrote first anatomical studies

K. Laid the ground work on asepsis

L. Started American Red Cross

M. Founder of modern nursing

N. Introduced ether as anesthetic

O. Discovered lens magnification

P. Discovered Xrays

Q. Founder of scientific surgery

R. Developed culture-plate method

S. Discovered insulin

T. First female physician in Britain

Investigation Activity

A. Make a list of the various ethnic, religious, and cultural groups you and your family members participate in, or are descended from.

B. Interview family members to determine how their ethnic, religious, or cultural beliefs impact the kind of medical care and treatment they expect to receive and how attitudes may have changed or evolved from generation to generation. Write a brief summary of your family's beliefs.

C. Write down any folk or home remedies used by your parents or grandparents that may or may not still be used by your family today. Why might these remedies have been more widely relied upon by previous generations? Is there a scientific basis for each remedy?

CASE STUDY

When fifty-two-year-old Margaret Thomas, Martin Gordon's younger sister, begins to experience mild hand tremors and balance problems, Martin suggests that Margaret go see Dr. Winston Lewis, Martin's primary care physician assisting in the treatment of his prostate cancer. Feeling more comfortable with a female physician, Margaret chooses to make an appointment with Dr. Lewis's associate in the group practice, Dr. Elizabeth King. On the day of the examination, she brings her twenty-five-year-old daughter with her to the physician's office.

After taking a detailed patient history and undertaking a thorough physical examination of Margaret Thomas, Dr. King makes note of signs and symptoms, including a resting tremor, shuffling gait, muscle rigidity, and difficulty in swallowing and speaking. Margaret also complains of a "hot feeling" and odd, uncharacteristic moments of defective judgment when "she just can't keep things straight." Dr. King suspects Parkinson's disease and tells Margaret and her daughter that she'd like to refer Margaret to a neurologist for more specific examination and medical tests. Dr. King explains that there are effective drug therapies for controlling the disease, although it has no known cure, and that the neurologist will outline Margaret's treatment options if a diagnosis of Parkinson's is made. Margaret seems to be shaken, but takes Dr. King's words in stride.

Dr. King leaves Margaret and her daughter in the examination room with Audrey Jones, CMA, who has assisted Dr. King throughout the examination and asks Audrey to be sure to give Mrs. Thomas the referral to the neurologist. Margaret's daughter asks Audrey if Parkinson's is the disease that has shown promise in fetal tissue research, and if her mother might be a candidate. Before Audrey can answer, Margaret becomes visibly distressed. "We're a good Catholic family, I could never consider that. Me, a grandmother." Looking to Audrey, she adds, "Please tell me I won't be involved with such a thing."

Discuss the following:

1. What part does the role of women in medicine and in society play in this situation?
2. How should medical assistant Audrey Jones reply to Mrs. Thomas and her daughter? What course of action, if any, should she take?
3. How do religious beliefs impact the attitude toward illness held by the patient? How might these beliefs affect a treatment plan?
4. Discuss the issues that arise when a potential medical breakthrough involves controversial or radical ideas that challenge long-held cultural viewpoints and beliefs.

SUPPLEMENTAL RESOURCES

Student Guide Disk: Additional practice exercises for this chapter are available on the Study Guide disk found in the back of the textbook.

Medical Assisting Videos: Appropriate content is available on Delmar's Medical Assisting Videos, 2nd ed., Tape 1, for the following topics:

Your Career as a Medical Assistant
Display Professionalism
Work as a Team Member
Career-Seeking Skills
Communication Skills

EVALUATION OF CHAPTER KNOWLEDGE

Skills achieved:

Skills	Instructor Evaluation *Good*	*Average*	*Poor*
Sensitivity to cultural, ethnic, or religious beliefs of others	_____	_____	_____
Understanding of the importance of mutual respect in physician-patient relationship	_____	_____	_____
Ability to identify attitudes toward illness	_____	_____	_____
Ability to trace major discoveries and contributions to history of medicine	_____	_____	_____
Recognizes major figures of medical history	_____	_____	_____
Shows patience and open-mindedness toward others	_____	_____	_____
Ability to describe the role of the medical assistant in the future of medicine	_____	_____	_____

Student's Initials:____ Instructor's Initials:____

Grade: _______

CHAPTER 4

Federal Regulations and Guidelines

PERFORMANCE OBJECTIVES

While treating patients in the medical facility, health care professionals, including medical assistants, come into contact with blood and body fluids that may be highly infectious. To protect patients and health care providers from infection, medical asepsis or infection control measures are practiced to prevent and/or limit the spread of infection. State and federal agencies such as the Centers for Disease Control and Prevention (CDC), the Clinical Laboratory Amendments of 1988 (CLIA '88), and the Occupational Safety and Health Administration (OSHA) establish guidelines and regulations for health care providers and employers to follow in order to reduce the risk of transmission of infectious diseases. Medical assistants must understand the regulations set forth by these government agencies and implement them in the ambulatory care setting for the health and safety of patients and health care professionals. Medical assistants should practice standard and universal precautions, guidelines designed to protect all health care providers, patients, and visitors from a wide range of communicable diseases, with meticulous care to reduce the risk of spreading infection in the ambulatory care setting.

EXERCISES AND ACTIVITIES

Vocabulary Builder

A. Solve the crossword puzzle on the following page to identify key vocabulary terms that are used in relation to federal guidelines and regulations set to safeguard both patients and health care professionals and to reduce the risk of transmission of infectious diseases.

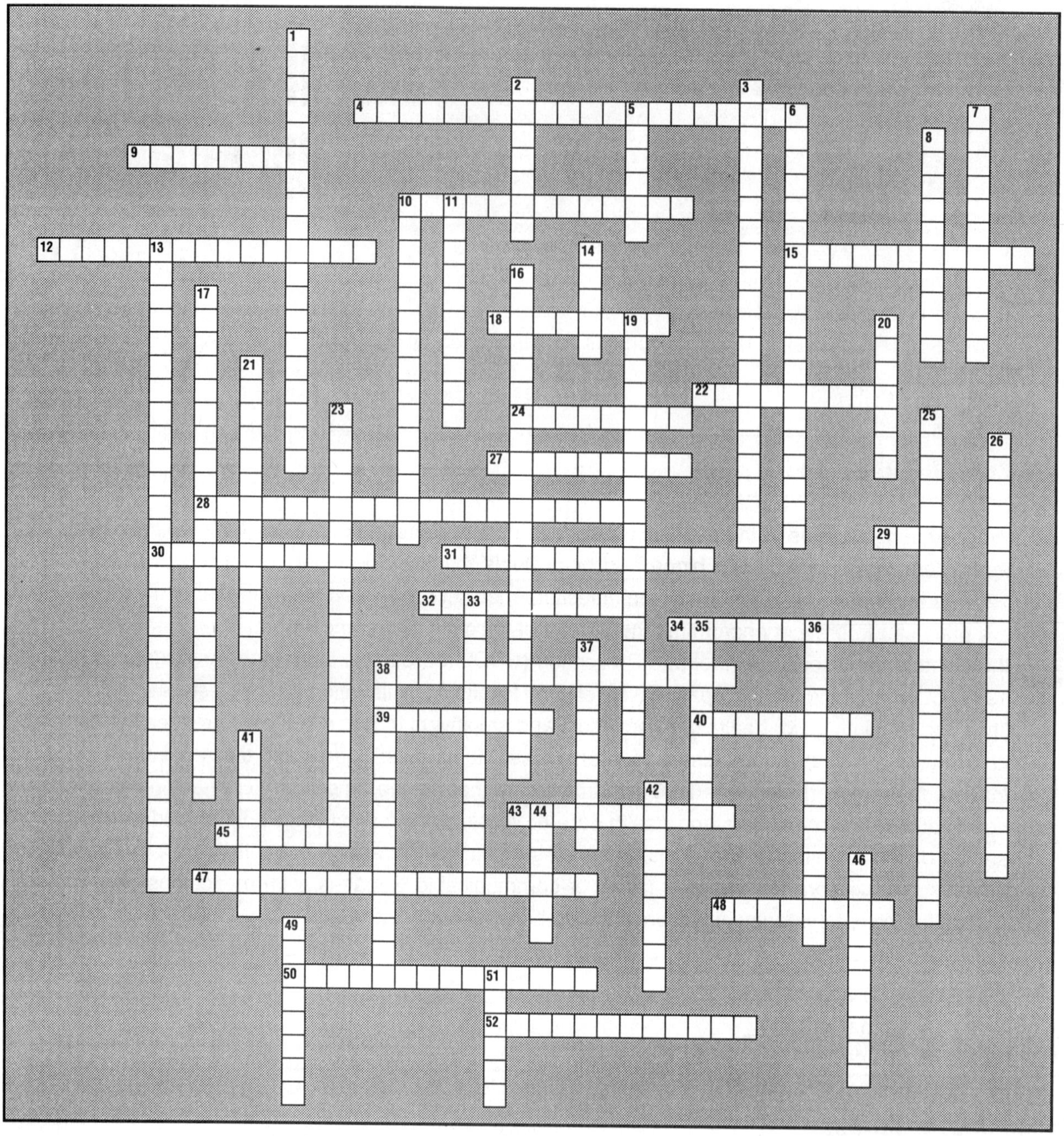

CLUES

Across

4. Guidelines established in 1985 by the Centers for Disease Control for the protection of health care workers from infectious diseases.
9. Term used to describe surgical techniques or procedures that penetrate healthy tissue.
10. Providing factual support through written information.
12. Contaminated items; items that have come in contact with patient blood and/or body fluids.
15. A written request for laboratory analysis to be performed on a specimen.
18. Commercially packaged materials containing supplies and equipment needed to clean a spill of biohazardous substances.
22. A material that has been in contact with body fluid and is capable of transmitting disease.

24. Rules set up and established to measure quality, weight, extent, or value.
27. The substance produced by the cells of glandular organs from materials in the blood.
28. A pathway of possible infection from pathogens present in the atmosphere.
29. Commercially packaged materials needed to perform laboratory tests.
30. Recognized as being outstanding.
32. To destroy by fire.
34. Federal government agency from which written CLIA '88 documents may be obtained.
38. Methods used to ensure reliable, accurate data.
39. To remove by suction.
40. To advance beyond established or proper limits.
43. A means of transmission of an infectious disease (such as HIV and HBV) via human blood.
45. Needles, scalpels, or other instruments capable of causing a penetrating or puncture wound of the skin.
47. Sample tests performed in a clinical laboratory to determine that a specific degree of accuracy is achieved.
48. To acquire through infection, as a disease.
50. Any refuse that contains infectious material that would pose a threat due to possible transmission of pathogenic microorganisms.
52. The body's strong line of defense against invading microorganisms.

Down

1. A pathway of possible infection from pathogens suspended in particles of liquid.
2. Personal protective equipment (PPE).
3. Measures used in the workplace that consist of physical equipment and mechanical devices to control employee exposure to bloodborne pathogens and OPIM.
5. A person who harbors a pathogenic organism and who is capable of transmitting the organism to others.
6. Guidelines released by the CDC in 1996, which represent the most current and comprehensive approach to infection control.
7. To make impure or unclean.
8. Conforming or adapting.
10. A written formal refusal.
11. Degree of difficulty.
13. Precautions issued by the CDC to be used in addition to standard precautions when caring for specific categories of patients.
14. A type of white blood cell that provides immunity.
16. An immune system unable to function normally due to the presence of a disease such as AIDS.
17. A system that maintains that personal protective equipment should be worn for contact with all body fluids whether or not blood is visible.
19. A system developed by CDC for grouping patients with infectious diseases, including strict, respiratory, protective, enteric, wound and skin, discharge, and blood.
20. A formal order to obey certain rules and regulations.
21. Payment.
23. Physical or mechanical devices that isolate or remove health hazards from the workplace.
25. Infections from any organisms that occur due to the possibility offered by the altered physiological state of the host.
26. A pathway of possible infection from pathogens present on surfaces.

33. The determination of the accuracy of an instrument by comparing the information provided with an accepted standard known to be accurate.
35. The elimination of waste products from the body.
36. Surgical puncture of the lumbar area of the intervertebral spaces to aspirate cerebral spinal fluid for laboratory analysis.
37. Removing a seriously ill patient or a patient with an infectious disease from others to reduce the risk of infection and to protect the patient.
38. Measures used to monitor the processing of laboratory specimens.
41. A barrier used in the laboratory to capture chemical vapors.
42. Any secretion or excretion from the human body.
44. An injury or wound.
46. Inspection with a microscope.
49. Infectious; able to overcome the host's defense mechanisms.
51. Used to describe a category of clinical laboratory tests that are simple, unvarying, and require a minimum of judgment and interpretation.

B. To test your spelling skill, unscramble the key vocabulary terms that follow. Then define each term in the space provided.

1. TANOECE ______________________________

____

____

2. SEGAI ______________________________

____

____

3. RADIQEUC CODMENIFIYMUNIEC MOREYNDS ______________________________

____

____

4. STONENCSEMIAI ______________________________

____

____

5. PATMIRHEEHCUTEOC TANGES ______________________________

____

____

6. RATMETDISI ______________________________

____

____

7. SONYEDPOC ______________________________

____

____

8. TELHY LOCOLAH ______________________________

____

____

9. RENCOSIF ______

10. DOYEFAMEDLRH ______

11. NUHAM FODENICIYIMUCENM SUVIR ______

12. BINOLUGMISMOLUN ______

13. CADIJUNE ______

14. RELORAKEUH ______

15. ALOHIC ______

16. LAMDCIE PASSISE ______

17. NESESM ______

18. ALPENARERT ______

19. GETNAPOH ______

20. BOPMEYOTLH ______

21. MOPLARYNU AMEDE ______

22. MOSIUD HEYPOCOHIRTL ______________________________

____

____

23. TUSMUP ______________________________

____

____

24. RENTSETCASOIH ______________________________

____

____

25. TEARIVUNAC ______________________________

____

____

Learning Review

Fill in the blanks.

1. A. Universal Blood and Body Fluid Precautions, or universal precautions, were issued by the CDC in 1985 as a means of infection control to minimize the possibility of infection from ______________________, ______________________, and other ______________________ diseases.

B. In 1996, the CDC released a new set of standard precautions, in addition to the universal precautions, for infection control that should now be used by all health care professionals for all patients. Standard precautions apply to what four sources of infection from the human body?

(1) ______________________________

(2) ______________________________

(3) ______________________________

(4) ______________________________

2. For each of the following situations, what guidelines of the universal and standard precautions should the medical assistant implement to practice effective medical asepsis?

A. Jaime Carrera, a construction worker, presents at Inner City Health Care with head wound that is bleeding profusely; his clothes and skin are covered with blood. Two workers accompany Jaime, and they are both covered with blood as well.

____

____

B. Lourdes Austen, a breast cancer survivor, presents for a flexible sigmoidoscopy, an endoscopy procedure.

____

____

C. (1) Audrey Jones, CMA, prepares to perform venipuncture on Maria Jover, a patient suspected of HIV infection.

____

____

(2) Audrey must dispose of the needle after performing venipuncture on Maria.

____

____

(3) Audrey properly disposes of gloves in a biohazard container.

____

____

D. Bruce Goldman, CMA, performs cardiopulmonary resuscitation (CPR) on a walk-in emergency patient at Inner City Health Care who collapses in the reception area.

____

____

E. Wanda Slawson, CMA, prepares to clean and sanitize the examination room after Dr. James Whitney completes emergency treatment of Jaime Carrera's head wound, an open laceration requiring stitches.

____

____

F. Karen Ritter, CMA, prepares urine and blood specimens collected for transport to an off-site laboratory for analysis.

____

____

G. While suffering a brief bout of dermatitis, administrative/clinical medical assistant Joe Guerrero is assigned to administrative office duties.

____

____

H. Ellen Armstrong, CMA, greets and correctly identifies patient Nora Fowler and prepares to initiate contact with the patient to obtain a blood pressure reading.

____

____

3. With the release of standard precautions in 1996, the CDC also introduced transmission-based precautions to be used in addition to standard precautions for patients diagnosed with or suspected of specific highly transmissible diseases.

For each of the following sets of symbols representing categories of transmission-based precautions, identify the pathway of infection for pathogens the precautions are designed to protect against. In each case, what special precautions are necessary to supplement standard precautions?

A. ______________________________ Precautions

____

____

____

B. ______________________ Precautions

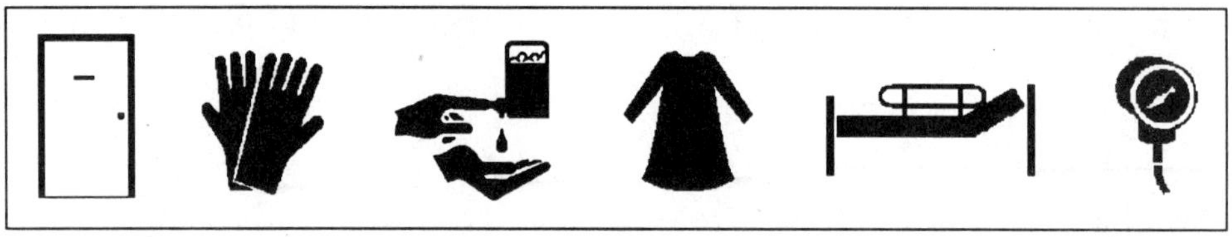

____

____

____

C. ______________________ Precautions

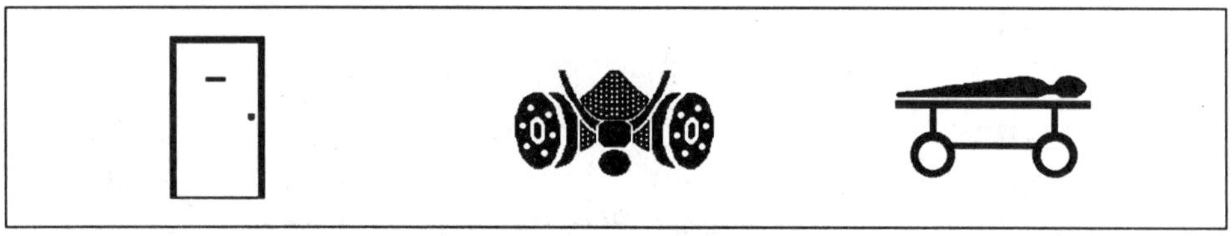

____

____

____

4. Persons infected with HIV or HBV remain infected for life. As carriers, infected persons are capable of transmitting the virus to others, even if they are asymptomatic. Name four ways these viruses are primarily transmitted:

(1) ____

____

(2) ____

____

(3) ____

____

(4) ____

____

5. The four categories of laboratory testing are waived, physician-performed microscopy tests (which are all waived tests), moderate-complexity tests, and high-complexity tests. All laboratories are required to register with CLIA '88 and receive certification to perform specific categories of tests within strict boundaries of compliance. Waived tests deliver simple unvarying results and require a minimum of judgment and interpretation. Name 10 waived tests.

(1) ____________________ (6) ____________________

(2) ____________________ (7) ____________________

(3) ____________________ (8) ____________________

(4) ____________________ (9) ____________________

(5) ____________________ (10) ____________________

6. CLIA '88 requires every facility that tests human specimens for diagnosis, treatment, and prevention of disease to meet specific federal requirements. Name five specific duties a medical assistant may perform that will impact the medical facility's compliance with CLIA '88 regulations.

(1) ____

____

(2) ____

____

(3) ____

____

(4) ____

____

(5) ____

____

7. A written chemical hygiene plan (CHP) is required of all medical facilities to comply with safety standards outlined by the Occupational Health and Safety Administration (OSHA). To comply with OSHA regulations, chemicals must be labeled using the National Fire Protection Association's color and number method.

A. *Match the colors below to the type of hazard each signifies.*

____ Blue — 1. Fire

____ White — 2. Reactivity

____ Yellow — 3. Use of personal protective equipment (PPE)

____ Red — 4. Health

B. *For each configuration listed, use the NFPA color and number method to describe the hazardous properties of each chemical.*

(1) CHEMICAL X: Red/2; Blue/3; Yellow/3; White/F.

____

____

____

(2) CHEMICAL Y: Red/0; Blue/1; Yellow/0; White/X.

____

____

____

(3) CHEMICAL Z: Red/1; Blue/2; Yellow/1; White/E.

____

____

____

8. The Bloodborne Pathogen Standard, effective in 1992, attempts to reduce the occupational-related cases of HIV and HBV infections among health care professionals. It covers all employees "reasonably anticipated" to come into contact with, as a result of performing their job duties, blood and other potentially infectious materials (OPIM) and seeks to limit exposure to pathogens.

Match each of the following components of the Bloodborne Pathogen Standard to a strategy used to implement it.

____ 1. Document exposure incident.
____ 2. Placed in a secondary container if the outside of the container is contaminated.
____ 3. Examples include needleless IVs, sharps disposal containers, and aerosol-free tubes.
____ 4. Go through training and cooperate; obey policies.
____ 5. Transported in bags that prevent soak-through or leakage.
____ 6. Epidemiology and symptoms of bloodborne disease.
____ 7. Records must be maintained for 30 years plus the duration of employment.
____ 8. Summary of contents of training program (kept for 3 years).
____ 9. Biohazard symbol and word *biohazard* must be visible.
____ 10. Prescription glasses may be fitted with solid side shields.
____ 11. Puncture-resistant, leak-proof, routinely replaced so there is no overflow.
____ 12. Training material must be appropriate for literacy and education level of employee.
____ 13. All human blood and OPIM are considered to be infectious.

A. Sharps containers
B. Protective clothing (component of PPE)
C. Labels
D. Work practice controls
E. Housekeeping
F. Methods of compliance
G. Medical records
H. Laundry
I. Training components
J. Exposure control plan
K. Engineering controls
L. Eye protection (component of PPE)

____ 14. Vinyl or latex are required for general use.
____ 15. Laundry personnel must use PPE and have a sharps container accessible.
____ 16. A list of job classifications where occupational exposure occurs.
____ 17. Contaminated equipment and surfaces must be cleaned as soon as feasible for obvious contamination or at the end of the work shift if no contamination has occurred.
____ 18. No eating, drinking, smoking, and so on in the work area.
____ 19. Lab coats are worn when a low-level risk for exposure is present.
____ 20. PPE, engineering and work practice controls, standard precautions, housekeeping.
____ 21. Given in accordance with the U. S. Public Health Service guidelines at no cost to employees. May be required for students to be admitted to college health programs as well as for externship.
____ 22. The standard applies to all occupational exposure to blood and OPIM, and includes part-time employees, designated first aiders, and mental health workers as well as exposed medical personnel.

M. Regulated waste containers (nonsharp)
N. Scope and application
O. Laundry facility
P. Training records
Q. Standard precautions
R. Gloves (component of PPE)
S. Hepatitis B vaccination
T. Employee responsibilities
U. Postexposure follow-up
V. Information and training

Investigation Activity

Material safety data sheets (MSDS) are compiled into a manual that must be kept on-site and made available to all employees. MSDS give information regarding any hazardous properties of chemical substances and are often supplied by the manufacturer when chemicals are ordered. MSDS manuals are required as a component of compliance with the OSHA standard for chemical exposure. In the ambulatory care setting, medical assistants come into contact with many substances that pose potential chemical hazards. Improper exposure to hazardous substances can cause illnesses, ranging from skin irritations to blindness to pulmonary edema. Substances range from ordinary office supplies (such as typewriter correction fluid) and essential cleansers (such as sodium hypochlorite or household bleach) to medical supplies (such as stains, ethyl alcohol, formaldehyde, fixatives, and preservatives), injectables (such as chemotherapeutic agents), and more.

As a class, come up with a list of chemical substances commonly found in the ambulatory care setting. Each student should select one substance. Then each student should perform research to identify a manufacturer who makes and supplies the substance. Write or call the manufacturer to obtain an MSDS and/or relevant information regarding the chemical substance's potential hazards. Using the National Fire Protection Association's color and number method for labeling to warn for potential hazards, configure a chemical hazard label for the substance based on the MSDS or hazard information supplied by the manufacturer.

Record information regarding the assigned chemical substance below.

Name of substance:____

Purpose of substance in the ambulatory care setting: ______________________

____

Name of manufacturer: ______________________

Address: ______________________

____

____

Telephone: ______________________

Suggested NFPA label coding for chemical hazards of the substance:

Red: ______________ Yellow: ______________

Blue: ______________ White: ______________

CASE STUDY

Annette Samuels comes to Inner City Health Care experiencing flulike symptoms. Her skin and the whites of her eyes have a yellowish tone. Dr. Mark Woo examines the patient, assisted by Liz Corbin, CMA. It is discovered that Annette had her navel pierced at a local piercing and tattoo salon that recently opened in town. Mark suspects hepatitis B and asks Liz to perform venipuncture to obtain a blood sample for analysis to confirm the diagnosis.

Discuss the following:

1. What standard precautions will Liz employ to protect against infection while performing the venipuncture procedure?
2. What might have caused Annette's HBV infection? How can Mark help prevent the further spread of the hepatitis B infection to others at potential risk?
3. What regulation helps protect health care workers from HBV infection?

SUPPLEMENTARY RESOURCES

Study Guide Disks: Additional practice exercises for this chapter are available on the Study Guide disk found in the back of the textbook.

Medical Assisting Videos: Appropriate content is available on Delmar's Medical Assisting Videos, 2nd ed., for the following topics:

Tape 5: Standard Precautions
Perform Medical Aseptic Procedure of Hand Washing
Use Disposable Single-Contact Gloves
Personal Protective Equipment
Perform Medical Aseptic Procedures
Infections in the Office

Tape 12: Completion Procedures Following Injections
OSHA Regulations for Needles and "Sharps"
Accidental Needlesticks

EVALUATION OF CHAPTER KNOWLEDGE

How has your instructor evaluated the knowledge you have achieved?

Knowledge	Instructor Evaluation *Good*	*Average*	*Poor*
Understands and can implement			
Universal precautions	_____	_____	_____
Standard precautions	_____	_____	_____
Transmission-based precautions	_____	_____	_____
Knows routes of transmission for HIV/AIDS and HBV	_____	_____	_____
Identifies body fluids and OPIM	_____	_____	_____
Can identify government regulatory agencies responsible for setting standards	_____	_____	_____
Knows categories of testing and understands CLIA '88 requirements	_____	_____	_____
Understands components of OSHA's bloodborne standard	_____	_____	_____
Can define and identify PPE	_____	_____	_____
Understands the purpose and requirements of a chemical hygiene plan	_____	_____	_____
Understands the purpose of the MSDS manual and can apply NFPA system of chemical hazard labeling	_____	_____	_____
Knows procedures for proper disposal of infectious waste	_____	_____	_____
Can identify situations of potential risk of exposure to pathogens in the ambulatory care setting	_____	_____	_____

Student's Initials:_______ Instructor's Initials:_______

Grade: _______

CHAPTER 5

Emergency Procedures and First Aid

PERFORMANCE OBJECTIVES

Medical assistants may encounter emergency situations and should be familiar with the various types of potential emergencies that may occur both within the ambulatory care setting and outside of the office environment. In the ambulatory care setting, primarily designed to see patients in non-emergency situations, a physician is usually available to provide emergency care. The ambulatory care setting also contains medical equipment and supplies to address emergency situations. The medical assistant, however, is often the first health care professional to interact with an emergency patient. The physician-employer will establish policies and procedures for emergency situations in an emergency policies and procedures manual for the ambulatory care setting that all employees, including medical assistants, will follow in emergency situations. The manual will be reviewed at regularly scheduled staff meetings. Emergency care is provided under the physician's instruction and according to the guidelines established in the emergency policies and procedures manual. Medical assistants must develop the essential skills of triaging emergency situations, that is, of recognizing emergency situations and correctly identifying the emergency measures that must be taken to provide immediate care. As with any health care professional, medical assistants should provide emergency care only within the scope of their knowledge and training. Medical assistants are encouraged to enroll in either a Red Cross or American Heart Association first aid and CPR program and take refresher courses at least every two years to update skills.

EXERCISES, EMERGENCY PROCEDURES, AND ACTIVITY

Vocabulary Builder

Identify each of the following key vocabulary terms as an emergency condition (EC), an emergency or first aid procedure performed by health care professionals (EP), emergency equipment (EQ), or an emergency service provided to assist in emergency situations (ES).

A. _____ A. First aid

_____ B. Triage

_____ C. Syncope

_____ D. Shock
_____ E. Wounds
_____ F. Crash tray or cart
_____ G. Heimlich maneuver
_____ H. Occlusion
_____ I. Universal emergency medical identification symbol and card
_____ J. Hypothermia
_____ K. Standard precautions
_____ L. Cardiopulmonary resuscitation (CPR)
_____ M. Sprain
_____ N. Emergency medical services (EMS)
_____ O. Fractures
_____ P. Splints
_____ Q. Strain
_____ R. Rescue breathing

B. Match each key vocabulary term given in part A with its definition listed below.

_____ 1. A break in a bone. There are several types, but all are classified as open or closed.

_____ 2. A tray or portable cart that contains medications and supplies needed for emergency and first aid procedures.

_____ 3. An injury to the soft tissue between joints, it involves the tearing of muscles or tendons and occurs often in the neck, back, or thigh muscles.

_____ 4. A break in the skin and/or underlying tissues, categorized as open or closed.

_____ 5. Closure of a passage.

_____ 6. An injury to a joint, often an ankle, knee, or wrist, that involves a tearing of the ligaments. Most are minor and heal quickly; others are more severe, include swelling, and may not heal properly if the patient continues to put stress on the affected joint.

_____ 7. A local network of police, fire, and medical personnel trained to respond to emergency situations. In most communities, the system is activated by calling 911.

_____ 8. Abdominal thrusts designed to overcome breathing difficulties in patients who are choking.

_____ 9. Identification sometimes carried by individuals to identify any health problems they might have.

_____10. Any device used to immobilize a body part. Often used by EMS personnel.

_____11. An extremely dangerous cold-related condition that can result in death if the individual does not receive care and if the progression of the condition is not reversed. Symptoms include shivering, cold skin, and confusion.

_____12. Fainting.

_____13. The immediate care provided to persons who are suddenly ill or injured, typically followed by more comprehensive care and treatment.

_____14. A condition in which the circulatory system is not providing enough blood to all parts of the body, causing the body's organs to fail to function properly.

_____15. The combination of rescue breathing and chest compressions performed by a trained individual on a patient experiencing cardiac arrest.

_____16. To assess patients' conditions and prioritize the need for care.

_____17. Performed in individuals in respiratory arrest, this is a mouth-to-mouth (using appropriate protective equipment) or mouth-to-nose procedure that provides oxygen to the patient until emergency personnel arrive.

_____18. Guidelines issued by the Centers for Disease Control and Prevention (CDC) in 1996 that combine many of the basic principles of universal precautions and body substance isolation techniques. These augmented 1996 guidelines represent the new requirements for infection control measures and are intended to protect health care professionals, patients, and visitors.

Learning Review

1. Keen observation skills are necessary to recognize potential emergency situations; medical assistants rely on sight, hearing, and even smell and must be acutely sensitive to unusual behaviors. To identify the nature of the emergency and respond effectively, what five things must the medical assistant do to triage, or assess, the patient's situation?

   (1) ____

   (2) ____

   (3) ____

   (4) ____

   (5) ____

2. In an urgent care setting, two or more patients may present with emergency symptoms. The order in which emergency patients will receive care depends on the health care professionals' abilities to triage patients' symptoms to determine who needs care most urgently.

   The following five patients present simultaneously on New Year's Eve at Inner City Health Care, an urgent care center. Office manager Walter Seals, CMA, is working the evening shift with Dr. Mark Woo. In what order will Walter and Mark triage the priority of treatment?

   Number the patients 1 through 5 to correspond to the urgency of their conditions. For each patient, list the emergency conditions he or she is suffering from, in order of severity, and name the emergency procedures the health care team will initiate to treat the patient.

   A. A patient presents with a gunshot wound to the leg that is bleeding severely. The patient is conscious but his pupils are dilated and he is unable to answer simple questions put to him by Walter and Dr. Woo. He cradles his right arm and will not let anyone touch it, though there is no immediate evidence of an open wound to the arm.

   Urgency of Condition: ____

   ____

   ____

   ____

   B. An elderly man, brought in by his grandson, complains of debilitating chest pains and nausea after eating a large family dinner. The man is a regular patient of Dr. Ray Reynolds, another physician at Inner City Health Care. The patient's medical record reveals that he suffers from a hiatal hernia, slipped disks, high blood pressure, and mild angina. His vital signs are within a normal range for his general physical condition. The man is walking and speaking with moderate distress and is extremely anxious.

Urgency of Condition: ____________________

____

____

C. A young woman presents with her boyfriend. She appears to have multiple abrasions on her right palm and knee, with damage to the right knee and ankle joints sustained after a fall on in-line skates. Both joints are swollen and painful. She received the skates as a Christmas gift from her boyfriend.

Urgency of Condition: ____________________

____

____

D. A man in his mid-thirties presents with the cotton tip of a cotton swab stuck in his ear canal. The tip became lodged in his ear while he was showering and dressing for a New Year's Eve party. Though the man feels a dull consistent pain in the ear, he says he has no trouble hearing. The outside of the ear appears normal and the man appears annoyed but not distressed.

Urgency of Condition: ____________________

____

____

E. A young woman presents with a group of friends, all college students, with an eye injury sustained by a champagne cork. The cork, which had a metal covering over its tip, hit the patient's eye; the students bring the cork with them. The young woman's eye is red and tearing and she is experiencing severe pain in the eye.

Urgency of Condition: ____________________

____

____

3. In administering emergency care in the ambulatory care setting, medical assistants and all health care professionals must follow standard precautions to protect themselves, their patients, and visitors. What five infection control measures can health care professionals follow to greatly reduce the risk of transmitting infectious disease when providing emergency care?

(1) ____________________

(2) ____________________

(3) ____________________

(4) ____________________

(5) ____________________

4. The medical crash cart or tray contains emergency or first aid supplies and medications health care professionals commonly use in treating emergencies. Using a medical encyclopedia or

reference such as the *Physician's Desk Reference* (PDR), describe the following emergency medications and identify potential uses for each. Remember that only a physician can order medications or treatment.

A. Lidocaine ____________________

B. Verapamil ____________________

C. Atropine ____________________

D. Insulin ____________________

E. Nitroglycerin ____________________

F. Marcaine ____________________

G. Diphenhydramine ____________________

H. Diazepam ____________________

5. Shock requires immediate medical attention. Progressive shock can reach an irreversible point and is life threatening. Shock occurs when the circulatory system is not providing enough blood to all parts of the body, causing the body's organs to function improperly.

For each of the patient symptoms or conditions below, identify the type of shock that is most likely.

____________________ A. Patient suffers heart attack.

_______________ B. Patient suffers severe infection following colon surgery.

_______________ C. Patient experiences syncope after witnessing a traumatic event.

_______________ D. Patient experiences reaction to food allergy.

_______________ E. Choking patient has extreme difficulty breathing.

_______________ F. A diabetic patient lapses into coma.

_______________ G. Patient suffers serious head trauma.

_______________ H. Accident victim suffers extreme loss of blood.

6. A common procedure for treating closed wounds is to RICE them. What do the letters of this acronym stand for?

R_______________ I_______________ C_______________ E_______________

7. A. Match each type of open wound to its defining characteristics.

A. Incision
B. Puncture
C. Laceration
D. Avulsion
E. Abrasion

_____ 1. A wound that pierces and penetrates the skin. This wound may appear insignificant but actually go quite deep.

_____ 2. These wounds commonly occur at exposed body parts such as the fingers, toes, and nose. Tissue is torn off and wounds may bleed profusely.

_____ 3. A wound that results from a sharp object such as a knife.

_____ 4. A painful wound that involves nerve endings. The epidermal layer of the skin is scraped away.

_____ 5. A wound that results in a jagged tear of body tissues and may contain debris.

B. For each type of wound, describe proper emergency concerns, care, and treatment.

Incision ____

____

____

Puncture ____

____

____

Laceration ____

____

____

Avulsion ____

____

____

Abrasion ______________________________

____

____

8. Name three sources other than heat that can cause burns. For each, describe the proper emergency concerns, care, and treatment.

(1) ______________________________

____

____

____

(2) ______________________________

____

____

____

(3) ______________________________

____

____

____

9. Musculoskeletal injuries, or injuries to muscles, bones, and joints, can be difficult to triage, especially for closed fractures. List five assessment techniques health care professionals can use to determine the seriousness of musculoskeletal injuries.

(1) ______________________________

(2) ______________________________

(3) ______________________________

(4) ______________________________

(5) ______________________________

10. For each set of symptoms that follows, identify the most likely emergency condition and describe emergency concerns, care, and treatment.

______________ A. Off-color, cold skin with a waxy appearance.

____

____

______________ B. Hives, itching, lightheadedness.

____

____

______________ C. Cold, clammy skin; profuse sweating; abdominal cramps; headache; general weakness.

____

____

________________ D. Lightheadedness, weakness, nausea, unsteadiness.

____

____

________________ E. Moist, pale skin; drooling; lack of appetite; diplopia; full pulse.

____

____

________________ F. Numbness in face, arm, and leg on one side of body; slurred speech; nausea and vomiting.

____

____

________________ G. Fever, convulsions, clenched teeth.

____

____

________________ H. Cold, clammy skin; anxiety; dilated pupils; weak pulse; rigid boardlike abdomen post-surgery for hysterectomy.

____

____

11. Identify the method of entry into the body for each of the following poisons:

________________ A. Carbon monoxide.

________________ B. Insect stingers.

________________ C. Chemical pesticides used in the garden.

________________ D. Spoiled food.

________________ E. Poison oak.

________________ F. Cleaning fluid fumes.

12. A. On a scale of 1 to 5, rate your personal comfort in regard to the following emergency situations medical assistants may find themselves involved with in an ambulatory or urgent care setting.

1. Extremely uncomfortable
2. Uncomfortable
3. Somewhat comfortable
4. Comfortable
5. Very comfortable

_____ Assisting in treatment of patients with injuries clearly sustained by an act of violence or abuse.

_____ Performing the Heimlich maneuver on an unconscious person.

_____ Administering CPR to a child.

_____ Administering back blows and thrusts to a conscious infant.

_____ Performing rescue breathing on someone who has poor personal hygiene.

_____ Bandaging the open wound of an HIV-infected person.

_____ Caring for a person experiencing a seizure.
_____ Administering care to a patient who faints after venipuncture.
_____ Administering care to a patient in extreme pain.
_____ Administering care to a patient who is verbally abusive or uncooperative.

B. On a scale of 1 to 5, rate your level of agreement with the statements that follow.

1. Never.
2. Occasionally.
3. Sometimes.
4. Most of the time.
5. All of the time.

_____ Life-threatening emergencies frighten me.
_____ I respond well under pressure.
_____ I am bothered by the sight of blood.
_____ I lose my temper easily, becoming openly frustrated and angry.
_____ I become frustrated and overwhelmed by feelings of helplessness in emergency situations.
_____ I remain calm and clear headed in emergency situations.
_____ I forget about myself completely and focus on the emergency victim.
_____ I am concerned about administering care in emergency situations where danger to myself may exist when giving such care.
_____ I am comfortable speaking to the family or friends of emergency victims.

Emergency Procedures

Emergency Procedure 1

Lenore McDonell, a wheelchair-bound woman in her early thirties, experiences a serious laceration to the right arm sustained from a fall while performing an independent transfer from the examination table to her wheelchair. Joe Guerrero, CMA, assists Dr. Winston Lewis in administering emergency care.

1. What standard precautions must the health care professionals follow before administering emergency treatment?

____

____

____

2. Joe and Dr. Lewis attempt to control Lenore's bleeding by applying a dressing and pressing firmly.

   A. When the bleeding does not stop, what two actions do the health care professionals perform?

   (1) ____

   (2) ____

B. In the unlikely event that bleeding continues, what piece of medical equipment will the health care team use in substitution of a tourniquet? Why is this alternative equipment effective and widely used today?

3. The bleeding stops, and Joe applies a pressure bandage over the dressing.

A. This patient is prone to fractures and will need to be Xrayed. What is the next emergency procedure Dr. Lewis will perform? Why is this procedure necessary and what equipment will the physician and medical assistant require?

B. Before applying a sling, what do the health care professionals check to be sure that the medical equipment used has not been too tightly applied?

4. What standard precautions will the health care team follow after the emergency treatment of the patient is successfully completed?

5. What information will the health care team include in documenting the procedure for the patient's medical record?

Emergency Procedure 2

New patient Grace Fisher comes to the offices of Drs. Lewis and King for a well baby visit with Dr. Elizabeth King for infant Joseph Michael. In the reception area, the baby is fussy, and Grace picks him up and holds him at her chest, rocking and gently patting the baby's back. Suddenly, the baby's face becomes red; it begins to cough and wheeze. When the baby does not quickly resume normal breathing, Ellen Armstrong, CMA, alerts Dr. King over the office intercom. As Ellen takes the baby from a bewildered and frightened Grace to begin rescue breathing in a nearby empty examination room, she motions to co-worker Joe Guerrero, CMA, to accompany them to attend to the mother's needs.

1. What four steps will Ellen perform to initiate rescue breathing?
   (1) ______
   (2) ______
   (3) ______
   (4) ______

2. Ellen checks for a pulse at the brachial artery. The pulse is present but the baby seems to have increased difficulty breathing. What sequence of actions will Ellen follow next? How long should Ellen continue this sequence?

______

______

______

3. After 3 minutes the baby is still conscious and has a pulse but is no longer able to cough, cry, or breathe. Dr. King has joined Grace and Ellen in the examination room.

   A. What procedure does Dr. King initiate at this time?

   ______

   B. What four steps does Dr. King follow to perform this procedure?
      (1) ______
      ______
      (2) ______
      ______
      (3) ______
      ______
      (4) ______
      ______

   C. How long will Dr. King continue this procedure?

   ______

4. The infant, Joseph Michael, loses consciousness. Grace becomes hysterical.

   A. As she shakes the infant to check for consciousness, Dr. King gives what two instructions to Joe?
   (1) ______
   (2) ______

   B. Dr. King begins to administer what procedure? How long will Dr. King administer this procedure? What happens if the baby loses a pulse?

   ______

   ______

5. On the second set of back blows and thrusts after the baby loses consciousness, Dr. King sweeps a bead out of the baby's mouth. Joseph Michael begins to cough and cry. A bead from Grace's sweater had come loose and lodged in the baby's trachea. "We've caught this just in time," Dr. King announces to a grateful and relieved mother.

   What follow-up procedures will the health care team initiate?

6. What information will the health care team include in documenting the procedure in the infant's medical record? in Grace's medical record?

   A. *Joseph Michael Fisher:*

   B. *Grace Fisher:*

Emergency Procedure 3

Edith Leonard, a frail widow in her early seventies, participates in the knitting club at the local senior center. As she knits, Edith becomes restless and begins to rub her chest and massage her jaw. Her breathing becomes shallow. Bruce Goldman, CMA, who volunteers at the senior center, remembers Edith as a patient at Inner City Health Care, where he works. When Edith slumps in her chair, Bruce rushes over.

1. When Bruce calls Edith's name, she nods her head. However, Edith seems to have extreme difficulty breathing and her face is contorted with pain. What is Bruce's first action?

2. Edith is no longer breathing. What procedure should Bruce initiate? What steps does Bruce follow in performing the procedure?

3. Edith is still not breathing and no pulse is present.

   A. What procedure does Bruce initiate?

   ___

   B. What is the correct method to administer chest compressions?

   ___

   C. How many slow breaths will Bruce administer after completing the chest compressions?

   ___

   D. How many times will Bruce repeat the sequence of chest compressions and rescue breathing before again checking Edith's pulse?

   ___

4. Under what four conditions is it acceptable for Bruce to stop administering this technique of chest compressions and rescue breathing?

   (1) ___

   (2) ___

   (3) ___

   (4) ___

5. After 10 minutes, EMS personnel arrive and transport Edith to a local hospital.

   A. What standard precautions will Bruce practice at the senior center after EMS personnel have transported the patient from the scene of the emergency?

   ___

   B. What supplies and equipment would the medical assistant have used if this emergency had taken place in an ambulatory care setting?

   ___

Investigation Activity

Educating patients and the general community about the responsibility to be prepared for addressing emergency situations is one role the medical assistant can perform in the ambulatory care setting. Health care professionals should encourage patients to keep complete emergency reference information in an easily accessible place in the home. Furthermore, patients should be encouraged to receive training in first aid and emergency procedures, including cardiopulmonary resuscitation (CPR), and to learn about strategies for creating a safer home environment. Complete the sample emergency information sheet below with the resources closest to your home and essential medical information relevant to your family.

As a class, designate one student to contact each of the six resources listed—fire department, poison control center, police department, ambulance service, local hospital emergency department, and primary care physician's office—to ask about emergency procedures and services each provides and to obtain any literature that is available about preventing or treating emergencies. Bring the information to class for discussion.

EMERGENCY INFORMATION FOR THE ______________________ FAMILY

Address: ______________________________

____

Telephone: ______________________________

Emergency Medical Services (EMS): Dial 911. If 911 is busy or does not answer, dial "0" (Operator) and ask for help. TDD/TTY for the Hearing Impaired, dial 311.

Fire Department

Address: ______________________________

Telephone: ______________________________

Poison Control Center

Address: ______________________________

Telephone: ______________________________

Police Department

Address: ______________________________

____

____

Telephone: ______________________________

Ambulance Service

Name: ______________________________

Address: ______________________________

____

Telephone: ______________________________

Local Hospital Emergency Department

Name: ______________________________

Address: ______________________________

Telephone: ______________________________

Primary Care Physician

Name: ______________________________

Address: ______________________________

Telephone: ______________________________

Names and ages of family members and any medical conditions or medications emergency medical professionals should know about.

1. ______________________________
2. ______________________________
3. ______________________________
4. ______________________________
5. ______________________________
6. ______________________________

Person, not at the household address, who should be contacted in case of emergency.

Name: ______________________________ Relationship to family: ______________________________

Address: ______________________________ Telephone: ______________________________

____

CASE STUDY

Mary O'Keefe calls Dr. King's office in a panic. Ellen Armstrong, CMA, answers the telephone. "Oh my God, help me. I need Dr. King."

"This is Ellen Armstrong, CMA. Who is this calling and what is the situation?"

"It's my baby, oh God, get Dr. King."

"Dr. King is unavailable, but we can help you. Now, tell me your name."

"It's Mary O'Keefe. Help me, I think my baby is dead."

"Are you at home?"

"Yes."

"Good. Tell me what's happened."

"My son Chris pried the plug off an outlet and he's electrocuted himself!" Mary cries. "He's just lying there. I'm so scared; if I touch him will I electrocute myself? Oh my God, my baby, my baby. What should I do?"

Ellen, who has been writing the details on a piece of paper motions to Joe Guerrero, another CMA in the office, and hands him her notes. Joe immediately accesses the O'Keefe's address from the patient database and uses another telephone line to call EMS with the nature of the emergency situation and directions to the O'Keefe's residence. Meanwhile, Ellen remains on the line with Mary. Dr. King is on rounds at the hospital this morning and won't be in the office for at least another hour.

"Mary, we're calling EMS and they will be there as soon as possible. In the meantime, I'm going to need you to focus and answer my questions. Okay?"

Discuss the following.

1. What steps does the medical assistant take to triage the emergency situation?
2. What questions should Ellen ask Mary regarding the emergency situation? Based on Mary's answers, what instructions should Ellen give Mary to begin emergency treatment?
3. What should the medical assistant do after EMS arrives and takes over emergency care? What follow-up procedures are necessary?

SUPPLEMENTARY RESOURCES

Study Guide Disks: Additional practice exercises for this chapter are available on the Study Guide Disk found in the back of the textbook.

Medical Assisting Videos: Appropriate content is available on Delmar's Medical Assisting Videos, 2nd ed., for the following topics:

Tape 2: Triage Skills
Tape 5: Standard Precautions
Infections in the Office
Tape 10: Recognize Emergencies
Workplace Hazards and Material Safety Data Sheets
Emergency Use of Oxygen in the Office
Introduction to Airway Obstruction
Abdominal Thrust (Heimlich maneuver)
Obstructed Airway in an Unconscious Patient
Diabetic Emergencies
Bandaging

EVALUATION OF CHAPTER KNOWLEDGE

How has your instructor evaluated the knowledge you have gained?

	Instructor Evaluation		
Knowledge	*Good*	*Average*	*Poor*
Recognizes emergency situations	____	____	____
Understands need for emergency preparation and the function of emergency medical services (EMS)	____	____	____
Possesses the ability to triage emergency cases in person and over the telephone	____	____	____
Understands legal and health considerations of emergency caregiving	____	____	____
Understands necessity of providing emergency care only within the scope of training and knowledge	____	____	____
Can assemble a medical crash tray or cart	____	____	____
Understands the use of standard precautions in emergency situations	____	____	____
Identifies signs and symptoms of shock, types of shock, and treatment of shock	____	____	____
Identifies classification and care of wounds	____	____	____
Identifies dressings, bandages, and their applications	____	____	____
Identifies first-, second-, and third-degree burns and burn care	____	____	____
Identifies musculoskeletal injuries, including types of fractures and strategies for care	____	____	____
Identifies heat- and cold-related illnesses and priorities for care	____	____	____
Understands how poisons enter the body	____	____	____
Identifies sudden illnesses such as syncope, seizures, diabetes, and hemorrhage	____	____	____
Recognizes cerebral vascular accident (CVA) and priorities for immediate emergency care	____	____	____
Recognizes heart attack and priorities for immediate emergency care	____	____	____
Can identify and name steps for performing these emergency procedures:			
Control of bleeding	____	____	____
Applying a splint	____	____	____
Heimlich maneuver	____	____	____
Rescue breathing	____	____	____
Cardiopulmonary resuscitation (CPR)	____	____	____

Student's Initials:_______ Instructor's Initials:____

Grade:_______

CHAPTER 6

Therapeutic Communication Skills

PERFORMANCE OBJECTIVES

The medical assistant is an important link in the communication process involving physicians, nurses, allied health care professionals, and patients. Communication forms the basis for every action performed by health care professionals in the care of their patients. Medical assisting students can use this workbook chapter to explore the many components of effective communication, cultivate the ability to learn and observe, recognize and respond to messages communicated both verbally and nonverbally, consider patients' needs with empathy and impartiality, and adapt messages sent to meet the receivers' abilities to understand. In personal, face-to-face communication as well as in telephone conversations, the medical assistant's goal is to achieve a level of therapeutic communication that enhances the patient's comfort level and eases the pathway of communication between the patient and the health care team.

EXERCISES AND ACTIVITIES

Vocabulary Builder

A. *Insert the key vocabulary terms that best fit the descriptions below.*

active listening	decode	kinesics
biases	encode	masking
body language	facial expressions	message
buffer words	feedback	modes of communication
closed questions	gestures/mannerisms	open-ended questions
cluster	hierarchy of needs	perception
communication cycle	indirect statements	position
congruency	interview techniques	posture

prejudices	sender	touch
receiver	territoriality	
roadblocks to communication	therapeutic communication	

1. ______________________ Communication that allows patients to feel comfortable, even when receiving difficult or unpleasant information, achieved through use of specific and well-defined professional communication skills.
2. ______________________ *"Good afternoon, this is* Inner City Health Care. *This is* Walter Seals. How may I help you?"
3. ______________________ Adept use of these methods encourages the best communication between health care professionals and patients, equalizing the relationship as much as possible.
4. ______________________ When she entered the room, medical assistant Audrey Jones's straight-backed pose, with arms at her side and head lifted, conveyed a message of confidence and professionalism.
5. ______________________ The specific order or rank within which a person's needs are met, moving from the most basic needs to self-actualization.
6. ______________________ These types of questions require only a yes or no answer: "Mrs. Leonard, are you feeling dizzy now?"
7. ______________________ These potential verbal or nonverbal messages that prevent a successful cycle of communication can be overcome by the medical assistant's sensitivity to patients' personalities and needs.
8. ______________________ Bruce Goldman, CMA, leans toward Louise Kipperley, maintaining face-to-face communication as he explains that he will be drawing blood as a part of her routine physical examination. His physical orientation toward the patient helps put her at ease.
9. ______________________ The study of body language explores methods of nonverbal communication that accompany speech.
10. ______________________ These statements turn a question into a topic of interest that allows the patient to speak without feeling directly questioned: "Mr. Taylor, tell me about any difficulties your father's dementia presents with daily living activities at home."
11. ______________________ Communication involves exchanges of information between two or more individuals; this process involves sending and receiving messages even when unconsciously aware of them.
12. ______________________ As Marilyn Johnson takes his family history for the patient record, Jim Marshall says repeatedly, "I am worried because my father died from a heart attack at a young age." Marilyn uses this kind of therapeutic communication to

rephrase the message by responding, "You are concerned about your cardiovascular health and your genetic risk?"

13. ______________________________ These personal preferences denote a predisposition for one particular belief or viewpoint over another.

14. ______________________________ These beliefs or viewpoints represent preconceived notions an individual may have formed before all the facts are known.

15. ______________________________ Communication requires this: content.

16. ______________________________ John O'Keefe sat with a sullen expression, eyes downcast, his arms folded across his chest, as he spoke to medical assistant Joe Guerrero about the financial hardships his family would face if his wife, Mary, were pregnant again. Joe relies on Mr. O'Keefe's nonverbal communication to convey his repressed feelings of anger.

17. ______________________________ Well-defined personal space sets physical boundaries where individuals feel comfortable while communicating with others.

18. ______________________________ These types of questions require more than a yes or no answer: "Ms. Johnson, how are you doing with the special diet Dr. Lewis suggested?"

19. ______________________________ Communication requires an individual to whom the sender's message is directed.

20. ______________________________ This aspect of body language involves the use of body parts, such as the hands and arms, during communication to enhance meaning or capture the attention of others.

21. ______________________________ Physical contact with others is a powerful way to communicate what cannot be articulated in words.

22. ______________________________ This attempt to hide from or repress obscures one's true feelings or real message.

23. ______________________________ Communication requires an individual who initiates the communication cycle.

24. ______________________________ Nonverbal messages grouped together to form, in aggregate, a statement or conclusion.

25. ______________________________ Medical assistant Karen Ritter nods her head yes as she explains to Annette Samuels that insurance will cover any medical tests related to her stomach cramps. Karen's nonverbal message agrees with her verbal message.

26. ______________________________ The receiver must interpret the meaning of the message in order to understand it.

27. ______________________________ The sender creates a message carefully crafted to match the receiver's ability to receive and interpret it properly.

28. ______________________________ The receiver uses this mode of communication to make sure that the message sent is the one the sender intended to give.

29. ____________________________ The channels of speaking, writing, listening, gestures or body language, and facial expressions are available to senders to use in formulating messages.

30. ____________________________ This kind of intuitive realization involves an active understanding of one's own feelings *and* the feelings of others.

31. ____________________________ Nonverbal messages are displayed on the face by moving facial muscles to convey emotion and feeling.

B. Individuals, in an effort to protect themselves from a painful or troubling message, often block effective communication by using defense mechanisms, behaviors that shield them from guilt, anxiety, or shame.

Insert the defense mechanisms that best fit the descriptions below.

denial	rationalization	sublimation
displacement	regression	
projection	repression	

1. ____________________________ This kind of rejection or refusal to acknowledge can lead to unfortunate consequences.

2. ____________________________ Herb Fowler stubbornly clings to the belief that his chronic cough is due to frequent colds and has nothing to do with his heavy smoking. This illogical justifying belief keeps him from facing the truth of his situation.

3. ____________________________ Individuals use this defense mechanism to move back to an earlier developmental stage, which allows them to escape conflict or fear.

4. ____________________________ Juanita Hansen complains that her building manager's refusal to make repairs to her apartment is a primary cause of her son Henry's frequent accidents. By placing the blame on the super, Juanita uses this defense mechanism to avoid taking responsibility for her son's well-being.

5. ____________________________ In the examination room, Cele Little yells at her sister, Dottie, for falling and injuring her back; minutes later, Cele tells Dr. Woo that Dottie's frequent falls are not serious and "don't mean anything." Cele is using this defense mechanism in regard to her sister's condition.

6. ____________________________ This defense mechanism redirects a socially unacceptable impulse into an acceptable one.

7. ____________________________ Wheelchair-bound Lenore McDonell works hardest in physical therapy when her therapist exhibits a healthy, athletic appearance. Lenore has placed her own treatment goals upon the therapist.

Learning Review

1. Culture presents a profound influence on successful therapeutic communication. For each of the seven cultural influences that follow, list one way in which therapeutic communication is impacted.

Ethnic heritage____

____

Geographic location and background ___________________________

____

Genetics ____

____

Economics ____

____

Educational experiences_______________________________________

____

Life experiences____

____

Personal value systems ____

____

2. Biases and prejudices common in today's society have the potential to create hostility. Match each difficult situation below to the corresponding bias or prejudice that motivates it.

   A. A preference for Western-style medicine.
   B. The tendency to choose female rather than male physicians.
   C. Prejudice related to a person's sexual preference.
   D. Discrimination based on race or religion.
   E. Hostile attitudes toward persons with a value system opposite your own.
   F. A belief that persons who cannot afford health care should receive less care than someone who can pay for full services.

   1. ____ Mr. Gordon refuses to accept a referral to an acupuncturist to help alleviate the chronic pain of advancing prostate cancer.
   2. ____ Medical assistant Bruce Goldman mistakenly assumes that patient Bill Schwartz has AIDS when he arrives at the clinic with a gentleman friend, seeking attention for a reoccuring black mole on this calf.
   3. ____ Rhoda and Lee Au fear they will not receive adequate medical care because they use Chinese as their first language and speak only broken English.
   4. ____ Corey Boyer resists his gym teacher's efforts to get him to the clinic to check out a recurring rash on his arm because his family has no health insurance.
   5. ____ Mary O'Keefe is relieved to find that the practice's OB/GYN is a female physician, Dr. Elizabeth King.
   6. ____ Edith Leonard, a widow in her seventies, counsels medical assistant Liz Corbin that she should settle down and get married instead of pursuing a dream to attend medical school and become a pediatrician.

3. In the following situation, the four elements of the communication cycle—Sender, Receiver, Message, and Feedback—are at work. Identify the Sender and Receiver and describe both the Message sent and Feedback received.

   Patient Martin Gordon, who has prostate cancer, calls the Northborough Family Medical Group to schedule a follow-up appointment with Dr. Lewis. Mr. Gordon's tone expresses anxiety and depression when medical assistant Ellen Armstrong informs him that Dr. Lewis is away at a medical convention for one week. Ellen acknowledges Mr. Gordon's concern over Dr. Lewis's absence and offers to schedule an appointment on the day of Dr. Lewis's return.

   Sender: ______________________________

   Receiver: ______________________________

   Message: ______________________________

   ____

   ____

   Feedback: ______________________________

   ____

   ____

4. The four modes of communication most pertinent in our everyday exchange are

   (1)______________________ (3)______________________

   (2)______________________ (4)______________________

5. Active listening is an important element of therapeutic communication. To practice active listening skills, rephrase each of the messages listed for verification from the sender; also include a therapeutic response.

   A. "I don't know what to do. My father takes so many pills he can't remember which is the right one, so he ends up refusing to take any of them."

   ____

   ____

   ____

   B. "I can't give you my insurance card; I lost it, and I don't remember the name of the company either. But you've always taken care of it before."

   ____

   ____

   ____

   C. "I can't help being worried. The doctor just suggested a referral for treatment at that hospital where somebody had their wrong foot operated on. What do you think?"

   ____

   ____

   ____

D. "I feel dizzy just thinking about having my blood taken. Do you really need to do it?"

____

____

6. Seventy percent of communication is nonverbal. By learning to recognize the emotions or feelings in patients' facial expressions, medical assistants greatly enhance their skill at therapeutic communication. Congruency occurs when verbal and nonverbal messages agree. Insert the correct emotions or physical states listed below for the facial expressions shown. Then fill in the appropriate emotion or physical state that is most likely congruent to the verbal message.

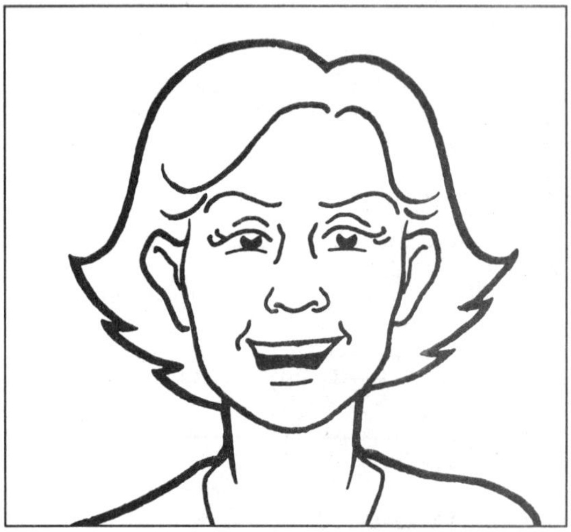

Happy

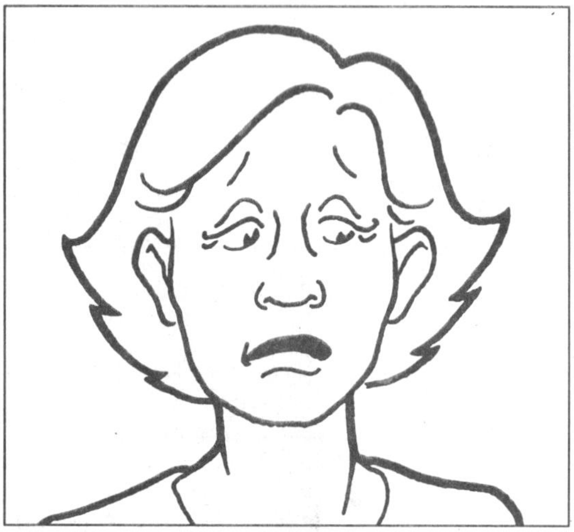

Sad

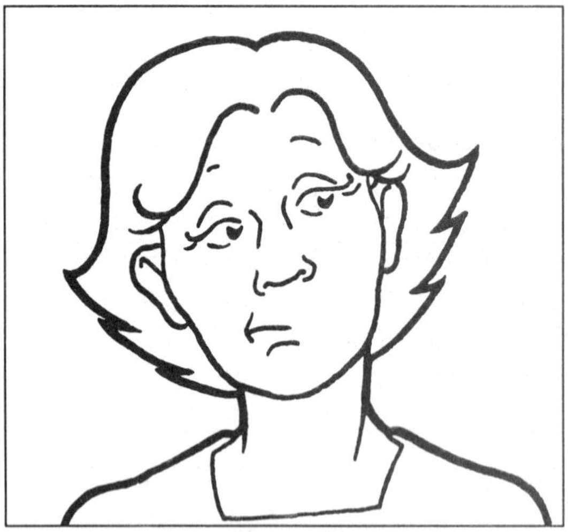

Confused

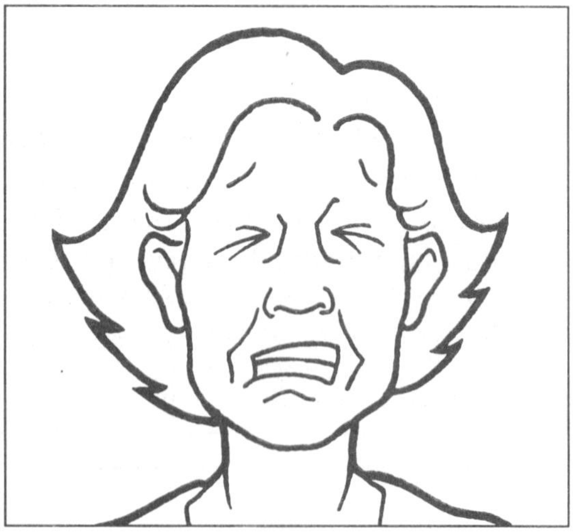

Pain

(1) ________________ "I've had stomach cramps for three days, and they keep getting worse."

(2) ________________ "The doctor said the biopsy results were negative. Is that good?"

(3) ________________ "I have to wear this awful knee brace another three weeks."

(4) ________________ "I'm excited; I think I might be pregnant again."

7. *Circle the five correct responses.*

The five Cs of communication are:

clear	complete	courteous
coherent	concise	credible
cohesive	constant	curious
comment	cooperative	curt

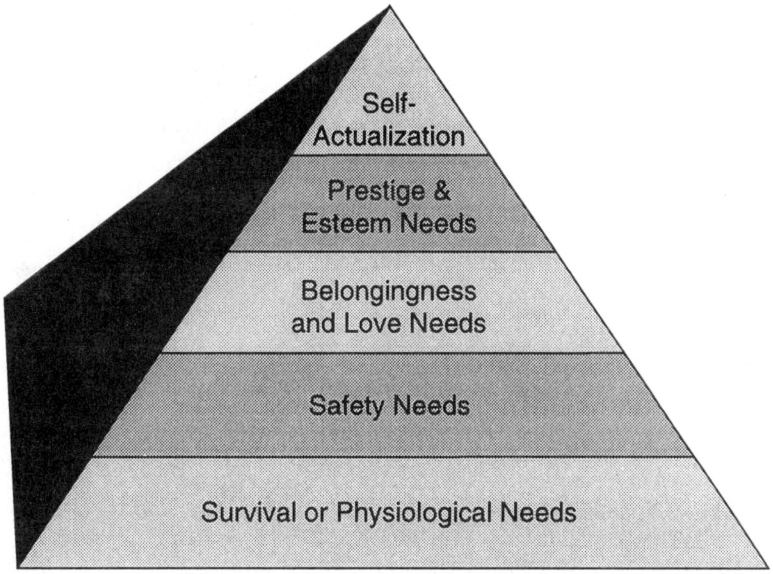

Maslow's Hierarchy of Needs

8. Abraham Maslow, the founder of humanistic psychology, postulated that a person's needs move from the most basic of survival to the state of self-actualization. Self-actualization occurs when the person realizes the maximum of human potential. Each level of need must be met before an individual can proceed successfully to the next level. Understanding Maslow's hierarchy will help medical assistants assess patients' needs and facilitate therapeutic communication. For each level, list a minimum of three needs that meet it.

Survival or physiological needs ______________________________

____

____

Safety needs ______________________________

____

Belongingness and love needs ______________________________

____

____

Prestige and esteem needs ______________________________

____

____

9. Identify eight significant roadblocks to communication:

(1)______________ (5)______________

(2)______________ (6)______________

(3)______________ (7)______________

(4)______________ (8)______________

10. Edith Leonard arrives at the clinic for a routine six-month follow-up examination. At her last visit, she had been referred to an ophthalmologist for removal of a cataract in her right eye. Compose a closed question, open-ended question, and indirect statement regarding Ms. Leonard's condition.

Closed question ______________________________

____

Open-ended question ______________________________

____

Indirect statement ______________________________

____

11. Telephone communication between medical assistants and patients is an important kind of therapeutic communication. Tone and pace of voice, along with word choice, carry the message when there is no visual feedback. List four tools of communication essential to conducting successful telephone conversations.

(1) ______________________________

____

(2) ______________________________

____

(3) ______________________________

____

(4) ______________________________

____

Investigation Activity

Learning to recognize and interpret nonverbal communication is a powerful tool to assist medical assistants in achieving the highest levels of therapeutic communication with patients. Clustering nonverbal cues into nonverbal statements enhances the ability to recognize patients' true feelings and emotions, which are often different from the words they speak out loud. The following exercises explore important body language or nonverbal communication behaviors: facial expressions, territoriality, position, posture, gestures/mannerisms, and touch.

A. Make a list of emotions or physical states and list each one on a separate index card. Some examples are thirst, frustration, fatigue, hot, cold, excitement, fear, grief, and surprise. In a group, or with a partner, have one student choose a card and portray the emotion or physical state listed on it using only nonverbal communication. The group or partner must correctly guess the emotion or physical state. On your own, practice recognizing emotions and physical states in front of a mirror; take the time to become physically aware of your own expressions and body language.

B. Now, again using the index cards from Exercise A, link the following verbal messages with a corresponding nonverbal message. For each verbal message below, choose a card and act out the verbal message, pairing it with the nonverbal emotion or physical state listed on the card. Note whether the verbal and nonverbal messages are congruent or incongruent. Practice this on your own in front of a mirror or have a partner identify the accompanying nonverbal message.

Patient

"My insurance company won't cover this entire procedure."
"How much longer will I have to wait to see the doctor?"
"My hand is bleeding. It's an emergency."
"The pain is sharp and steady; it hurts when you touch it."

Medical Assistant

"I understand that you feel grief over your loss."
"The tests results will be ready next week."
"Mr. Smith will need to fill out a new patient data sheet at his next appointment."
"The physician will be in to see you in a few minutes."

CASE STUDY

Wayne Elder arrives at the clinic for an examination to check on a recurrent ear infection that has been treated with antibiotics. Wayne, who is slightly retarded and lives in a group home, is still complaining of dizziness and pain in his ear. He has come to the clinic by himself, taking a bus from his job as a part-time dishwasher. Wayne's boss asked him to return to the clinic because Wayne could not concentrate at work.

Clinical medical assistant Wanda Slawson discovers from Wayne that he has not been taking his medication properly; he stopped taking pills once his ear began to feel better. She must politely ask Wayne to repeat himself several times before she can clearly understand his slurred speech, and she has difficulty holding his attention or maintaining eye contact.

Wanda conveys Wayne's situation to Dr. Ray Reynolds, who examines Wayne and gives him a new prescription for antibiotics, gently explaining the need to finish the entire prescription in order to get well. After Dr. Reynolds leaves the examination room, however, it is clear to Wanda that Wayne is still confused about why he must take the medication even after he begins to feel better. Wanda carefully explains to Wayne that the infection will continue to heal even though he no longer feels sick. To be sure he understands, Wanda asks Wayne to repeat to her what he must do and why; she then asks Dr. Reynolds to step in briefly to remind Wayne once more to complete the prescription.

Discuss the following issues:

1. How is the therapeutic communication between physician, medical assistant, and patient impacted by the unequal relationship that exists between patients and health care professionals?
2. How must medical assistant Wanda Slawson tailor her verbal and nonverbal messages to meet the abilities of her receivers: the physician (Dr. Ray Reynolds) and the patient (Wayne Elder)?
3. How does Wanda use active listening? Which interview techniques are the most effective in facilitating therapeutic communication? Does nonverbal communication play a role?
4. Using Maslow's hierarchy of needs, discuss how the health care team meets Wayne's special needs resulting from his disability.
5. Do you think the medical assistant acted appropriately? What else could she have done? What should she not do in this situation?

SUPPLEMENTARY RESOURCES

Study Guide Disk: Additional practice exercises for this chapter are available on the study guide disk found in the back of the textbook.

Medical Assisting Videos: Appropriate content is available on Delmar's Medical Assisting Videos, 2nd ed., Tape 1, for the following topics:

Your Career as a Medical Assistant
Display Professionalism
Work as a Team Member
Career-Seeking Skills
Communication Skills

EVALUATION OF CHAPTER KNOWLEDGE

Skills achieved:

Skills	Instructor Evaluation *Good*	*Average*	*Poor*
Identifies personal communication strengths	_____	_____	_____
Identifies areas for improvement in personal communication style	_____	_____	_____
Listens well	_____	_____	_____
Cultivates sharp observation skills	_____	_____	_____
Recognizes and responds to verbal and nonverbal communication	_____	_____	_____
Understands the communication cycle	_____	_____	_____
Adapts communication to individuals' abilities to understand	_____	_____	_____
Considers patients' needs with empathy and impartiality	_____	_____	_____
Ability to identify roadblocks to communication and defense mechanisms	_____	_____	_____
Uses proper telephone technique	_____	_____	_____
Practices successful therapeutic communication	_____	_____	_____

Student's Initials:_____ Instructor's Initials:_____

Grade: ______

CHAPTER 7

Coping Skills for the Medical Assistant

PERFORMANCE OBJECTIVES

Medical assistants and other health care professionals occasionally feel the stress of working in the demanding and challenging field of medicine and health care. Health care professionals must maintain a high level of skill and proficiency and possess knowledge about new technologies and medical advances. Whether juggling a full patient schedule, facing difficult—and sometimes life-or-death—situations with patients, or balancing administrative duties with a constant flow of paperwork, medical assistants take part in every phase of patient care. Students learning about medical assisting can use this workbook chapter to: learn about handling stress in the workplace environment of the ambulatory care setting; discover how the body adapts to stress and how to use techniques for coping with stress and avoiding burnout; and consider possible short- and long-range career goals that can act as a centering and motivating influence, further reducing stress and increasing confidence.

EXERCISES AND ACTIVITIES

Vocabulary Builder

Select the key vocabulary term listed below that best illustrates each of the following situations.

A. burnout	D. long-range goals	G. short-range goals
B. goal	E. outer-directed people	H. stress
C. inner-directed people	F. self-actualization	I. stressors

___ 1. James Whitney is a physician at Inner City Health Care. He hopes to go into private practice after gaining a few more years' experience at the urgent care center where he now works. James would like eventually to practice family medicine.

___ 2. Mark Woo, a physician at Inner City Health Care, prefers emergency medicine and often pulls double shifts working with emergency patients. Although he loves the work, Mark is experiencing chronic fatigue, frequently becomes angry at co-workers, and is prone to hair-trigger displays of emotion.

___ 3. Ellen Armstrong, CMA, is usually a calming influence in the offices of Drs. Lewis & King. Lately, however, it seems to Ellen that circumstances beyond her control are threatening to pull her down. An influx of new patients into the group practice has Ellen continually backed up with filing and paperwork, her steady baby-sitter announced she'll be unavailable for the summer months, and today her car broke down on the way to work.

___ 4. When Dr. Mark Woo tells emergency patient Annette Samuels that her severe stomach cramps may be caused by problems with her ovaries or appendix, she begins to feel panicky. Annette's blood pressure goes up, her breathing becomes rapid as her pulse quickens, and her eyes grow wide.

___ 5. Audrey Jones, CMA, enrolls at a local college for a night-school biology class as a first step toward her goal of obtaining a bachelor's degree.

___ 6. Dr. Elizabeth King, now in her mid-thirties, always knew what she wanted to do with her life. After graduating from Kansas University and Stanford University Medical School, Beth searched for a physician with whom to begin a group practice and found the perfect partner in Winston Lewis.

___ 7. Marilyn Johnson, CMA, office manager at the offices of Lewis & King, MD, enjoys her work and her life. Her children are grown and successful. With a masters degree in education, Marilyn teaches part-time at a local community college and is active in her town's music and art circles. She is a past president of the local chapter of the AAMA. Marilyn has worked hard to achieve the full potential of her abilities and talents and is now reaping the benefits of effort well spent.

___ 8. Maria Jover takes what life gives her, deeply believing that she has no power to change her circumstances or take charge of her life. Now, Dr. King says her chronic fatigue and gynecology problems may be symptoms of AIDS, contracted from a blood transfusion she received after a severe car accident that happened several years ago. "This horrible disease will take over my life," Maria tells Dr. King.

___ 9. Leo McKay is an elderly Irish Catholic man who has been laid off from his manufacturing job of twenty years. Leo asks easygoing Bruce Goldman, CMA, as he prepares Leo for a routine physical examination, "Don't you have something you're working toward, some ambition for yourself—big or small?"

Learning Review

1. Homeostasis is the general constancy of the body's internal environment, a delicate balance maintained as the body adjusts or adapts to enhance its ability to survive. Name five ways the body uses to restore homeostasis.

   (1)______________________ (4)______________________

   (2)______________________ (5)______________________

   (3)______________________

2. Han Selye's general adaptation syndrome (GAS) thery proposes that adaptation to stress occurs in four stages. Identify each stage in the order in which it is manifested and describe the physiological changes that occur during each one.

(1) ____

____

____

(2) ____

____

____

(3) ____

____

____

(4) ____

____

____

3. Match each of the following activities to its correct approach for coping with stress in the workplace.

A. Plan ahead
B. Arrive early
C. Personal assessment
D. Laugh
E. Music/Color/Light
F. Breaks
G. Work smarter, not harder

____ 1. Soothe and promote relaxation by softly playing a calming classical CD in the reception area.

____ 2. Go to the gym for an engergizing yoga class twice a week after work.

____ 3. Keep up an ability to see the humor in life's events.

____ 4. Join your local chapter of the AAMA and participate in continuing education activities.

____ 5. Keep a list of any special patient problems or needs by reviewing patient charts before formal office hours begin.

____ 6. Take a walk in a local park during a scheduled morning break.

____ 7. Learn how to practice self-motivation on tasks performed independently; feel free to contribute ideas and comments on group projects.

4. A. List the five considerations important in determining a goal. Define each one.

(1) ____

____

(2) ____

____

(3) ____

____

(4) ____

____

(5) ____

____

B. For each consideration, list a personal goal of your own that meets its particular requirements. Choose different goals for each answer; do not use the same goal twice.

(1) ____

____

(2) ____

____

(3) ____

____

(4) ____

____

(5) ____

____

5. A. Burnout is stress-related energy depletion that takes place in the working world. In the military world, burnout is called *battle fatigue.* Burnout occurs gradually over a period of continued stress.

Place a "P" next to those items that promote burnout and an "R" next to those that reduce the risk of burnout.

____ 1. Keep work separate from your home life.

____ 2. Have regular physical examinations.

____ 3. Work harder than anyone else in the office.

____ 4. Feel a greater need than others to do a job well for its own sake.

____ 5. Prioritize tasks and perform the most difficult ones first.

____ 6. Prefer to tackle projects yourself rather than consult a supervisor.

____ 7. Never stop until you achieve your goals, regardless of the personal cost to yourself or loved ones.

____ 8. Postpone vacation time.

____ 9. Give up unrealistic goals and expectations.

____ 10. Maintain a positive self-image and your self-esteem.

____ 11. Develop interests outside your profession.

____ 12. Procrastinate.

____ 13. Wear loose-fitting, comfortable clothes and shoes.

____ 14. Stretch or change positions. Walk around and deliver charts or laboratory specimens.

____ 15. Know your limits and be aware of your body's needs.

6. When filing patients' claims for insurance reimbursement for diagnoses or procedures related to stress, medical assistants may use some of the following codes.

Identify the diagnosis or procedure associated with each code.

90880 ____________________ 308.0 ____________________

307.81 ____________________ 90841-52 ____________________

306.8 ____________________

Investigation Activity: Stress Self-Test

Determining how well you now handle stress will help you to identify personal strengths and weaknesses and point you toward the skills you'll need to develop to be successful on the job as a medical assistant.

For each question, circle the response that best describes you.

1. I exercise
   A. Three times a week.
   B. Less than three times a week.
   C. Only if I am forced to.

2. When something stressful happens in my life, I
   A. Eat too much.
   B. Make sure I eat regular meals.
   C. Stop eating for days.

3. If I am struggling with a problem or project, I am most likely to
   A. Consult someone who may be able to help.
   B. Become determined to solve the problem or finish the project on my own.
   C. Abandon the project or just hope the problem goes away.

4. When I encounter difficult personalities, I
   A. Leave the scene and avoid the person in the future.
   B. Lose my temper and get into arguments.
   C. Practice the art of the diplomatic response.

5. When offered a new challenge or responsibility that requires obtaining new skills or training, I
   A. Get tension headaches.
   B. Respond with enthusiasm and an open mind.
   C. Express concern about taking on a new duty.

6. In emergency situations, I
   A. React calmly and efficiently.
   B. Feel paralyzed.
   C. Wait for someone else to take charge.

7. I feel confident and competent in group situations
   A. Only when I know everyone present.
   B. Most of the time.
   C. Hardly ever. Conversations with others make me uncomfortable.

8. I think meditating or taking time to be quiet and calm during a busy day is
   A. A terrific waste of time. I always have to be doing something.
   B. Good for other people. I've tried it more than once, but I can't seem to get into meditation.
   C. A great way to relax and refocus my mind.

9. The key to handling stressful situations lies in
   A. Staying out of stressful situations.
   B. Examining my view of the situation from a new direction.
   C. Insisting that everyone agree with my point of view.

10. To accomplish my personal goals, I
    A. Am willing to get up an hour earlier each day.
    B. Will give up sleep altogether.
    C. Find myself losing sleep because I am worrying about how I am going to get everything done.

11. I usually complete projects
    A. On time.
    B. At the last minute.
    C. Late—but only by a day.

12. As I prepare for a day's activities, I
    A. Prioritize and use time management skills to budget time carefully.
    B. Don't prepare. I like to be spontaneous.
    C. Find myself overwhelmed and unable to complete anything.

13. When I focus on setting a long-range goal, I
    A. Think through the short-range goals necessary to achieve it.
    B. Become impatient.
    C. Talk constantly about the goal without making plans to achieve it.

14. I volunteer to take on
    A. More tasks than any one person can easily accomplish—then amaze everyone by pulling them off.
    B. Only what I know I can reasonably accomplish.
    C. Only what is required to get the job done.

15. After a stressful day, the best way to unwind is to
    A. Talk all night with family or friends about what happened.
    B. Rent a funny movie.
    C. Work late to prepare for tomorrow.

16. People think of me as
    A. A person who is unpredicable. No one knows what I'll do next.
    B. Someone fixed in life roles.
    C. Someone who is confident about who I am, but who also is willing to grow and change as worthy opportunities arise.

Scoring: In the "My Score" column, record the number of points earned for each of your answers. The higher your score, the less you are prone to stress. The highest possible score is 160 points. If your score is low, consider the areas you need to focus on to reduce stress in your life.

		My Score
1.	A. 10 points B. 5 points C. 0 points Regular exercise reduces stress.	_______
2.	A. 0 points B. 10 points C. 0 points Eating regular meals reduces stress.	_______
3.	A. 10 points B. 5 points C. 0 points Problems rarely just go away; ask for help before struggling on your own.	_______
4.	A. 5 points B. 0 points C. 10 points You won't always be able to avoid a difficult person, and argument leads to stress. Tact and grace are needed.	_______
5.	A. 0 points B. 10 points C. 5 points Worrying to the point of causing physical symptoms is not productive. Close-mindedness could keep you from enjoying something new and cause stressful reactions.	_______
6.	A. 10 points B. 0 points C. 5 points Feelings of helplessness increase stress.	_______
7.	A. 5 points B. 10 points C. 0 points The ability to interact comfortably with others in group situations reduces stress.	_______
8.	A. 0 points B. 5 points C. 10 points The more you can separate your sense of well-being from daily events by taking time to relax and refocus, the less stress you will experience.	_______
9.	A. 0 points B. 10 points C. 0 points Stressful situations can't always be avoided; keeping a flexible instead of a rigid viewpoint will reduce stress.	_______
10.	A. 10 points B. 0 points C. 0 points Sleep is important in reducing stress. However, making time by getting up earlier is a good time-management technique.	_______
11.	A. 10 points B. 5 points C. 0 points Lateness causes stress for everyone.	_______
12.	A. 10 points B. 0 points C. 0 points Unexpected things can always happen, but prioritizing and budgeting time can help keep a handle on the day's events and reduce stress.	_______
13.	A. 10 points B. 5 points C. 0 points Achieving long-range goals takes perseverance and determination. Being realistic about goals reduces stress.	_______
14.	A. 0 points B. 10 points C. 5 points Taking on too much responsibility leads to stress.	_______
15.	A. 0 points B. 10 points C. 0 points Humor is an effective stress reducer—so is separating work from your home life.	_______
16.	A. 0 points B. 0 points C. 10 points Being grounded but open to new experiences reduces stress.	_______
	Total	_______

CASE STUDY

Angie Esposito is a physician at Inner City Health Care. It was her dream, even as a child, to become a physician and work in an environment where she could help people and benefit the community as well. Proud of her accomplishments, she is the first woman in her family to attend college and got herself through medical school with scholarships and student loans. Angie works hard, often pulling double shifts. Liz Corbin, CMA, has a similar dream and is working to save money to attend medical school to become a pediatrician. Dr. Esposito does her best to encourage Liz's ambitions and has taken Liz under her wing.

Late one night, Liz assists Dr. Esposito in treating three difficult emergency patients in a row. "That's it," Angie Esposito says. "We're taking a 15-minute break. Ask Dr. Woo if he can cover for a short time." When Liz catches up with Dr. Esposito in the employee lounge, she finds Angie in frustrated tears. "These double shifts," Angie says. "I'm so tired. And the patients just keep coming. I want to help them all," she sighs and her voice trails off, "I just can't help them all..."

Discuss the following:

1. Dr. Angie Esposito is experiencing burnout. What personality traits are promoting her burnout? Identify the stressors in Angie's life.
2. Liz Corbin, CMA, sees her mentor breaking down under stress. Should Liz reevaluate her own long-range goals?
3. Discuss the importance of keeping goals in perspective.
4. What is Liz's best therapeutic response to Dr. Esposito?

SUPPLEMENTARY RESOURCES

Study Guide Disk: Additional practice exercises for this chapter are available on the Study Guide disk found in the back of the textbook.

Medical Assisting Videos: Appropriate content is available on Delmar's Medical Assisting Videos, 2nd ed., for the following topics:

Tape 1: Your Career as a Medical Assistant
Display Professionalism
Work as a Team Member
Career-Seeking Skills
Communication Skills

Tape 3: Perform Administrative Duties
Triage Skills

EVALUATION OF CHAPTER KNOWLEDGE

Skills achieved:

Skills	Instructor Evaluation *Good*	*Average*	*Poor*
Can identify personal short-range and long-range goals	_____	_____	_____
Recognizes personal strengths and weaknesses in responding to stress	_____	_____	_____
Recognizes inner- and outer-directed qualities of personal character	_____	_____	_____
Ability to describe physiological effects of stress	_____	_____	_____
Understands behaviors that promote or reduce the risk of burnout	_____	_____	_____
Differentiates between stress and stressors	_____	_____	_____
Can identify stressors common in the ambulatory care setting	_____	_____	_____

Student's initials: ________ Instructor's initials ________

Grade:____________

CHAPTER 8

The Therapeutic Approach to the Patient with AIDS

PERFORMANCE OBJECTIVES

As a member of the health care team, the medical assistant will be involved in the care of patients with severe infectious diseases, including AIDS. In addition to providing medical, surgical, and psychological care, the health care team relies on the assets of empathy and compassion in building a strong therapeutic approach to the treatment and care of AIDS patients. As a source of information for AIDS patients and their families and significant others, medical assistants need to be sensitive, supportive, and respectful of people who are suffering from a controversial disease that challenges many strongly held cultural beliefs and attitudes. Medical assistants should strive to promote AIDS education and awareness by informing patients at high risk for contracting AIDS about preventive measures. It is important for medical assistants to remain impartial and professional, making AIDS patients as comfortable and confident as possible in the ambulatory care setting.

EXERCISES AND ACTIVITIES

Vocabulary Builder

Insert the proper key vocabulary terms into the paragraph on the following page.

acquired immunodeficiency syndrome (AIDS)
dementia
hemophilia
human immunodeficiency virus (HIV)
libido
living will
opportunistic infections
pathogens
physician's directive
psychomotor retardation
retroviruses
ribonucleic acid (RNA)

The incurable infectious disease ______________________ involves a flaw in cell-mediated immunity; diagnosis depends on a number of indicator conditions, including a T4 cell count that has dropped below 200. The disease is caused by a virus transmitted from the secretions and excretions of blood from an infected person to the bloodstream of an uninfected person. The transmittor virus, ____________________, is a member of the class of ____________________ that carry genetic material in their ____________________. As T4 cells are destroyed, the body is left open to ____________________ such as toxoplasmosis and tuberculosis, that exist from an altered physiological state of the host and are caused by disease-producing microorganisms called ____________________. Two groups of people at high risk for infection are those suffering from ____________________ or another coagulation disorder, and those who have received transfusions with infected blood or blood products. As the disease progresses, the central nervous system is involved, which causes many symptoms, including a loss of sexual drive, or ____________________; mental disorientation and confusion, called ____________________; and/or a slowing of motor activity, called ____________________. Many patients with this devastating disease choose to protect their treatment preferences at end-of-life by completing a ____________________. This legal document is considered a ____________________, a document that gives physicians advance instructions regarding patients' treatment wishes in emergency and end-of-life situations, when they may not be able to speak for themselves.

Learning Review

1. For each of the stages of progression from HIV infection to a diagnosis of AIDS listed, describe the defining factors contributing to the presence or absence of disease, or epidemiology, of each.

   (1) Initial infection with HIV ____________________

   ____

   ____

   ____

   ____

   ____

   (2) Asymptomatic stage ____________________

   ____

   ____

   ____

   ____

   ____

(3) Symptomatic stage ______________________________

(4) Diagnosis of AIDS ______________________________

2. Name the three methods of transmission of HIV.

(1) ______________________________

(2) ______________________________

(3) ______________________________

3. List the five population groups in which AIDS is most commonly diagnosed.

(1) ______________________________

(2) ______________________________

(3) ______________________________

(4) ______________________________

(5) ______________________________

4. A. Common conditions appearing in people with AIDS include immunologic (IM), integumentary (IT), respiratory (R), gastrointestinal (GI), and central nervous system (CNS) manifestations. Identify the conditions listed below according to their categories of manifestation by placing the proper abbreviation ("IM," "IT," "R," "GI," or "CNS") in the spaces provided.

___ Night sweats
___ Visual changes
___ Poor wound healing
___ Fatigue
___ Low white blood cell count
___ Nausea and vomiting
___ Lymphadenopathy
___ Shortness of breath
___ Memory loss
___ Headache

B. Opportunistic infections appearing in people with AIDS include these types: protozoal (P), fungal (F), bacterial (B), and viral (V). AIDS patients can also develop various malignancies (M). Identify each of the following conditions by its correct classification as an infection or malignancy by placing the proper abbreviation ("P," "F," "B," "V," or "M") in the spaces provided.

___ Candidiasis
___ Herpes simplex
___ Nocardiosis
___ Cryptosporidiosis
___ Kaposi's sarcoma
___ Hodgkin's lymphoma
___ *Pneumocystis carinii*
___ Tuberculosis
___ Cryptococcosis
___ Cytomegalovirus

5. Name six physical symptoms of the psychological suffering experienced by AIDS patients.

(1)______________________
(2)______________________
(3)______________________
(4)______________________
(5)______________________
(6)______________________

6. On a scale of 1 to 5, rate your personal comfort in regard to the following situations medical assistants may find themselves involved with in an ambulatory care setting.

1. Extremely uncomfortable 2. Uncomfortable 3. Somewhat comfortable
4. Comfortable 5. Very comfortable

____ Assisting in the care of substance abusers and drug-addicted patients.
____ Performing venipuncture on patients with high-risk lifestyles.
____ Touching HIV-infected individuals during the course of routine physical examinations.
____ Educating high-risk patients about preventive measures.
____ Maintaining a professional and nonjudgmental attitude about patient lifestyles and potential behaviors.
____ Following standard precautions for infection control.
____ Assessing your openness about homosexuality and acceptance of homosexual patients or co-workers.
____ Discussing AIDS in an open and frank manner with patients and their family members and significant others.
____ Facing your own fears and concerns about HIV infection and AIDS.

Investigaton Activity

One nonmedical form of assistance that medical assistants can provide to AIDS patients is the referral to national and community-based AIDS organizations, programs, hotlines, and service groups where AIDS patients can gather information and explore resources on topics ranging from insurance, legal, and financial concerns to better communications with family members, friends, and significant others.

A. Write or call an AIDS organization or hotline to request information available to AIDS patients and to the general public about coping with the disease. Bring the information to class. As a class, or in smaller groups, examine the brochures you are sent and discuss their content. Decide which brochures contain the best information and seem to be the most effective to recommend to patients and their families and significant others. Here are two national sources:

National Health Information Center
Office of Disease Prevention and Promotion
U. S. Department of Human Services
P. O. Box 1133
Washington, DC 20013-1133
800-336-4797

National AIDS Hotline
Centers for Disease Control and Prevention
Atlanta, GA 30333
800-342-AIDS

B. List two community-based groups located in the area where you live that supply information and services to AIDS patients.

Name: ______________________	Name: ______________________
Address: ______________________	Address: ______________________
______________________	______________________
______________________	______________________
Phone: ______________________	Phone: ______________________

CASE STUDIES

In working with AIDS patients, medical assistants hone their personal coping skills, capitalizing on strengths, maintaining hope, and showing continued human care and concern. For each case scenario presented, answer the following questions:

1. What is the best therapeutic response of the medical assistant?
2. On what criteria do you base this response as the best therapeutic approach?

Case 1

Jaime Carrera, a Hispanic man in his late twenties, is brought to Inner City Health Care, an urgent care center, by co-workers when he injures his head in an accident at a construction site where he is working. His head is bleeding profusely. As Jaime's co-workers watch the health care team implement standard precautions for infection control, one of them, his own shirt and hands covered with Jaime's blood, pulls the medical assistant aside and whispers frantically, "What are you doing? Does he have AIDS?"

Case 2

Mary O'Keefe is a new patient of Dr. Elizabeth King. Mary is undergoing prenatal care. After several office visits, Mary approaches administrative medical assistant Ellen Armstrong, CMA, and sheepishly apologizes for asking what Mary calls a "paranoid" question. "Ellen, do Doctors Lewis and King treat AIDS patients at this practice? Normally, I wouldn't be concerned about the risk, but I'm pregnant, you know, and I worry about the baby being exposed."

Case 3

A. Liz Corbin, CMA, a young African-American woman, works part-time at Inner City Health Care, an urgent care center that sponsors a treatment program for AIDS patients. Liz works professionally and compassionately with the AIDS patients she encounters during her hours at the clinic. On one stressful afternoon, however, Liz seeks out office manager Walter Seals, CMA. Liz breaks down and cries after assisting in the examination of a patient infected with HIV who discovered that she is pregnant and may pass HIV to her unborn child. Liz's ambition is to someday attend medical school to become a pediatrician. "Walter, this disease is so unfair," Liz says passionately. "I just can't take it any more."

B. About a month later, Liz is again assisting in the examination of the pregnant female HIV-infected patient. After the physician leaves the examination room, the woman turns to Liz, takes her hand, and says, "How can I afford this medicine? Why is this happening to me and to my baby?"

SUPPLEMENTARY RESOURCES

Study Guide Disk: Additional practice exercises for this chapter are available on the study guide disk found in the back of the textbook.

Medical Assisting Videos: Appropriate content is available on Delmar's Medical Assisting Videos, 2nd ed., for the following topics:

Tape 1: Communication Skills
Tape 5: Infection Control and Universal Precautions
Apply Principles of Aseptic Technique and Infection Control
Standard Precautions
Infections in the Office
Tape 8: Taking a Patient History
Introduction to Health Promotion, Disease Prevention, and Self-Responsibility
Tape 12: OSHA Regulations for Needles and "Sharps"
Accidental Needlesticks

EVALUATION OF CHAPTER KNOWLEDGE

Evaluate your own strengths and weaknesses in administering a therapeutic approach to the patient with AIDS. Compare this evaluation to the one provided by your instructor.

Skills achieved:

	Student Self-Evaluation			Instructor Evaluation		
Skills	*Good*	*Average*	*Poor*	*Good*	*Average*	*Poor*
Ability to describe the epidemiology of HIV and AIDS in lay terms	___	___	___	___	___	___
Identifies population groups in which the AIDS diagnosis is commonly found	___	___	___	___	___	___
Recognizes psychological problems that accompany AIDS	___	___	___	___	___	___
Identifies personal fears or concerns about assisting in the care and treatment of AIDS patients	___	___	___	___	___	___
Ability to treat AIDS patients with empathy, impartiality, and respect	___	___	___	___	___	___
Possesses working knowledge of conditions, manifestations, opportunistic infections, and malignancies that may appear in AIDS patients	___	___	___	___	___	___
Recognizes the demands of providing therapeutic care for AIDS patients in the ambulatory care setting	___	___	___	___	___	___
Ability to avoid emotional burnout when caring for AIDS patients	___	___	___	___	___	___
Understands the use of standard precautions for infection control in protecting themselves from AIDS infection	___	___	___	___	___	___
Advocates AIDS education and methods of disease prevention for high-risk individuals	___	___	___	___	___	___

Student's Initials:____ Instructor's Initials:_____

Grade:________

CHAPTER 9

Applied Legal Concepts

PERFORMANCE OBJECTIVES

Medical assistants and other health care professionals are employed in the medical profession where laws regulate medical and business practices on both the state and the federal levels. Regulatory agencies act to investigate the quality of health care, control health care costs while providing equitable access to care, and protect the patient. Medical assistants need to be aware of the laws and regulations that govern the practices and procedures followed by health care professionals in the ambulatory care setting. In a society that strongly advocates the individual's right to seek redress in a court of law, the potential for litigation in medical settings must be considered. As responsible health care professionals, medical assistants need to understand the regulations and laws that affect their daily experiences on the job and to behave appropriately within the scope of their training and knowledge.

EXERCISES AND ACTIVITIES

Vocabulary Builder

Match the key vocabulary terms that follow with the example appropriate to each.

___ **1.** To require or dictate by law.

___ **2.** Designation of health care surrogate.

___ **3.** An unconscious heart attack victim at a baseball game receives emergency CPR from an off-duty health professional seated in the same section.

___ **4.** A 17-year-old person serving in the U. S. Armed Forces.

___ **5.** Medical practice acts, or laws, that regulate the practice of law, such as licensure and standards of care.

A. Agents

B. Civil law

C. Criminal law

D. Defendants

E. Doctrines

F. Durable power of attorney for health care

G. Emancipated minor

___ 6. A patient who refuses needed care, such as a cancer patient who will not complete a series of chemotherapy treatments.

___ 7. A physician or health care professional who testifies in court to establish a reasonable and expected standard of care with respect to a specific medical situation so that jurors can understand the nature of medical information.

___ 8. The failure to exercise the standard of care that a reasonable person would exercise in similar circumstances.

___ 9. A patient sues a laboratory for money damages for delivering an incorrect analysis of a specimen that results in misdiagnosis by a physician.

___ 10. In a state where medical assistants must be licensed to perform venipuncture, charges are brought against a person who is performing this invasive procedure without the proper licensure.

___ 11. Persons who bring charges in a civil case.

___ 12. Employees of physician-employers.

___ 13. A written lease for office space.

___ 14. A patient tilts her head back and opens her eyes wide for instillation of medicated eyedrops from a medical assistant without any verbal instructions to do so.

___ 15. Professional negligence.

___ 16. *Respondeat superior* and *res ipsa loquitur.*

___ 17. Though the patient, a competent adult, forcibly draws back, the medical assistant proceeds to administer an injection.

___ 18. Court order.

___ 19. Persons against whom charges are brought.

___ 20. A medical assistant writes in the patient's record, "Jim Marshall is a ruthless, rude man who is very full of himself. Be careful around him."

___ 21. A patient says loudly in the reception area of Inner City Health Care, filled to capacity with waiting patients, "Dr. Reynolds should retire. I know he's not up on the latest medical techniques."

___ 22. Lawsuit.

___ 23. A 17-year-old student who lives with his or her parents.

___ 24. A person found by the court to be insane, inadequate, or not an adult.

___ 25. Actions that make the medical assistant and the physician-employer less vulnerable to lawsuits.

H. Expert witness

I. Expressed contract

J. Implied consent

K. Implied contract by law

L. Incompetent

M. Libel

N. Litigation

O. Malpractice

P. Mandate

Q. Minor

R. Negligence

S. Noncompliant

T. Plaintiffs

U. Risk management

V. Slander

W. Statutes

X. Subpoena

Y. Tort

Learning Review

1. Civil law is a branch of the law where restitution is awarded to individuals, usually in monetary form, when a civil wrong is committed. Crimes against the safety and welfare of society as a whole, however, are addressed by criminal law, where the punishment is usually incarceration and/or a fine.

Identify whether the following actions fall under the domain of civil law (CV) or criminal law (CM) and explain why.

____ A. A physician is siphoning off narcotics from an urgent care center's locked drug cabinet and continuing to treat patients while under the influence of the drugs.

____

____

____

____ B. A woman sues her insurer when it refuses to provide benefits for a bone marrow transplant in the advanced stages of breast cancer.

____

____

____

____ C. An office manager steals, or embezzles, funds from the medical practice.

____

____

____

2. Contracts are expressed or implied. Expressed contracts are written or verbal agreements that specify the exact duties of each party. Implied contracts depend on the power of action and circumstance; the actions performed would have been intended had an expressed contract existed.

Identify each of the following as an expressed (E), implied (I), or invalid (X) contract.

____ A. Marriage ceremony.

____ B. Living will.

____ C. Rescue breathing.

____ D. Patient appointment scheduled over the telephone.

____ E. A purchase order for office supplies.

____ F. Colposcopy performed by a gynecologist when visual inspection reveals an abnormal appearance of the cervix during a physical examination.

____ G. A will signed by an Alzheimer's patient with progressive disease.

____ H. A medical decision made by a health care surrogate for a patient suffering a debilitating cerebral vascular accident (CVA).

____ I. Setting the fractured arm of a child rushed to the emergency room after a playground fall.

____ J. Confirming verbal acceptance of a job offer as a clinical medical assistant by a handshake with the office manager of the medical practice.

3. (For this exercise, consult Figures 9–2, 9–3, and 9–4 from the textbook.) A physician-patient contract is terminated when the patient discharges the physician, the physician formally withdraws from patient care, or the patient no longer needs treatment and is formally discharged by the physician. What is the appropriate legal and ethical action when each patient responds as follows to receipt of a letter terminating the patient-physician relationship?

   A. After telephoning Dr. Winston Lewis to complain about his treatment and to threaten to find a new doctor, Jim Marshall receives a letter from Winston confirming that Jim has discharged him as his physician. Jim is outraged. He calls office manager Marilyn Johnson, CMA, to insist on making an appointment, claiming he never intended to find a new doctor but only to get Dr. Lewis to prescribe a more effective medication to control his high blood pressure.

   Action: ____

   ____

   ____

   ____

   ____

   B. Two months after receiving the letter confirming that Dr. James Whitney has withdrawn from Lenny Taylor's case because the patient will not follow the medical plan for his care, Lenny, who suffers mild dementia, still refuses to contact a gerontologist or to take the medications James had prescribed previously. In desperation, his son, George Taylor, calls James to plead with him to take his father back as a patient.

   Action: ____

   ____

   ____

   ____

   ____

   C. Rhoda Au writes to Dr. Mark Woo to inform him that she has found a physician trained in both Western and traditional Chinese medicine, who is more willing to integrate both approaches into a treatment plan for her. She cites Mark's skepticism in pursuing alternative treatments and his sole reliance on Western drug therapies to treat her diagnosed case of lupus erythematosus as the reason why she refused to follow his treatment plan. Rhoda goes further to say that she feels Mark has forgotten his heritage; she supplies the new physician's name and address.

Action: ____

____

____

____

____

4. List and define the 4 Ds of negligence:

(1) ____

____

(2) ____

____

(3) ____

____

(4) ____

____

5. List 11 strategies for risk management in an ambulatory care setting that will lessen the potential for litigation.

(1) ____

____

(2) ____

____

(3) ____

____

(4) ____

____

(5) ____

____

(6) ____

____

(7) ____

____

(8) ____

____

(9) ______________________________

____

(10) ______________________________

____

(11) ______________________________

____

6. The patient's chart is the legal record of medical care administered. An action not recorded in the chart is generally considered an action not performed. Before any invasive or surgical procedure is performed, patients are asked to sign consent forms, which become a permanent part of the medical record. What four things must the patient know in order to give *informed* consent?

   (1) ______________________________

   (2) ______________________________

   (3) ______________________________

   (4) ______________________________

7. A tort is a wrongful act that results in injury to one person by another. Malpractice is the unintentional tort of negligence; that is, a health care professional either failed to act in a reasonable and prudent manner and caused harm to the patient or did what a reasonable and prudent person would not have done and caused harm to a patient.

   A. Define the following three examples of torts common in the ambulatory care setting.

   Battery: ______________________________

   ____

   ____

   Defamation of character: ______________________________

   ____

   ____

   Invasion of privacy: ______________________________

   ____

   ____

   B. There are two doctrines of negligence. Define each.

   Res ipsa loquitur: ______________________________

   ____

   Respondeat superior: ______________________________

   ____

8. Advance directives, living wills, and durable powers of attorney for health care are legal documents patients can execute to protect their treatment wishes in the event that they cannot communicate for themselves due to serious illness or injury. Medical assistants are asked to attach these documents as a permanent part of the patient's medical record. Most states have their own forms, and legal requirements vary from state to state. These documents should be initialed and updated periodically to ensure their enforceability.

The decision to withdraw or administer treatment is intensely personal and will differ vastly from patient to patient. Individuals hold strong beliefs regarding medical treatment and life-saving measures that must be respected by medical assistants and all health care professionals. The form below is an excerpt from a generic living will document supplied by Choice in Dying. Explore your own feelings and preferences by completing the form below.* This page may be removed from the workbook and kept confidential; your instructor will not review it.

INSTRUCTIONS

CHOICE IN DYING LIVING WILL

PRINT YOUR NAME

I, ______________________________, being of sound mind, make this statement as a directive to be followed if I become permanently unable to participate in decisions regarding my medical care. These instructions reflect my firm and settled commitment to decline medical treatment under the circumstances indicated below:

I direct my attending physician to withhold or withdraw treatment that merely prolongs my dying, if I should be in an **incurable or irreversible mental or physical condition with no reasonable expectation of recovery,** including but not limited to: (a) **a terminal condition;** (b) **a permanently unconscious condition;** or (c) **a minimally conscious condition in which I am permanently unable to make decisions or express my wishes.**

I direct that treatment be limited to measures to keep me comfortable and to relieve pain, including any pain that might occur by withholding or withdrawing treatment.

While I understand that I am not legally required to be specific about future treatments, **if I am in the condition(s) described above I feel especially strongly about the following forms of treatment:**

CROSS OUT ANY STATEMENTS THAT DO NOT REFLECT YOUR WISHES

I do not want cardiac resuscitation.
I do not want mechanical respiration.
I do not want tube feeding.
I do not want antibiotics.

However, **I do want** maximum pain relief, even if it may hasten my death.

**Note: This workbook activity is not to be construed as a legal document, but is used for teaching purposes only.*

Add personal instructions (if any)

Other directions (insert personal instructions):

These directions express my legal right to refuse treatment under federal and state law. I intend my instructions to be carried out, unless I have revoked them in a new writing or by clearly indicating that I have changed my mind.

Sign and date the document and print your address

Signed: ______________________ Date: ______________

Address: ______________________________________

____

Witnessing Procedure

I declare that the person who signed this document appeared to execute the living will willingly and free from duress. He or she signed (or asked another to sign for him or her) this document in my presence.

Two witnesses must sign and print their addresses

Witness: ______________________________________

Address: ______________________________________

____

Witness: ______________________________________

Address: ______________________________________

____

Courtesy of **Choice in Dying, Inc.**
200 Varick Street, New York, NY 10014 212-366-5540
Reprinted by permission.

6/96

INVESTIGATION ACTIVITIES

Activity 1

Child abuse, spousal abuse, and elder abuse are all too common in our society today. Physician-patient confidentiality does not apply in cases of abuse; health care professionals must report suspected abuse to the appropriate authorities or face criminal or civil charges for the failure to do so. Careful charting and maintenance of the medical record in each case of abuse is critical, as the medical record becomes the legal document of care that will be considered by a court of law.

Medical assistants have a responsibility to the patients they serve and to the community at large to respond with professionalism, empathy, and compassion to the victims of domestic violence. Patient education and community awareness are two ways medical assistants can help become involved.

1. List one organization in the community where you live that provides information and services as a strong advocate for the protection of children, the elderly, and battered women.

   Children

   Name: ______________________________

   Address: ______________________________

   ____

   ____

   Phone: ______________________________

   Elderly

   Name: ______________________________

   Address: ______________________________

   ____

   ____

   Phone: ______________________________

   Battered Women

   Name: ______________________________

   Address: ______________________________

   ____

   ____

   Phone: ______________________________

2. Contact one of the organizations above for literature and information about the services provided. Obtain information about the services provided to the organizations by community volunteers. Bring the information to class and discuss ways that health care professionals can contribute to community awareness. Discuss the legal responsibilities of health care professionals to victims of abuse.

Activity 2

Statutes, or laws, govern licensure, standards of care, professional liability and negligence, confidentiality, and torts. Some states regulate personnel who may be employed in the ambulatory care setting. For example, the scope of practice of medical assistants can vary from state to state. Some states require additional certification or licensure to perform certain clinical duties. Investigate the laws in your state regarding the scope of practice, or duty of care, of medical assistants. As a class, have each student choose one other state to investigate any scope of practice for medical assistants identified in that state. Bring the information to class and discuss how state requirements differ and how the requirements might affect employment opportunities in the medical assisting profession. Two places to begin your research are the AAMA and your state's licensure board.

CASE STUDIES

For each of the following cases, what errors are made that could leave the medical assistants and/or physician-employers vulnerable to litigation? How might the errors leave the health care professionals open to potential lawsuits? How could the errors have been avoided through effective risk management techniques?

Case 1

On a busy afternoon at Inner City Health Care, the reception area is filled with walk-in patients and the staff struggles to keep up with the patient load. Administrative medical assistant Liz Corbin, CMA, gives the patient file for Edith Leonard to clinical medical assistant Bruce Goldman, CMA. "Dr. Reynolds wants a CBC done stat on the elderly woman in exam room 1," she tells Bruce, handing him the file.

Bruce proceeds to examination room 1; without identifying the patient, he performs a venipuncture on Cele Little, who has come to the clinic for a hearing problem. Cele asks Bruce why the procedure needs to be performed and doesn't want to have it. Bruce insists that the physician has ordered the procedure and performs the venipuncture anyway. The procedure frightens Cele, and she begins to fear her hearing loss is indicative of a more serious illness.

Case 2

Dr. Elizabeth King has just completed a routine physical examination of Abigail Johnson. Elizabeth asks Anna Preciado, CMA, to administer a flu shot to Abigail before she leaves the office. Abigail, an elderly African-American woman, is accompanied by her daughter. When Anna attempts to administer the flu vaccine, Abigail says, "Is that a flu shot? They make me sick; I don't want it."

Abigail's daughter says, "Yes, she does want it. Go ahead and give it to her."

Abigail begins to laugh. "Okay," Anna says, "May I give you the vaccination?"

Abigail says nothing, but she rolls up her sleeve. As Anne administers the parenteral injection, the older woman looks up at her seriously and says, "I didn't want any flu shot. My daughter makes me get it every year." However, Abigail does not withdraw physically.

Case 3

Dr. Elizabeth King is going over the daily list of scheduled patients with Ellen Armstrong, CMA. They are standing at the front desk close to the reception area; several patients are waiting for the first appointments of the day. Elizabeth's eye moves down the list and stops over the name Mary O'Keefe. "Mary O'Keefe," she mutters, "she's so neurotic and pestering. It's a small wonder her husband hasn't left her yet; just wait till they have that third child. ...I don't think I have the patience for Mary today."

Case 4

Lydia Renzi, a deaf woman with some residual hearing, comes to Inner City Health Care with a recurrent vaginal discharge. Lydia is diagnosed by Dr. Angie Esposito with candidiasis, a yeast infection caused by the fungus *Candida albicans;* Angie prescribes a vaginal suppository and asks Wanda Slawson, CMA, to give Lydia instructions for using the prescription. Lydia wears a hearing aid and has chosen not to be accompanied to the clinic by a sign language interpreter. Lydia has trouble understanding Wanda, who is soft spoken; Wanda is also standing against a brightly lit window, and Lydia has trouble seeing her face. Lydia writes on a pad she has brought with her, "Is this a sexually transmitted illness?"

In frustration, Wanda begins shouting, "You just have a yeast infection; it's not like you have herpes or anything." At that moment, Bruce Goldman, CMA, is escorting a male patient past the open door of the examination room. Both men turn their heads away, though it is clear they have overheard.

Case 5

Construction workers Jaime Carrera and Ralph Samson are required to take a pre-employment drug-screening test before they can be hired to work on a new site to which they have applied. Jaime and Ralph come to Inner City Health Care where urine specimens are collected for examination. The test comes back positive for Jaime, and his potential employer does not give him the job. Ralph tests negative. Two weeks later, Ralph returns to Inner City Health Care for a routine physical examination.

"Whatever happened to Jaime Carrera?" Ralph asks Bruce Goldman, CMA. "I haven't seen him around the site."

"Oh," Bruce replies, "he tested positive for chemical substance abuse, and now he's in a rehab program Dr. Whitney suggested."

SUPPLEMENTARY RESOURCES

Study Guide Disk: Additional practice exercises for this chapter are available on the Study Guide disk found in the back of the textbook.

Medical Assisting Videos: Appropriate content is available on Delmar's Medical Assisting Videos, 2nd ed., Tape 2, for the following topics:

Apply Legal Concepts to Practice
Legal Aspects and Confidentiality of Medical Records
Practice Risk Management to Prevent Professional Liability
Perform within Ethical Boundaries

SKILLS PROFICIENCY EVALUATION

How has your instructor evaluated the skills you have achieved?

Skills	Instructor Evaluation *Good*	 *Average*	 *Poor*
Can apply legal concepts to the ambulatory care setting	_____	_____	_____
Understands the concept of standard of care	_____	_____	_____
Can identify expressed and implied contracts	_____	_____	_____
Understands informed consent	_____	_____	_____
Recognizes the need to practice effective risk management techniques	_____	_____	_____
Understands the doctrine of *respondeat superior*	_____	_____	_____
Can identify common torts in the ambulatory care setting	_____	_____	_____
Can define malpractice, or professional negligence	_____	_____	_____
Working knowledge of Good Samaritan laws, physician's directive, and the ADA	_____	_____	_____
Understands accurately documenting and reporting abuse	_____	_____	_____

Student's Initials:______ Instructor's Initials:______

Grade: _____

CHAPTER 10

Applied Ethical Concepts

PERFORMANCE OBJECTIVES

Laws and regulations that govern the practice of medicine ensure that basic requirements and guidelines for protecting both patients and providers are observed. Medical assistants and all health care professionals are charged with the ethical responsibility to follow the law and to perform their duties within the scope of their training and practice. Laws and regulations find their origins in a system of ethics, what is considered to be right and wrong behavior. As medical technology advances, ethical dilemmas are created that challenge traditional codes of behavior. Medical ethics often confront ethical issues of great social controversy, such as in the field of bioethics. Medical assistants need to examine carefully their own deeply held values and beliefs, their system of personal ethics, to build a strong foundation with which to face the ethical dilemmas encountered in the ambulatory care setting.

EXERCISES AND ACTIVITY

Vocabulary Builder

A. Ethics are defined in terms of what is morally right and wrong. Personal ethics will vary from person to person. There are many ethical issues related to health care and medicine, however, that are shared across the lifespan. For each life passage below, list one problem or issue of concern relating to medical ethics. Then pose your own solution to the ethical problem.

Infants or Children

Ethical Issue: ____

____

Ethical Solution: ____

____

Adults

Ethical Issue: ____________________

____

Ethical Solution: ____________________

____

Senior Adults

Ethical Issue: ____________________

____

Ethical Solution: ____________________

____

B. Bioethics is a branch of medical ethics concerned with moral issues resulting from high technology and sophisticated medical research. Name six important bioethical issues that are challenging the medical profession today.

(1) ____________________

(2) ____________________

(3) ____________________

(4) ____________________

(5) ____________________

(6) ____________________

C. Define *surrogacy*. What deeply held societal beliefs does the bioethical issue of surrogacy challenge in our society?

____

____

____

____

____

D. Define *genetic engineering*. Name one medical benefit and one potential danger of genetic manipulation. In your personal opinion, are the benefits of genetic engineering greater than the risks and dangers? Why?

____

____

____

____

____

Learning Review

1. The AAMA Code of Ethics presents five basic principles that medical assistants must pledge to honor as members of the medical assisting profession.

For each situation presented, identify the AAMA ethical principle that applies.

1. Render service with full respect for the dignity of humanity.
2. Respect confidential information.
3. Uphold the honor and integrity of the profession.
4. Pursue continuing education activities and improve knowledge and skills.
5. Participate in community services and education.

____ A. Marilyn Johnson, CMA, in conversation with co-office manager Shirley Brooks, CMA, refuses to speculate about whether a diagnosis of AIDS will be confirmed for patient Maria Jover.

____ B. Administrative medical assistant Karen Ritter joins a study group to prepare for the CMA certification examination as a method of securing her recertification of credentials, which is required every 5 years.

____ C. Clinical medical assistant Anna Preciado agrees to speak to a group of high school students who are interested in pursuing a career in the medical assisting profession.

____ D. Liz Corbin, CMA, politely reminds elderly patient Edith Leonard that she is a medical assistant, not a nurse, but assures Edith that she is qualified to perform the instillation of medicated eyedrops ordered by Dr. Susan Rice.

____ E. When patient Dottie Tate makes an appointment at Inner City Health Care for follow-up treatment of chronic back pain and a recent history of frequent falls, Bruce Goldman, CMA, prearranges for a wheelchair to accommodate Dottie's office visit.

____ F. Karen Ritter, CMA, volunteers at the local community office of Planned Parenthood on weekends.

____ G. Jane O'Hara, CMA, gently and kindly guides patient Wayne Elder, whose mild retardation often causes him to become confused in unfamiliar settings, back to the proper examination room when she finds him wandering down the hallway in search of Dr. Ray Reynolds.

____ H. When filing a group of recent laboratory reports into the correct patient files, Ellen Armstrong, CMA, takes care to complete the task quickly and efficiently. She performs the task at a private office station away from the general reception area and does not leave the charts open or unattended as she works.

____ I. Audrey Jones, CMA, approaches office manager Shirley Brooks, CMA, about opportunities for obtaining advanced training in order to become qualified to perform a wider array of clinical procedures in the ambulatory care setting.

____ J. Clinical medical assistant Wanda Slawson, who assisted Dr. Mark Woo in the treatment of patient Rhoda Au, diagnosed with lupus erythematosus, feels the patient is foolhardy when she rejects Mark's treatment plan of Western drug therapy in favor of an approach that integrates Chinese medicine. However, she respects the patient's heritage and right to choose her own health care.

2. The American Medical Association publishes the Principles of Medical Ethics, a list of standards of conduct that define the essentials of honorable behavior required of physicians. *For each situation listed below, identify whether the physician's action is ethical or unethical according to the AMA code of ethics. Explain why.*

    ____A. Drs. Winston Lewis and Elizabeth King hold a monthly staff meeting to discuss ways the practice can involve itself in community outreach programs and encourage all employees to perform volunteer services.

    ____B. Dr. Susan Rice is actively involved in a national research project studying the long-term effects of estrogen replacement therapy on postmenopausal women.

    ____C. Dr. Angie Esposito confirms the diagnosis of child abuse in the case of patient Juanita Hansen and her son Henry. Angie informs Juanita that she will respect her privacy for now, but will report the abuse if Henry's condition does not improve at a follow-up examination in one month.

    ____D. After formally withdrawing from the care of Lenny Taylor, an elderly man suffering mild dementia who will not follow his treatment plan, Dr. James Whitney refuses to accept Lenny back as a patient despite the desperate request of Lenny's son, George.

    ____E. When Mary O'Keefe's pregnancy test results come back positive, Dr. Elizabeth King immediately telephones Mary's husband, John O'Keefe, to tell him the good news.

    ____F. When patient Lourdes Austen breaks down and cries during a physical examination one year after she has completed treatment for breast cancer, Dr. Elizabeth King takes her hand and acknowledges the stress of living with cancer.

    ____G. Dr. Winston Lewis declines to refer patients to a local urologist who also owns a controlling interest in a medical laboratory to which all patient specimens are sent for analysis.

3. According to the *Current Opinions of the Council on Ethical and Judicial Affairs of the AMA*, advertising by physicians is considered ethical if the ad follows certain requirements. Which of the following are appropriate types of physician advertisements? *Circle each correct response.*

    A. Testimonials from patients cured of serious illnesses or whose conditions were reversed or controlled under the care and treatment of the physician.

    B. Physicians' credentials, along with physicians' hospital or community affiliations.

    C. A description of the practice, facility hours of operation, and the types of services available to health care consumers.

    D. Photographs of health care professionals performing their duties at a medical facility. For example, a physical therapist applying ultrasound, a deep tissue modality, to a patient suffering chronic lower back pain.

    E. Guarantees of cure promised within a specific time frame.

    F. Word-of-mouth advertisement from patients.

4. Without the patient's expressed approval, health care professionals are not allowed to discuss that patient's medical condition with members of the media. Only information that is in the public domain can be released to any media representative without patient approval.

   A. Define *public domain.* ______________________________

   B. For each of the following four types of information considered to be in the public domain, write a one-sentence public announcement suitable for release to the media, naming the patient "John Jones" or "Jane Jones." What details are appropriate to the announcement?

   Birth: ______________________________

   ____

   ____

   Death: ______________________________

   ____

   ____

   Accident: ______________________________

   ____

   ____

   Police Record: ______________________________

   ____

   ____

5. Patient medical records are confidential legal documents. Name three instances, however, where health professionals are allowed or required to reveal confidential patient information by law.

   (1) ______________________________

   (2) ______________________________

   (3) ______________________________

6. *Circle each item that follows which represents an ethical practice in regard to the professional fees and charges appropriate in the ambulatory care setting.*

   A. Patients are notified that a $10 fee will be charged for appointments that are not canceled within 24 hours of the scheduled appointment time.

   B. Physicians agree to include a diagnosis and procedure code on the insurance claim form for a routine physical examination, so that the insurance policy will cover the charges.

   C. Fees for comparable services are often higher in busy, metropolitan areas.

   D. A surcharge is attached for submitting difficult or complicated insurance claims.

   E. A $100 surcharge is attached to any emergency medical procedure performed in an ambulatory care setting.

F. Patient fees are split between the physician-employers of a large group practice.

G. Interest is charged on overdue patient account balances after 90 days.

Investigation Activity

Bioethical Dilemmas: A Self-exploration

Bioethical issues in the field of medicine have a powerful impact on the lives of patients. Many of these issues engage the highly charged emotions and deeply held beliefs of patients, caregivers, and health care professionals. As a medical assistant, you will participate in situations involving bioethical dilemmas. By answering the questions that follow, you will begin to explore your own comfort levels with bioethical dilemmas such as allocation of scarce medical resources, abortion and fetal tissue research, genetic engineering and manipulation, artificial insemination and surrogacy, end-of-life treatment, and HIV/AIDS. The system of medical ethics involving these issues is constantly changing and evolving as society comes to grips with the implications and challenges of bioethical dilemmas. Many of the questions listed have not yet been resolved; there is often no one right or wrong answer. Circle the response that most closely matches your own personal ethical position. If you hold a differing opinion, write it in.

1. I believe Medicare/Medicaid patients should

   A. Receive the lowest level of competent care medically necessary.

   B. Receive the full benefit of treatments made possible by costly medical technology.

   C. Receive the same care as any other patient, regardless of their Medicare/Medicaid status.

   D. ______________________________

   ____

2. I believe the only unscheduled patient appointment of the day should be

   A. Given to the first patient who asks for it.

   B. Reserved for emergency patients only.

   C. Reserved for rescheduling purposes if patient appointments need to be shuffled in the course of the day.

   D. ______________________________

   ____

3. I believe life begins

   A. At the moment of conception.

   B. At some point during the development of the fetus in the womb.

   C. At birth.

   D. ______________________________

   ____

4. I believe fetal tissue research and transplantation should

   A. Be allowed as a potentially life-saving treatment for patients with serious, life-threatening illnesses.

   B. Encourage women to have abortions and should not be allowed.

   C. Be allowed, but only under certain conditions and with close government regulation.

   D. ______________________________

   ____

5. I believe that the results of laboratory blood tests to screen for the presence of genes associated with certain serious life-threatening illnesses should

   A. Be used to establish pre-existing conditions if the results are positive; test results should be accessible to insurance companies to determine individual coverage of benefits.

   B. Be held in strict confidence between physician and patient with no authorized legal release of information to any third party.

   C. Be used to encourage preventive health measures without any penalty or restriction of coverage imposed by insurers.

   D. ______________________________

   ____

6. I believe genetic manipulation

   A. Holds the potential to prevent or cure disease and prolong the lifespan.

   B. Is humankind's dangerous attempt to manipulate nature and determine the course of its own evolution.

   C. Holds too many possibilities for abuse and destructive purposes.

   D. ______________________________

   ____

7. I believe adoptive parents should have the right

   A. To information regarding the medical history of the biological parents.

   B. To adopt an infant even if one or both spouses is over the age of 50.

   C. To choose surrogacy as a viable alternative to parenthood.

   D. ______________________________

   ____

8. I believe artificial insemination should be performed

   A. For heterosexual couples only.

   B. For heterosexual couples and single women only.

C. For heterosexual couples, single women, and lesbians.

D. ____

____

9. I believe that elderly people with chronic and serious health problems should

A. Live with and be cared for by their children.

B. Be cared for in long-term care facilities that provide assistance and skilled nursing services.

C. Be allowed to stay in their own homes with the assistance of qualified home health aides.

D. ____

____

10. I believe physician-assisted suicide

A. Violates the medical code of ethics dedicated to upholding life.

B. Is a responsible answer to the unnecessary prolonging of life made possible through advances in medical technology.

C. Is acceptable only in the most extreme cases of human pain and suffering.

D. ____

____

11. I believe that physicians and health care providers who are HIV positive should

A. Be entitled to the same right to confidentiality as patients who are HIV positive.

B. Be required to reveal their HIV positive status to patients and co-workers.

C. Be required to register their HIV positive status with OSHA, with the guarantee that information will be held confidential from any third party.

D. ____

____

12. I believe experimental drug therapies for AIDS patients should

A. Be accessible to any patient whose case qualifies for their use, with full coverage guaranteed by insurers.

B. Be restricted only to participants in federal- or state-approved research studies.

C. Be covered by Medicare and Medicaid to make treatments accessible on a wider scale to an increased number of patients.

D. ____

____

Conclusion:

As health care providers, medical assistants must deal with difficult situations and bioethical issues about which they hold strong and individual personal opinions. As professionals, however, medical assistants must remain impartial and nonjudgmental in providing care, learning to consider and respect the morals and values of patients and co-workers even though those morals and values may be different from their own.

CASE STUDY

Lourdes Austen arrives at the offices of Drs. Winston Lewis and Elizabeth King for her annual physical examination. It is one year since Lourdes had surgery to remove a tumor in her breast by lumpectomy with axillary lymph node dissection, followed by a course of radiation. Lourdes's one-year mammogram and follow-up examinations with her surgeon and radiologist find no evidence of a recurrence of the cancer. Lourdes is a single woman in her late thirties. As Elizabeth begins the routine physical examination, assisted by Anna Preciado, CMA, Lourdes begins to cry. "I'm so happy to be alive," Lourdes says. "And so afraid of the cancer coming back. But, I want to celebrate life. I've talked to my boyfriend about it and we want to get pregnant. What should I do?"

Elizabeth takes Lourdes's hand. "I know that living with cancer is hard. You are doing well. But there are many things we need to consider..."

Discuss the following:

1. What bioethical dilemma exists in Lourdes's situation? In your opinion, is Lourdes's choice to become pregnant an ethical one?
2. How do deeply held beliefs and attitudes about parenthood and the role of women in our society impact on the patient's decision? How could these beliefs impact the health care team's response to Lourdes?
3. What is Elizabeth's best therapeutic response to Lourdes? What medical issues should the health care team consider if Lourdes becomes pregnant?
4. What is the role of the medical assistant in this situation?

SUPPLEMENTARY RESOURCES

Study Guide Disk: Additional practice exercises for this chapter are available on the study guide disk found in the back of the textbook.

Medical Assisting Videos: Appropriate content is available on Delmar's Medical Assisting Videos, 2nd ed., Tape 2, on the following topics:

Legal Aspects and Confidentiality of Medical Records
Use Appropriate Guidelines When Releasing Records
Perform within Ethical Boundaries

SKILLS PROFICIENCY EVALUATION

How has your instructor evaluated the skills you have achieved?

	Instructor Evaluation		
Skills	*Good*	*Average*	*Poor*
Open to exploring and building a strong personal ethic	____	____	____
Has respect for the morals and values of others	____	____	____
Understands the need to maintain confidentiality of patient records	____	____	____
Understands and can apply the AAMA Code of Ethics and creed to the ambulatory care setting	____	____	____
Recognizes the seven standards of conduct outlined by the AMA for physicians	____	____	____
Recognizes common ethical issues across the lifespan	____	____	____
Identifies sensitive bioethical dilemmas	____	____	____
Will uphold the honor, integrity, and professionalism of the medical assisting profession	____	____	____

Student's Initials:_____ Instructor's Initials:______

Grade: ___________

CHAPTER 11

Creating the Facility Environment

PERFORMANCE OBJECTIVES

Medical assistants are employed in ambulatory care settings, for example, the medical practice or clinic. The physical environment of the health care facility is an important contributing factor to patient comfort. Effective facility design and layout can also increase efficiency and boost the medical facility's functional utility. Medical assistants recognize that maintaining a professional, welcoming environment for patient care promotes health and increases patient confidence in the physician and in the entire health care team. Complying with the Americans with Disabilities Act (ADA) also ensures that the physically challenged have equal access to care.

EXERCISES AND ACTIVITIES

Vocabulary Builder

A. What is the purpose of the Americans with Disabilities Act (ADA)?

____

____

____

____

B. When creating the facility environment, why is accessibility a major consideration?

____

____

____

____

C. Name four ways an ambulatory care setting can accommodate the physically challenged.

(1) ____________________

(2) ____________________

(3) ____________________

(4) ____________________

Learning Review

1. The physical office environment can contribute to the patient's sense of confidence and comfort or can be viewed by the patient as intimidating or anxiety-producing. For each office area below, describe why the area could be perceived by patients as a frightening place. What can be done to make each area a more comforting environment for patients?

Reception area: ____________________

Corridors: ____________________

Examination rooms: ____________________

2. Health care professionals should strive to empower the patient with as much control and dignity as possible. For each of the following situations listed, identify strategies that health care professionals can use to respect the patient's dignity and/or to lessen the sense of disproportion between health care providers and the patient.

A. Bill Schwartz is referred to a dermatologist by Dr. Ray Reynolds for examination of a recurring mole on his calf. The dermatologist tells Bill that a full-body inspection will need to be done to ensure that no other areas of the skin are affected. Bill must appear disrobed in front of the dermatologist and medical assistant, who are both female.

____

B. Martin Gordon, diagnosed with prostate cancer, begins a series of radiation treatments. At the radiation clinic, he is required to disrobe from the waist down and put on a hospital gown. While waiting for access to the treatment room, Martin must sit in a common area with other patients, male and female, who are also waiting for radiation treatments.

____

____

____

C. Ellen Armstrong, CMA, places a Holter monitor on patient Charles Williams. After the Holter monitor is in place, Charles has several questions about the patient activity diary that he would prefer to discuss with Dr. Winston Lewis.

____

____

____

3. The medical receptionist, often a medical assistant with other duties to perform as well, is the person who sets the social climate for the interchange between the patient and the health care team. A friendly, reassuring demeanor and an ability to triage situations are essential skills. For each situation listed, what is the best action or response of the medical receptionist?

   A. A patient with intense stomach pain doubles over and then bolts up to the reception desk, saying, "I'm going to throw up."

   ____

   ____

   ____

   ____

   B. When presented with a bill, the patient exclaims, "I can't pay for all of this now! Every time I come here it seems like the doctor bill goes up a hundred dollars."

   ____

   ____

   ____

   ____

   C. A patient is looking for the correct exit from the examination area to the waiting area and makes a wrong turn into the receptionist's area. He asks, "Where do I go?"

   ____

   ____

   ____

   ____

D. A patient new to an HMO plan does not realize that a separate referral form is needed for a follow-up visit with the gastroenterologist one week after a colonoscopy test has been performed. She says, "I drove an hour to get to this appointment. No one told me I needed another form."

____

____

____

____

4. *Match the color(s) to the appropriate psychological effect in the ambulatory care setting.*

A. Blue.	____	1. Increases alertness and outward orientation.
B. Pastel yellow and blue.	____	2. Overwhelms, threatens, or intimidates.
C. Bright red and orange.	____	3. Promotes quiet and extended concentration.
D. Earthy green tone.	____	4. Presents difficulty in distinguishing colors for elderly patients
E. Warm mauve.	____	5. Causes individuals to underestimate time.

5. A. Create a checklist of five activities to perform upon opening a medical facility.

(1) ✔ ____

(2) ✔ ____

(3) ✔ ____

(4) ✔ ____

(5) ✔ ____

B. Create a checklist of five activities to perform upon closing a medical facility.

(1) ✔ ____

(2) ✔ ____

(3) ✔ ____

(4) ✔ ____

(5) ✔ ____

Investigation Activity

A well-designed reception area allows for patient comfort, along with a functional and efficient use of space. The reception area should be well lit; should not be too bright or too dark; and should have clearly defined areas that are accessible, roomy, and comfortable. If a practice includes several patient populations, from children to the elderly, sections of the reception area

A. Templates

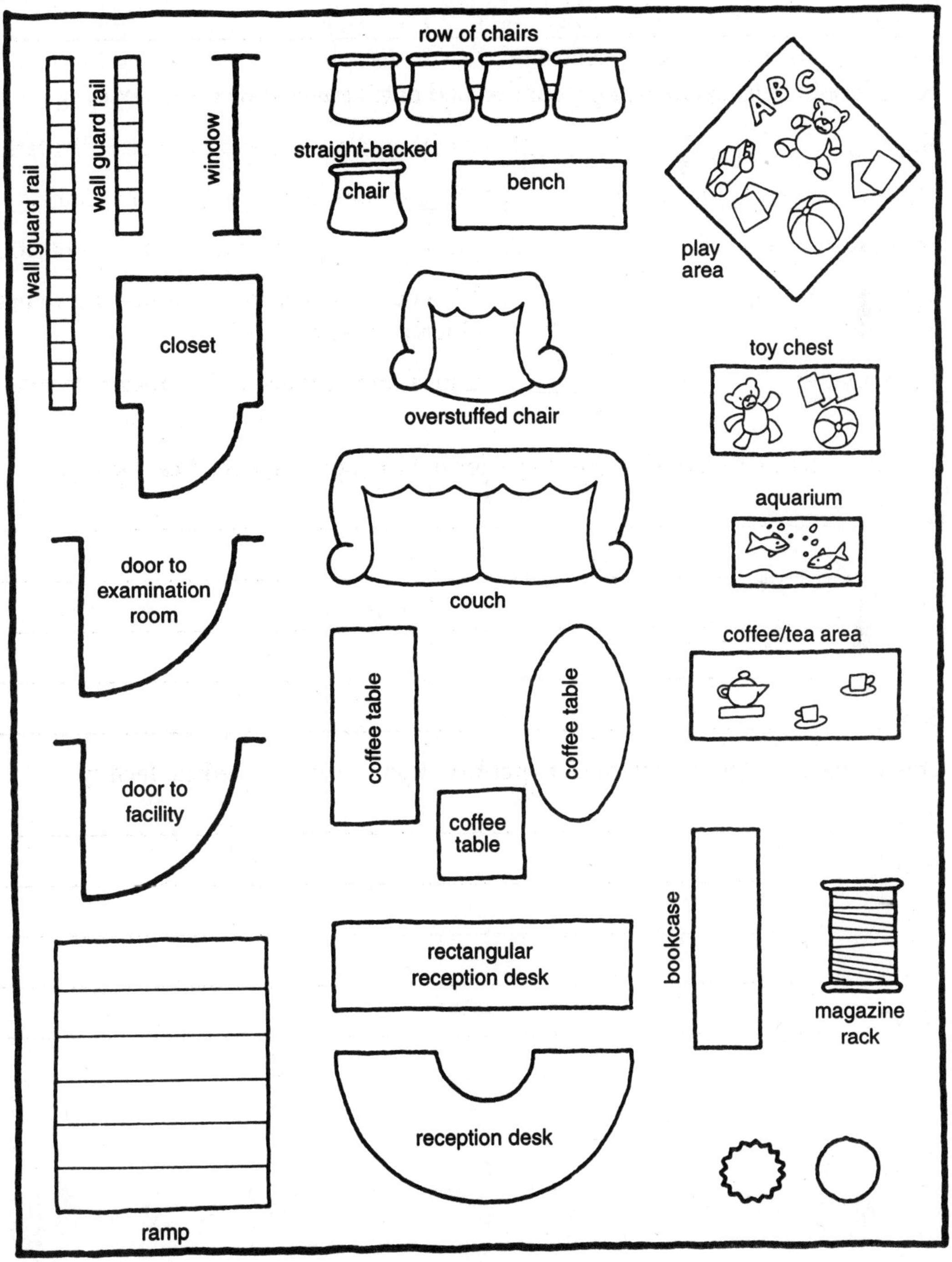

can be designed to accommodate each group's special requirements. The medical receptionist should have a clear view of patients who are waiting to see the physician. All areas should be fully accessible to the physically challenged, in compliance with the ADA.

Using the templates on the previous page, design a functional reception area. Move the templates around on the floor plan; use tracing paper to experiment with different placements and configurations. Visualize your experience of the space, both as a patient of the practice who is waiting for service and as a medical professional who must work in the space. Use only those templates that you determine are the most functional and efficient for the space you are designing; you do not have to incorporate each element into your design. Once you have decided on an arrangement, copy the final configuration onto the floor plan in section B. When you have completed your design, write a brief description of the nature of the medical practice the reception area is intended for (for example, pediatrician, gerontologist, or family practitioner) and of the patients who will be using the space.

B. Final Reception Area Design

C. Description of the Medical Practice and Its Patients

___

___

___

___

___

___

___

___

___

___

___

___

CASE STUDY

Lydia Renzi, a deaf woman with some residual hearing, is a patient of Dr. Angie Esposito's at Inner City Health Care. Lydia is fluent in American Sign Language (ASL) and usually wears a hearing aid when she is away from home.

Lydia calls to make her appointment at Inner City Health Care using a telecommunications device for the deaf (TDD) and the services of a government-funded relay operator. Though Lydia often chooses not to be accompanied by an interpreter, Inner City Health Care always provides the option to supply the services of a qualified professional sign language interpreter in compliance with the ADA. When Lydia arrives at Inner City Health Care with a high fever and a suspected case of the flu, the staff accommodates Lydia's special needs in several simple ways. Remembering that deaf people rely on visual images to receive and to convey messages, Liz Corbin, CMA, always faces Lydia directly so that the patient can see her facial expressions and lip movements. Liz holds eye contact with Lydia and does not break it until she is sure that Lydia understands her message and has time to think and respond. Special care is taken to provide Lydia with written instructions for prescriptions and for following through on home care.

Discuss the following:

1. What are the special communication needs of the hearing-impaired patient in the ambulatory care setting?
2. How can the medical assistant's actions impact directly upon the quality of care given to hearing-impaired patients?
3. Suppose that Lydia is an elderly woman who is embarrassed and sensitive about her hearing loss and will not admit that she has trouble hearing others. How might the medical assistant accommodate the special needs of this patient?

SUPPLEMENTARY RESOURCES

Study Guide Disk: Additional practice exercises for this chapter are available on the Study Guide disk found in the back of the textbook.

Medical Assisting Videos: Appropriate content is available on Delmar's Medical Assisting Videos, 2nd ed., for the following topics:

Tape 1: Communication Skills
Tape 2: Confidentiality in the Reception Area
Tape 3: Triage Skills

SKILLS PROFICIENCY EVALUATION

How has your instructor evaluated the skills you have achieved?

	Instructor Evaluation		
Skills	*Good*	*Average*	*Poor*
Identifies tasks in opening and closing facility	_____	_____	_____
Recognizes importance of the medical receptionist	_____	_____	_____
Relates the physical environment of the facility to the patient's care and comfort	_____	_____	_____
Relates the physical environment of the facility to optimal functionality and efficiency	_____	_____	_____
Safeguards patient privacy			
Understands the purpose of the ADA and can describe methods of compliance	_____	_____	_____
Empathizes with the patient experience of the health care facility	_____	_____	_____

Student's Initials: _____ Instructor's Initials: _____

Grade: _____

CHAPTER 12

Computer Use in the Ambulatory Care Setting

PERFORMANCE OBJECTIVES

Ambulatory care settings are making the transition from manual to computerized systems. Medical assistants with a knowledge of computer equipment, or hardware, and computer programs, or software, are a strong asset to the medical office. Today, computers are used in complex clinical applications such as assisting in performing sensitive surgeries, diagnosing illnesses, and developing patient treatment strategies. In the ambulatory care setting, physician-employers purchase computer systems to perform administrative tasks, such as patient data collection, correspondence, reports, billing, and insurance claim filing. Confidentiality of computerized patient records must be strictly maintained. Medical assistants are expected to be able to learn and use office computer applications. Often, medical assistants are involved in researching and implementing computer applications for specific administrative office functions. Medical assisting students are encouraged to explore the potential of computers. Seemingly intimidating, computers—with a little experience—become user-friendly tools that offer valuable methods for streamlining tasks and increasing efficiency in the ambulatory care setting.

EXERCISES AND ACTIVITY

Vocabulary Builder

As more ambulatory care facilities are purchasing computer hardware and software to perform office tasks from correspondence to billing and accounting to maintaining a database of patient information, medical assistants need to become familiar with computer operations and software applications.

Match the key vocabulary terms listed below with the correct definitions.

A. Hardware

A. Ergonomics
B. Hardware
C. Internet
D. Mainframe computer
E. Microcomputer
F. Minicomputer
G. Modem
H. Personal computer
I. RAM
J. Supercomputer
K. System

______ 1. A device used by a computer to communicate to a remote computer through phone lines.

______ 2. The scientific study of work and space, including factors that influence workers' productivity and that affect workers' health.

______ 3. A large computer system capable of processing massive volumes of data.

______ 4. A personal, or desktop, computer.

______ 5. Acronym for random access memory, a type of computer memory that can be written to and read from.

______ 6. The physical equipment used by the computer system to process data.

______ 7. Larger than a microcomputer and smaller than a mainframe.

______ 8. A worldwide computer network available via modem.

______ 9. The fastest, largest, and most expensive computers currently being manufactured.

______ 10. Also known as microcomputer.

______ 11. A unit composed of a number of parts that function together to perform a particular task.

B. Software

A. Applications software
B. Bit
C. Byte
D. Communications software
E. Data
F. Database management software
G. Documentation
H. Electronic mail
I. Fields
J. Footers
K. Graphics software
L. Headers
M. Information retrieval systems
N. Macros
O. Merge operations
P. Operating system
Q. Orphan
R. Record
S. Software
T. Sort
U. Spreadsheet software
V. Systems software
W. Widow
X. Word processing software

_____ 1. A page formatting feature that allows the bottom of all pages to be marked with keyed-in data.

_____ 2. The raw material; the collection of characters and numbers entered into a computer.

_____ 3. A word processing operation designed to produce form letters.

_____ 4. Software that provides instructions to the computer hardware.

_____ 5. Systems that allow electronic access to very large databases for the retrieval of information.

_____ 6. Related fields, grouped together and organized in the same order.

_____ 7. Smallest unit of data a computer can process.

_____ 8. Applications software used to create pictorial representations.

_____ 9. A frequently used data processing operation that arranges data in a particular sequence or order.

_____ 10. In typesetting, a term describing the situation where a new paragraph begins on the last line of a printed page.

_____ 11. Communications that take place on-line from computer to computer by means of a modem.

_____ 12. Equivalent of a computer program or programs.

_____ 13. Amount of memory needed to store one character.

_____ 14. A page formatting feature that allows the top of a page to be printed with identifying information.

_____ 15. A series of keystrokes that have been saved under a separate file name that can be used and inserted repeatedly into a document or documents.

_____ 16. Software that performs a specific data processing function.

_____ 17. A computer application that allows the user to format and edit documents before printing.

_____ 18. The software that controls the hardware and also runs computer programs.

_____ 19. A basic data category within the database.

_____ 20. Computer applications packages that act as "number crunchers" because of their mathematical processing capabilities.

_____ 21. Written material that accompanies purchased software, containing the information necessary for using the software appropriately.

_____ 22. Applications software used for the transfer of data from one computer system to another.

_____ 23. In typesetting, a term describing the situation where a line of text that is the end of a paragraph ends on a new page of printed text.

_____ 24. Applications software designed for the manipulation of data within a database.

Learning Review

1. Medical assistants may encounter many types of software in the ambulatory care setting including scheduling (S); word processing (WP); clinical (C); accounting (A); billing, collecting, and insurance (BCI); and practice management (PM).

Identify the tasks listed below according to the type of software used to perform them by placing the proper letters in the spaces provided.

_____ A. Inventories and drug supplies

_____ B. Medical records

_____ C. Aging accounts receivable

_____ D. Patient reminders

_____ E. Employee vacation records

_____ F. Charge slips

_____ G. Insurance claim processing

_____ H. Check writing

_____ I. Labels and addressing

_____ J. Prescription writing

_____ K. Payroll

_____ L. Thank-you letters

_____ M. Consultation reports

_____ N. Treatment plans

2. Computer systems are great assets to any ambulatory care setting in streamlining tasks and increasing productivity. Special steps need to be taken to keep the systems operating at peak efficiency. Name five steps medical assistants should take in the care and handling of computer components.

(1) ______________________________

(2) ______________________________

(3) ______________________________

(4) ______________________________

(5) ______________________________

3. There are six operations that are fundamental to the operation of any computer software. Identify the proper operation in the examples below.

______________________________ A. Administrative medical assistant Ellen Armstrong, CMA, working in the offices of Drs. Lewis and King, makes adjustments in format and corrects spelling and punctuation errors in a thank-you letter the practice sends to new patients.

______________________________ B. Ellen prepares a hard copy of Martin Gordon's treatment plan for Dr. Winston Lewis.

______________________________ C. Office manager Marilyn Johnson, CMA, asks Ellen to add columns to the existing drug inventory spreadsheet.

______________________________ D. Ellen enters data on employee vacation and sick time into the new spreadsheet software.

________________ E. After entering all of the patient addresses into a single file, Ellen makes sure that the file will be retained permanently.

________________ F. On request from Dr. Elizabeth King, Ellen produces the most recent correspondence sent to patient Maria Jover.

4. Word processing is largely concerned with the production of textual material and is an integral part of the ambulatory care setting. Match the following common word processing features with the correct descriptions.

A. Multicolumn output
B. Macros
C. Page formatting
D. Sorting
E. Import and export
F. Block operations

____ 1. These allow the user to highlight and move text to another position within the document.

____ 2. This refers to the rearrangement of information.

____ 3. Allows users to carry a text file into another applications program.

____ 4. Keystrokes that have been saved separately so the saved keystrokes may be inserted into any document.

____ 5. The arrangement of text on a page in two or more columns.

____ 6. This is used to create a variety of looks for the printed page.

5. Spreadsheet software "crunches," or calculates, numbers. Define the following elements of spreadsheet programs.

A. Cell location ________________

B. Worksheet ________________

C. Values ________________

D. Labels ________________

Name three tasks for which spreadsheet software is particularly useful.

(1) ________________

(2) ________________

(3) ________________

6. A. Databases or database management systems (DBMS) are built from the concept of data organization. Name four elements that comprise the organization of data.

(1) ________________ (3) ________________

(2) ________________ (4) ________________

B. Ellen Armstrong, CMA, is creating a patient database for the offices of Drs. Lewis and King. The office currently maintains information on one thousand patients. List ten fields of information the database should contain to track the patients.

(1) ______________________________

(2) ______________________________

(3) ______________________________

(4) ______________________________

(5) ______________________________

(6) ______________________________

(7) ______________________________

(8) ______________________________

(9) ______________________________

(10) ______________________________

7. The use of computerized databases in the delivery of health care services is becoming an established methodology for patient care. However, the trend toward computerizing medical records and the electronic processing of insurance claims presents challenges in preserving patient confidentiality.

A. Name the federal legislation that protects against unauthorized access or interception of data communication:

____

B. The ______________________________ has put forth guidelines to follow for the enactment of laws that protect individual privacy and confidentiality.

8. The American Medical Association (AMA) has published computer confidentiality guidelines to assist physicians and computer service organizations in maintaining the confidentiality of information in medical records when that information is stored in computerized databases.

A. Confidential medical information should be entered into the computer-based patient record only by ______________________.

B. The person making any additions to the record should be ______________________.

C. The computerized medical database should be on-line to the computer terminal only when ______________________ are being used.

D. Name three security measures that can be used to control access to the computerized data base.

(1) ______________________________

(2) ______________________________

(3) ______________________________

Investigation Activity

Computers are used at work, in school, and at home by more and more people each year. The electronic Information Age has become a part of everyday life. In the ambulatory care setting, computers perform simple tasks, but they also make possible an array of more complex tasks that would have been difficult or time-consuming to execute manually, such as compiling information for and extracting information from databases and executing mail merges and sorts. New software applications are continually released that are user-friendly and perform tasks quickly and efficiently. The potential of computers seems endless, and now the Internet is opening up whole new areas of communication and information access via the computer.

Discover the range of resources, services, and products available to today's computer user. The more savvy administrative medical assistants are about new and existing applications and resources, the more they can contribute to getting the most out of the office's computerized systems. Go to your local library, bookstore, and computer superstore to research and identify the following.

A. Name five magazines devoted to computer hardware, software, or computer issues and applications. Give a one-sentence description of the main focus of each periodical.

(1) ______________________________

____

(2) ______________________________

____

(3) ______________________________

____

(4) ______________________________

____

(5) ______________________________

____

B. List five computer programs that each perform a different function. Give the name of the program and describe the function it performs.

(1) ______________________________

____

(2) ______________________________

____

(3) ______________________________

____

(4) ______________________________

____

(5) ____

____

C. Name three resources that provide medical information on-line. Give the Internet or World Wide Web addresses and a brief description of the nature and type of information available. A librarian is a good person to help you find this information. Two examples of on-line resources are MEDLINE, a bibliographic database of articles from medical journals, and the National Institutes of Health.

(1) ____

____

____

(2) ____

____

____

(3) ____

____

____

CASE STUDY

The offices of Drs. Lewis and King recently experienced a pronounced surge in patient load when the physician-employers agreed to accept patients from several HMOs operating in the area. The group practice added two new staff members, co-office manager Shirley Brooks, CMA, and clinical medical assistant Anna Preciado, CMA. To handle the increased load of paperwork, Dr. Winston Lewis asks Shirley to devise a database to identify patient insurance variables. The practice already has a functional database of patient information.

Discuss the following.

1. What strategies will Shirley use to research the proper database software and to determine the desired organization of information within the new patient insurance database?
2. What information will the patient insurance database need to contain to allow for the streamlining of paperwork and claims processing?
3. What will the office manager do when she has completed her research and has devised a plan for assembling the patient insurance database?

SUPPLEMENTARY RESOURCES

Study Guide Disk: Additional practice exercises for this chapter are available on the Study Guide disk found in the back of the textbook.

Medical Assisting Videos: Appropriate content is available on Delmar's Medical Assisting Videos, 2nd ed., for the following topics:

Tape 2

Control of and Access to the Computerized Medical Record

Tape 3

Use Basic Office Equipment
Apply Computer Concepts for Office Procedures
Computerized Medical Records
Billing Cycle and Collections
Manage Physician's Professional and Hospital Schedule

Tape 4

Computerized Management of Reimbursement Systems

SKILLS COMPETENCY ASSESSMENT

Procedure 12-1: Selecting Appropriate Software

Student's Name: ______________________________ Date: ____________

Objective: To determine software a computer system is capable of running prior to purchase.

Conditions: The student demonstrates the ability to determine what software a computer system is capable of running using the following equipment and information: documentation or manual for hardware components, including computer central processing unit (CPU), memory, hard disk size and available space, printer, monitor, sound board, and CD-ROM if applicable.

Time Requirements and Accuracy Standards: 45 minutes. Points assigned reflect importance of step to meeting objective: Important = (5) Essential = (10) Critical = (15). Automatic failure results if any of the **critical** tasks are omitted or performed incorrectly.

SKILLS ASSESSMENT CHECKLIST

Task Performed	Possible Points	TASKS
❑	10	Determines the type of microprocessor the computer system uses.
❑	10	Determines the type of operating system (and operating environment) the system currently uses.
❑	5	Identifies the type of printer and monitor.
❑	10	Identifies the amount of primary or random access memory (RAM) the system currently has available and the amount of secondary storage the system has free.
❑	5	Determines if the computer has the capability to generate sound as required by software.
❑	5	Completed the tasks within 45 minutes.
❑	15	Results obtained were accurate.

______	Earned	ADD POINTS OF TASKS CHECKED
60	Points	TOTAL POINTS POSSIBLE
______	SCORE	DETERMINE SCORE (divide points earned by total points possible, multiply results by 100)

Actual Student Time Needed to Complete Procedure: ____________

Student's Initials: ____________ Instructor's Initials: ____________ Grade: ____________

Suggestions for Improvement: ______________________________

Evaluator's Name (print) ______________________________

Evaluator's Signature ______________________________

Comments ______________________________

SKILLS COMPETENCY ASSESSMENT

Procedure 12–2: Basic Computer Operations

Student's Name: ______________________________ Date: ____________

Objective: To demonstrate knowledge of computer concepts, including operating systems, operating environments, and applications.

Conditions: The student demonstrates a knowledge of computer concepts using the following equipment: computer hardware and software.

Time Requirements and Accuracy Standards: 45 minutes. Points assigned reflect importance of step to meeting objective: Important = (5) Essential = (10) Critical = (15). Automatic failure results if any of the **critical** tasks are omitted or performed incorrectly.

SKILLS ASSESSMENT CHECKLIST

Task Performed	Possible Points	TASKS
❑	5	Turns on the computer's system unit and all system input and output devices.
❑	5	Accesses the operating system or the operating environment.
❑	15	Uses the operating system (or the operating environment) to format a floppy disk in the A-drive.
❑	10	Uses the operating system (or the operating environment) to copy or make a backup copy of a file from the current drive.
❑	10	Uses the operating system (or the operating environment) to copy a disk from the A-drive to the B-drive.
❑	5	Uses the operating system (or the operating environment) to view the directory (all file names).
❑	10	Uses the operating system (or the operating environment) to delete a file from the current drive.
❑	10	Uses the operating system (or the operating environment) to make or create a directory from the current drive.
❑	10	Uses the operating system (or the operating environment) to change the directory path from current drive to new directory.
❑	10	Uses the operating system (or the operating environment) to remove or delete a directory.
❑	5	Completed the tasks within 45 minutes.

SKILLS COMPETENCY ASSESSMENT — continued

Procedure 12–2: Basic Computer Operations

Task Performed	Possible Points	TASKS
❑	15	Results obtained were accurate.

________		Earned	ADD POINTS OF TASKS CHECKED
	110	Points	TOTAL POINTS POSSIBLE
________		SCORE	DETERMINE SCORE (divide points earned by total points possible, multiply results by 100)

Actual Student Time Needed to Complete Procedure: ____________

Student's Initials: ____________ Instructor's Initials: ____________ Grade: ____________

Suggestions for Improvement: ____

____

____

____

Evaluator's Name (print) ____

Evaluator's Signature ____

Comments ____

EVALUATION OF CHAPTER KNOWLEDGE

How has your instructor evaluated the knowledge you have gained?

	Instructor Evaluation		
Knowledge	*Good*	*Average*	*Poor*
Understands how computers enhance office efficiency and can give examples of specific methods	_____	_____	_____
Identifies types of computer hardware	_____	_____	_____
Can distinguish between systems and applications software	_____	_____	_____
Identifies categories of applications software and can describe the purpose of each	_____	_____	_____
Applies database management concepts to ambulatory care setting	_____	_____	_____
Understands issue of preserving patient confidentiality and can identify guidelines for maintaining confidentiality	_____	_____	_____
Recognizes potential of computer for locating resources and information	_____	_____	_____
Can relate relevant ergonomic theories and give guidelines for setting up ergonomic workstations	_____	_____	_____
Recognizes growing role of medical assistant as information manager	_____	_____	_____
Can discuss increasing role of computers in medicine for both clinical and administrative tasks	_____	_____	_____

Student's Initials: ____ Instructor's Initials: ____

Grade: _______

CHAPTER 13

Telephone Techniques

PERFORMANCE OBJECTIVES

Telephone communication, including facsimile (fax) and electronic mail (e-mail) transmission, is crucial to the effective management of the ambulatory care setting. Medical assistants will use the telephone to speak with patients; schedule appointments; respond to emergencies; and communicate with physicians, health care professionals, and others. To become efficient, successful communicators, medical assistants must be familiar with proper telephone etiquette, understand the extent of their authority when answering questions and releasing information, and develop proficiency in the use of various telephone systems and technologies. Upholding patient confidentiality and maintaining a professional telephone manner are essential skills of the medical assistant.

EXERCISES AND ACTIVITY

Vocabulary Builder

A. *Insert the proper key vocabulary terms into the paragraph below.*

Empathy	Jargon	Posture	Etiquette
Ethical	Screen	Enunciate	Fluent
Triage	Obfuscation	Diaphragm	Slang
Good Samaritan laws	Confidentiality		

When speaking on the telephone, medical assistants must employ proper telephone ______________________________, which means being courteous and professional to others. To ensure that listeners understand what is said, it is important to ______________________________, or say the words clearly. The tone of voice is affected by one's ______________________________. Slouching can compress or restrict the

________________________ and make the voice sound tense and tired. Simple terms rather than medical ________________________ promotes mutual understanding rather than confusion or ________________________. The use of ________________________ words and expressions is considered unprofessional and disrespectful. When speaking with a caller who is not ________________________ in English, it is helpful to speak slowly and use short sentences. Responding with ________________________ conveys an appreciation for the caller's concerns and needs. Medical assistants will ________________________ calls that come into the medical facility to ensure that callers speak to the appropriate staff member and to ________________________ their medical problems. Because complete patient ________________________ is considered a legal and ________________________ obligation, medical assistants must not discuss patients outside of the professional environment or share any patient information with others without written patient permission. When providing emergency medical aid, it is important to remember that ________________________ provide protection to medical assistants who act to provide assistance or care within the scope of their training and expertise.

B. Match the following devices or services listed in Column A with corresponding descriptions in Column B.

Column A	Column B
1. Pager ______	a Takes calls when the office is closed.
2. Answering service ______	b. Sends a document via phone lines to an electronic mailbox located in another person's computer.
3. Cellular service ______	c. A one-way communication device used to contact staff when away from the office.
4. Automated routing unit ______	d. A portable telephone.
5. Fax ______	e. A document sent over telephone lines from one facsimile machine or modem to another.
6. E-mail ______	f. A system that allows callers to reach specific people or departments by pressing a specified number on a touch-tone telephone.

Learning Review

1. Effective telephone communication requires prompt and professional responses from medical assistants. For each of the scenarios listed below, what should the medical assistant say to give the best telephone response?

   A. Karen Ritter, CMA, answers the first call of the morning at Inner City Health Care.

   Medical assistant: ____________________

   ____

   ____

   B. Patient Nora Fowler calls with a question about medication prescribed for her rheumatoid arthritis and insists on a call back from Dr. Elizabeth King. Dr. King is presently on rounds at the hospital and will not be available until 4:30 P.M. Nora's tone of voice reveals that she is distrustful of the medication and of the physician's reliability, and it is clear from the conversation that Nora has discontinued taking her medication.

   Medical assistant: ____________________

   ____

   ____

   C. While speaking on telephone line 1 with patient Bill Schwartz, who is calling to schedule a physical examination, medical assistant Wanda Slawson receives another call on line 2 from a laboratory with a summary of emergency test results for another patient. Wanda knows Dr. Susan Rice is waiting for the results.

   Medical assistant: ____________________

   ____

   ____

   D. Bruce Goldman, CMA, takes a call from patient Juanita Hansen. Juanita is inquiring about a bill and indicating that her insurance carrier, Blue Cross, did not pay the entire fee for her son's last examination, which left her with a balance owed to Inner City Health Care. Office manager Walter Seals is responsible for managing insurance claims and inquiries.

   Medical assistant: ____________________

   ____

   ____

2. Showing compassion and concern for the well-being of the caller allows both potential and established patients to feel confident about the high quality of care they receive.

   A. Name four reasons why a potential patient will contact an ambulatory care facility by telephone.

   (1) ____________________

(2) ______________________________

(3) ______________________________

(4) ______________________________

B. What nine pieces of information should a medical assistant record in the appointment book when scheduling an initial appointment with the physician?

(1) ______________ (6) ______________

(2) ______________ (7) ______________

(3) ______________ (8) ______________

(4) ______________ (9) ______________

(5) ______________

3. Indicate the calls described below that fall within the scope of practice for a medical assistant (MA) to respond to and the calls that should be directed to the physician (P). For each call handled by a medical assistant, describe the information needed to address the needs of the caller. For each call referred to the physician, give reasons why a physician must handle the call.

____ A. Insurance questions.

____

____

____ B. Scheduling patient testing and office appointments.

____

____

____ C. Medical emergencies.

____

____

____ D. Requests for prescription refills.

____

____

____ E. Complaints.

____

____

____ F. General information about the practice.

____

____

____ G. Poor progress reports from patient.

____

____

____ H. Requests for medications other than prescription refills.

____

____

____ I. Medical questions.

____

____

____ J. Salespeople.

____

____

4. Answering services and answering machines are two methods of taking calls after hours. Answering services are staffed by live operators who take messages for the physician and medical practice when the office is closed. Answering machines can also be used for taking the majority of after-hours calls, with a telephone number given in the outgoing message that will connect callers with a live operator in the event of an emergency.

A. Compose an appropriate outgoing message for the offices of Drs. Lewis and King.

____

____

____

____

____

B. Each morning, administrative medical assistant Ellen Armstrong is responsible for transcribing messages left on the medical practice's answering machine the evening before. Using the message pad slips below, transcribe each message completely and appropriately. In the space for "Attachments," list any records, files, or documents that should be attached to the message slip for the recipient's review.

Message #1. "Ellen, this is Anna Preciado. Can you tell the office manager, Marilyn Johnson, that I won't be in tomorrow for the afternoon shift? I've got a 101 degree temperature and bad flu symptoms. Maybe Joe Guerrero can come in to sub for me as the clinical medical assistant; yesterday, he said he might be available if I wasn't feeling well enough to come in. I know Dr. Lewis has several patients scheduled for clinical testing in the afternoon. I'm at 555-6622. Thanks."

Message #2. "This is Heidi from Dr. Kwiczola's office calling for Dr. Lewis. We have a new patient, Marsha Beckman, in our psychiatric practice who is experiencing symptoms of fatigue, anxiety, palpitations, and weight loss whom Dr. Kwiczola suspects may be suffering from hyperthyroidism. Dr. Kwiczola will be in the office tomorrow from 2 P.M. to 7 P.M. and can be reached at 555-7181."

Message #3. "This is Martin Gordon, a patient of Dr. Lewis's. I need to talk to Shirley Brooks, the office manager who handles insurance. I've got a question about my out-of-pocket maximum."

Message #4. "This is Charles Williams. Dr. Lewis put me on a Holter monitor today. It's about 11 P.M. and one of the leads came off. I put it back on but I'm worried about whether I'll have to do this test again. Can you call me at home before 8 at 555-6124 or at the office after 9 at 555-8125?"

Message #1	**Message #2**
To: ______________ Date: ______	To: ______________ Date: ______
From: ______________ Time: ______	From: ______________ Time: ______
Telephone #: ______________	Telephone #: ______________
Message: ______________	Message: ______________
______________	______________
______________	______________
______________	______________
Initials: ______	Initials: ______
Attachments: ______________	Attachments: ______________
______________	______________
______________	______________
______________	______________

Message #3	
To: ______	Date: ______
From: ______	Time: ______
Telephone #: ______	
Message: ______	
______	
______	
______	
	Initials: ______
Attachments: ______	
______	
______	
______	

Message #4	
To: ______	Date: ______
From: ______	Time: ______
Telephone #: ______	
Message: ______	
______	
______	
______	
	Initials: ______
Attachments: ______	
______	
______	
______	

5. Medical assistants must observe laws regarding patient confidentiality and the patient's right to privacy.

Indicate which people and under what restrictions a medical assistant may discuss a patient's medical condition or reveal details from the medical record.

Person	**Yes**	**No**	**Yes, w/Signed Release**
Patient's spouse or family	❑	❑	❑

______

______

______

Patient's employer	❑	❑	❑

______

______

______

Patient's attorney	❑	❑	❑

______

______

______

Person	Yes	No	Yes, w/Signed Release
Another health care provider	☐	☐	☐
Insurance carrier or HMOs	☐	☐	☐
Referring physician's office	☐	☐	☐
Credit bureaus and/or collection agencies	☐	☐	☐
Members of the office staff, as necessary for patient care	☐	☐	☐
Patient's insurance carrier	☐	☐	☐
Other patients	☐	☐	☐

Person	Yes	No	Yes, w/Signed Release
People outside the office (friends, family, acquaintances of the medical assistant)	❑	❑	❑

____

____

____

Person	Yes	No	Yes, w/Signed Release
Patient's parent or legal guardian, except concerning issues of birth control, abortion, or sexually transmitted diseases	❑	❑	❑

____

____

____

6. Many physicians and health care professionals use paging systems. Paging systems allow the medical assistant to alert a physician or other health care professional who is not on site to call in for an important message. Name and describe four paging system options.

   (1) ____

   ____

   ____

   (2) ____

   ____

   ____

   (3) ____

   ____

   ____

   (4) ____

   ____

   ____

Investigation Activity

The medical assistant's tone of voice while speaking on the telephone is as important as the specific words that are said to others. Practice can help medical assisting students develop a pleasant telephone personality and improve the clarity and sound of their voices so callers will trust and understand what is said.

For each telephone scenario listed, students form pairs to role-play the parts of the medical assistant and the patient or caller. Use nonworking phones as props to approximate the experience of a real telephone call; callers and call recipients should not be able to see each other. Use a tape recorder to record the role-playing exercise for each scenario. Medical assistants should always demonstrate professionalism. Other characters in each scenario can be role-played as broadly and creatively as possible to challenge the student who takes the role of the medical assistant. Create additional scenarios for role-playing.

Telephone Scenarios

A. Medical assistant answers a call from Jaime Carrera who has been diagnosed by Dr. James Whitney with back strain from heavy lifting at his construction job. Jaime is taking a prescription for Tylenol with codeine. He reveals that he is dizzy, has a severe pounding headache, and feels like he will faint if he tries to walk. Jaime slurs his words and seems "out of it." Dr. Whitney is currently with another patient. Jaime recently completed a substance abuse rehabilitation program.

B. Medical assistant takes a call from Mr. Richards, a very aggressive medical supply salesperson, who requests the earliest possible appointment with Dr. Elizabeth King.

C. Medical assistant calls Cele Little, an elderly woman who is hard of hearing, to confirm her 3:00 P.M. appointment with Dr. Susan Rice on Friday, January 15. Cele does not remember making the appointment.

Play back the taped telephone conversations and evaluate the following elements of the medical assistant's telephone techniques and etiquette.

1. Enunciation: Are the words spoken clearly?
2. Tone of voice: Does the tone convey enthusiasm, warmth, empathy, and interest in the caller?
3. Speed: Is the rate of the speech fast, slow, or normal?
4. Volume: Is the volume such that the patient can hear without difficulty, but is not so loud that others can overhear or is irritating to the caller?
5. Etiquette: Is the medical assistant courteous, considerate, patient, and responsive?
6. Professionalism: Does the medical assistant respond appropriately?

Identify the techniques that need improvement and how they can be improved.

____

____

____

____

____

____

____

CASE STUDY

As Inner City Health Care, an urgent care center, continues to grow, increasing both patient load and staff, the existing telephone system consisting of a simple intercom and four telephone lines is no longer sufficient to handle the call volume and allow for full, immediate accessibility for all staff members. Callers are frustrated by the length of time it takes to get through and by long amounts of time spent on hold. Messages are often late in getting properly routed. Administrative medical assistant Karen Ritter suggests to office manager Jane O'Hara that an automated routing unit (ARU) might be more efficient for the growing clinic's needs. At the next regularly scheduled staff meeting, the physician-employers give the go-ahead to research an automated routing system.

Discuss the following:

1. ARU systems provide several options for callers that identify specific departments or services that callers can be connected with directly. What kinds of caller options might be appropriate for Inner City Health Care?
2. What can be done so emergency patients or hearing-impaired patients can speak automatically to a "live" operator?
3. How can an automated system help staff members receive their calls more efficiently?
4. How can the office manager and medical assistant implement the ARU system with a minimum of disruption to physicians, staff, and patients?

SUPPLEMENTARY RESOURCES

Study Guide Disk: Additional practice exercises for this chapter are available on the Study Guide disk found in the back of the textbook.

Medical Assisting Videos: Appropriate content is available on Delmar's Medical Assisting Videos, 2nd ed., for the following topics:

Tape 1
- Communication Skills

Tape 2
- Complete Medical Records
- Confidentiality on the Telephone

Tape 3
- Use Basic Office Equipment
- Triage Skills

SKILLS COMPETENCY ASSESSMENT

Procedure 13–1: Answering Incoming Calls

Student's Name: ______________________________ Date: __________

Objective: To answer telephone calls professionally, acquiring all necessary information from the caller, documenting it correctly, and properly acting on it.

Conditions: The student demonstrates the ability to answer incoming calls using the following equipment and supplies: telephone, telephone message pad, appointment calendar, and pen or pencil.

Time Requirements and Accuracy Standards: 10 minutes. Points assigned reflect importance of step to meeting objective: Important = (5) Essential = (10) Critical = (15). Automatic failure results if any of the **critical** tasks are omitted or performed incorrectly.

SKILLS ASSESSMENT CHECKLIST

Task Performed	Possible Points	TASKS
❑	15	Answers telephone promptly (no more than three rings).
❑	5	Answers with preferred office greeting.
❑	15	Asks name of caller as quickly as possible.
❑	15	Focuses on call.
❑	10	Expresses warmth and interest in tone of voice.
❑	15	Is prepared with appropriate materials, such as notepad or appointment calendar.
❑	10	Uses notepad to record caller's name and phone line and notes on the content of the call if using a multi-line telephone system.
❑	15	Documents information on a message pad and/or the patient's chart as required and records appropriate future actions necessary.
❑	10	Repeats information back to the caller.
❑	5	Asks if caller has further questions.
❑	10	Ends the call courteously.
❑	5	Lets the caller hang up first before disconnecting.
❑	5	Completed the tasks within 10 minutes.

Task Performed	Possible Points	TASKS
❑	15	Results obtained were accurate.

________	Earned	ADD POINTS OF TASKS CHECKED
150	Points	TOTAL POINTS POSSIBLE
________	SCORE	DETERMINE SCORE (divide points earned by total points possible, multiply results by 100)

Actual Student Time Needed to Complete Procedure: ____________

Student's Initials: ____________ Instructor's Initials: ____________ Grade: ____________

Suggestions for Improvement: ____

____

____

____

Evaluator's Name (print) ____

Evaluator's Signature ____

Comments ____

DOCUMENTATION

Chart the procedure for the patient's medical record using the following conditions: The patient has called to cancel an appointment for an annual physical examination and will call back to reschedule at a later time.

Date: ________________

Charting: ____

____

____

____

Student's Initials: __________

SKILLS COMPETENCY ASSESSMENT

Procedure 13–2: Handling Problem Calls

Student's Name: ______________________________ Date: ____________

Objective: To handle calls in a positive and professional manner while providing necessary comfort, empathy, and information to the caller to resolve the problem.

Conditions: The student demonstrates the ability to handle difficult calls using telephone, message pad, and pen or pencil.

Time Requirements and Accuracy Standards: 15 minutes. Points assigned reflect importance of step to meeting objective: Important = (5) Essential = (10) Critical = (15). Automatic failure results if any of the **critical** tasks are omitted or performed incorrectly.

SKILLS ASSESSMENT CHECKLIST

Task Performed	Possible Points	TASKS
❑	15	Remains calm and professional.
❑	10	Allows caller to finish speaking thoughts without interruption (unless it is a medical emergency requiring immediate attention).
❑	10	Listens to what the caller is upset about.
❑	15	Asks questions when appropriate during pauses.
❑	15	Handles the situation objectively, without taking the caller's words personally.
❑	10	Offers assistance.
❑	15	Documents the call accurately and promptly.
For a frightened or hysterical caller:		
❑	15	Speaks in a soothing voice and a slower, lower tone than normal.
❑	15	If an emergency, begins triage procedures as needed.
❑	15	Has caller repeat back any instructions given.
❑	10	Finalizes and follows through on action to be taken.
❑	15	Reports problem calls immediately to physician or office manager.
For an angry or a hostile caller:		
❑	10	Lowers pitch and volume of voice.
❑	10	Uses the words *I understand* to express an interest in and empathy with the caller's concerns.

Task Performed	Possible Points	TASKS
❑	15	Finalizes and follows through on action to be taken.
❑	15	Reports problem calls immediately to physician or office manager.
❑	10	If caller becomes abusive, politely but firmly tells caller the conversation must be ended and immediately terminates call.
❑	5	Completed the tasks within 15 minutes.
❑	15	Results obtained were accurate.

_______	Earned	ADD POINTS OF TASKS CHECKED
240	Points	TOTAL POINTS POSSIBLE
_______	SCORE	DETERMINE SCORE (divide points earned by total points possible, multiply results by 100)

Actual Student Time Needed to Complete Procedure: ____________

Student's Initials: ____________ Instructor's Initials: ____________ Grade: ____________

Suggestions for Improvement: ______________________________

____

____

____

Evaluator's Name (print) ______________________________

Evaluator's Signature ______________________________

Comments ______________________________

DOCUMENTATION

Chart the procedure for the patient's medical record using the following conditions: A patient calls to complain after receiving a letter from the physician stating that the physician is withdrawing from treatment of the patient because the patient is not following the physician's treatment plan. The physician is currently at a meeting out of the office.

Date: ______________

Charting: ______________________________

____

____

____

Student's Initials: __________

SKILLS COMPETENCY ASSESSMENT

Procedure 13–3: Placing Outgoing Calls

Student's Name: ______________________________ Date: ____________

Objective: To place outgoing calls efficiently and effectively.

Conditions: The student demonstrates the ability to place outgoing calls using telephone, message pad, pen or pencil, and any materials specifically applicable to the call.

Time Requirements and Accuracy Standards: 10 minutes. Points assigned reflect importance of step to meeting objective: Important = (5) Essential = (10) Critical = (15). Automatic failure results if any of the **critical** tasks are omitted or performed incorrectly.

SKILLS ASSESSMENT CHECKLIST

Task Performed	Possible Points	TASKS
❑	15	Prepares all appropriate materials, including telephone number, chart, financial information, appointment book, and notes of questions or information.
❑	5	Makes calls from quiet location.
❑	10	*Rationale:* Understands necessity of preserving patient confidentiality.
❑	10	Makes calls at a time when there is no interference with other office duties.
❑	10	Makes calls at appropriate time for the needs of the caller (e.g., considers time zones and business hours).
❑	15	Uses appropriate language, tone, and communication techniques to ensure that the message is understood.
❑	15	Knows and follows legal guidelines for collection calls.
❑	5	Completed the tasks within 10 minutes.
❑	15	Results obtained were accurate.

________	Earned	ADD POINTS OF TASKS CHECKED
100	Points	TOTAL POINTS POSSIBLE
________	SCORE	DETERMINE SCORE (divide points earned by total points possible, multiply results by 100)

Actual Student Time Needed to Complete Procedure: ____________

Student's Initials: ____________ Instructor's Initials: ____________ Grade: ____________

Suggestions for Improvement: ____

____

____

____

Evaluator's Name (print) ____

Evaluator's Signature ____

Comments ____

DOCUMENTATION

Chart the procedure for the patient's medical record using the following conditions: The medical assistant places an outgoing call to a long-standing established patient regarding an overdue balance. The patient reveals a recent job lay-off. The medical assistant offers the patient the option of an extended payment plan, in accordance with office policies and procedures.

Date: ________________

Charting: ____

____

____

____

Student's Initials: __________

EVALUATION OF CHAPTER KNOWLEDGE

Evaluate your own strengths and weaknesses in communicating with others on the telephone, performing triage, directing calls, and understanding telephone systems and technology. Compare this evaluation to the one provided by your instructor.

	Student Self-Evaluation			Instructor Evaluation		
Knowledge	*Good*	*Average*	*Poor*	*Good*	*Average*	*Poor*
Adheres to the principles of preserving patient confidentiality	____	____	____	____	____	____
Projects empathy and enthusiasm	____	____	____	____	____	____
Understands telephone procedures for new and existing patient appointments	____	____	____	____	____	____
Ability to triage and respond to medical emergencies	____	____	____	____	____	____
Possesses good listening skills	____	____	____	____	____	____
Ability to receive, prioritize, organize, and transmit information	____	____	____	____	____	____
Understands the principles of successful telephone communication	____	____	____	____	____	____
Performs effective telephone triage	____	____	____	____	____	____
Understands use of communication technology such as fax machine, automated routing units, and e-mail	____	____	____	____	____	____
Ability to communicate effectively with people at their levels of understanding	____	____	____	____	____	____
Demonstrates ability to make outgoing calls	____	____	____	____	____	____
Serves as an effective liaison between physician and others	____	____	____	____	____	____
Performs within ethical boundaries	____	____	____	____	____	____
Practices within the scope of training and expertise	____	____	____	____	____	____

Student's Initials: _____ Instructor's Initials: _____

Grade: _______

CHAPTER 14

Patient Scheduling

PERFORMANCE OBJECTIVES

The effective scheduling of patient appointments is an essential skill of the medical assistant. Achieving efficient patient flow requires that the medical assistant coordinate the schedules of physicians, staff, and patients. Use of staff and physical facilities are also considered in selecting the proper scheduling system. When scheduling appointments, medical assistants draw on administrative and computer skills as well as communication skills. By considering and respecting the needs, time, and comfort of the patient, the medical assistant creates a positive impression of the physician and the medical practice.

EXERCISES AND ACTIVITIES

Vocabulary Builder

Insert the key vocabulary terms that best fit the descriptions below.

Clustering	Open hours
Double booking	Practice-based
Established patient	Slack time
Matrix	Stream
Modified wave	Triage
New patient	Wave
No-show	

1. ______________________________ Inner City Health Care reserves 9 A.M. to 12 P.M. on Thursday mornings for walk-in patients who are seen on a first-come, first-served basis within that time frame.

2. ______________________ At the offices of Drs. Lewis and King, Ellen Armstrong, CMA, schedules Mary O'Keefe for a 1:00 P.M. appointment with Dr. Elizabeth King and Martin Gordon for a 1:00 P.M. appointment with Dr. Winston Lewis.

3. ______________________ Lenny Taylor, an elderly man who suffers mild dementia, forgets his third appointment with Dr. James Whitney.

4. ______________________ At Inner City Health Care, vaccinations are scheduled every 10 minutes from 10 A.M. to 12:20 P.M. on Mondays; Tuesday office hours are reserved for new patients only.

5. ______________________ Five patients are scheduled to receive radiation treatments in the first half hour of every hour and are seen throughout the hour.

6. ______________________ Ellen Armstrong, CMA, takes a complete current medical history from patient Lourdes Austen on her first visit to Dr. Elizabeth King.

7. ______________________ Joe Guerrero, CMA, asks patient Martin Gordon if the personal information in his medical chart is complete and up-to-date before escorting him to the examination room to be seen by Dr. Winston Lewis.

8. ______________________ Dr. Elizabeth King prefers to see patients for regular gynecological examinations in consecutive appointments from 8:30 A.M. to 11:30 A.M. and patients who are pregnant from 1:00 P.M. to 3:30 P.M.

9. ______________________ When patient Herb Fowler calls to set up an appointment with Dr. Winston Lewis for his chronic cough, Ellen Armstrong, CMA, asks Herb a series of screening questions to ascertain the nature, extent, and urgency of his condition.

10. ______________________ Dr. Winston Lewis prefers patients to be scheduled on a continuous basis throughout the day at 30- or 60-minute intervals, with each patient having a distinct appointment time.

11. ______________________ An ophthalmologist schedules three patients at the beginning of each hour for comprehensive examinations, followed by single appointments every 10 to 20 minutes during the rest of the hour for quick, follow-up procedures such as removing eye patches or instilling eyedrops.

12. ______________________ Ellen Armstrong, CMA, uses empty or unscheduled periods for dictation or processing paperwork.

13. ______________________ On the fifteenth day of each month, office manager Walter Seals, CMA, who is responsible for efficient patient flow at Inner City Health Care, asks each of the urgent care center's five physicians to confirm their scheduling commitments for the upcoming month to block off unavailable times in the appointment book.

Appointment Book Matrix and Scheduling Activity

Student's Name: ______________________________ Date: ____________

Complete the appointment book for Drs. Lewis and King according to the instructions in the appropriate Learning Review exercises.

LEWIS & KING, MD
2501 CENTER STREET
NORTHBOROUGH, OH 12345

Friday, Feb. 7		Dr. Lewis	Dr. King
7	30		
	45		
8	00		
	15		
	30		
	45		
9	00		
	15		
	30		
	45		
10	00		
	15		
	30		
	45		

11	00		
	15		
	30		
	45		
12	00		
	15		
	30		
	45		
1	00		
	15		
	30		
	45		
2	00		
	15		
	30		
	45		
3	00		
	15		
	30		
	45		
4	00		

Learning Review

1. The first step in scheduling appointments is to establish an appointment matrix. The matrix blocks off time during the day that is used for purposes other than patient appointments and is unavailable for patient scheduling. Using the information below, complete Figure 14–1 to establish an appointment matrix for the offices of Drs. Lewis & King on Friday, February 7. Physicians' commitments should be entered with a red pen.

   Dr. King's commitments: Aerobics 7:30–8:00 A.M.; hospital rounds 8:00–9:00 A.M.; 12:30–1:30 P.M. lunch for local chapter of American Medical Women's Association; 2:45–3:15 P.M. weekly meeting with office managers Marilyn Johnson and Shirley Brooks; 3:45–5:00 P.M. community lecture sponsored by Planned Parenthood.

   Dr. Lewis's commitments: 7:30–8:30 A.M. breakfast meeting with current president of the State Medical Society; 1:00–1:30 P.M. lunch in office; 3:30 P.M. golf with Dr. Wilson.

2. A. Appointment books are legal documents recording patient flow. For example, the Internal Revenue Service (IRS) can legally demand records from the beginning of a practice. For a manual appointment system, where pencil is used for ease in rescheduling, what can the medical assistant do to ensure that a permanent record is secured?

   ____

   ____

   For a computerized appointment system, what can a medical assistant do to ensure that a permanent record of patient flow is secured?

   ____

   ____

   B. Name two primary goals in determining the best method for scheduling patient appointments:

   (1) ____

   ____

   (2) ____

   ____

   C. What is the typical scheduling time for each of the following types of office visits for an internal medicine practice?

   (1) Patient consultation ____________________

   (2) Established patient routine follow-up ____________________

   (3) New patient ____________________

   (4) Complete physical examination ____________________

   (5) Cold/flu symptoms ____________________

   (6) Vaccination ____________________

D. Using Figure 14–1, schedule the following appointments for Drs. Lewis and King for Friday, February 7.

Dr. King

Lourdes Austen; 651-8282; HMO insurance; complete physical exam and consultation regarding pregnancy after breast cancer; 1 hour, checkup and lab work.

Margaret Thomas; 651-0020; PPO insurance; chief complaint: Parkinson's disease; routine follow-up and vitamin B12 injection; 45 minutes.

Abigail Johnson; 389-2631; chief complaint: hypertension, diabetes mellitus, and angina; routine follow-up examination, ½ hour.

Susan Marshall; 628-9981; PPO insurance; chief complaint: intense emotional stress, heart palpitations; complete examination and ECG; 1 hour.

Herb Fowler; 639-1134; chief complaint: ankle sprain from recent fall in garage; recheck, 15 minutes.

Dr. Lewis

Charles Williams; 689-1144; Blue Cross Blue Shield; chief complaint: recurrent chest pain; physical examination and administer Holter monitor; 1 hour.

Rowena Lawrence; 628-3485; HMO insurance; chief complaint: hoarseness and bloody sputum; physical examination and lab, 1 hour.

Mark Johnson; 635-1111; HMO insurance; chief complaint: chronic lower back pain; recheck, 15 minutes.

Helen Armstrong; 628-9967; PPO insurance; new patient, self-referred; chief complaint: mild edema in right leg; physical exam, 1 hour.

Larry Melnick; 635-7721; accountant; 1 hour to discuss income statement for previous year and preparation of tax returns for the medical practice.

Marsha Lewis; 628-9986; representative of pharmaceutical company; sales meeting; 15 minutes.

Martin Gordon; 635-9834; HMO insurance; chief complaint: prostate cancer; routine follow-up; ½ hour.

Veronica Hallett; 635-4432; PPO insurance; chief complaint: persistent dermatitis; follow-up, 15 minutes.

Anne Ortiz; 628-5467; new patient, referred by Dr. John Elmos; Blue Cross Blue Shield; chief complaint: recurring stomach problems; 45 minutes.

3. Daily appointment sheets provide permanent records for legal risk management and are excellent tools for quality management of patient flow. Appointment sheets can be used to check off shows, no-shows, and cancellations. A pocket-sized edition of the daily appointment sheet is often given to the physician for easy referral. Compile a daily patient appointment sheet for Dr. Winston Lewis based on your scheduling of his appointments into the appointment matrix in Figure 14–1.

Daily Appointment Sheet **Dr. Lewis Friday, February 7**

Appointment Time	Patient Name	Time Allotted	Reason for Visit

4. Daily worksheets include not only patient appointments but all other physician and/or staff appointments as well. Daily worksheets are helpful tools that indicate blocks of time in any given day that are booked for any purpose and so are not available as scheduling time to see patients. Compile a daily worksheet based on Dr. Elizabeth King's schedule for Friday, February 7.

Daily Worksheet **Dr. King Friday, February 7**

Time	Appointment	Expected Length of Appointment	Reason for Appointment

Daily Worksheet (continued)

Time	Appointment	Expected Length of Appointment	Reason for Appointment

5. A. What are six variables involved in the process of scheduling appointments for patients and other visitors to the ambulatory care setting?

(1) ______________________________

(2) ______________________________

(3) ______________________________

(4) ______________________________

(5) ______________________________

(6) ______________________________

B. Patient Flow Analysis sheets help medical practices determine the effectiveness of patient scheduling and devise plans for improving a smooth patient flow through the ambulatory care setting. What kinds of problems can a study of these data reveal?

____

____

____

____

____

6. A. What are the five steps of scheduling a specific appointment time for a patient?

(1) ______________________________

(2) ______________________________

(3) ______________________________

(4) ______________________________

(5) ______________________________

B. Describe the process for scheduling an appointment for a patient using a computerized scheduling program.

____

____

____

____

____

7. Cancellations, emergencies, no-shows, and appointment changes can affect the appointment scheduling for any given day in the ambulatory care setting. Photocopy the appointment schedule for Drs. Lewis and King completed in Figure 14–1. Use the photocopy to make scheduling adjustments for the following.

A. Mary O'Keefe calls at 8:45 A.M. when her 3-year-old son Chris wakes with severe ear pain. The child is pulling on his right ear and has screamed uncontrollably for 45 minutes. Chris and Mary are established patients of Dr. King.

This telephone call is triaged as an emergency requiring immediate attention. Reschedule appointments as necessary to give the patient an emergency 9:00 A.M. appointment with Dr. King; about ½ hour should be reserved for the emergency. Describe your logic in determining how Dr. King's appointment schedule will be adjusted to handle the emergency situation.

____

____

____

____

____

B. Patient Mark Johnson is a no-show on Dr. Lewis's schedule. Mark the no-show appropriately on the appointment schedule. What other action must be taken to document Mr. Johnson's no-show status? Why is it important to accurately and completely document patient no-shows and cancellations?

____

____

____

____

C. Patient Martin Gordon calls to cancel his appointment with Dr. Lewis. He has rescheduled his appointment two weeks later at the same time.

(1) Mark the cancellation appropriately on the appointment schedule.

(2) A. After documenting the appointment change in the patient chart, the medical assistant completes an appointment card and mails it to Mr. Gordon as a reminder of his new appointment time.

L&K LEWIS & KING, MD
2501 CENTER STREET
NORTHBOROUGH, OH 12345

M ______________________________

has an appointment on

Mon. ____________ at ____________

Tues. ____________ at ____________

Wed. ____________ at ____________

Thurs. ____________ at ____________

Fri. ____________ at ____________

If unable to keep appointment, kindly give 24 hours notice.

B. Two ways of reminding patients of upcoming appointments are to give the appointment card personally to the patient and to mail the card to the patient. Identify a third reminder system. What procedures must be observed to protect patient confidentiality when employing this third method?

____

____

____

8. The best scheduling system for a practice is the one that effects good patient flow and proper use of staff and physical facilities.

A. Identify seven scheduling systems.

(1) ______________________________

(2) ______________________________

(3) ______________________________

(4) ______________________________

(5) ____________________

(6) ____________________

(7) ____________________

B. For each medical practice or facility below, identify the best scheduling system and explain the reasoning behind your choice.

(1) Hospital emergency room: ____________________

____

____

(2) Laboratory for blood testing: ____________________

____

____

(3) Two-physician group practice: ____________________

____

____

(4) Urgent care center with emergency and clinic facilities: ____________________

____

____

INVESTIGATION ACTIVITY

Many ambulatory care settings produce information brochures. These brochures describe the nature of medical practices and their services and provide a wide range of information about the facilities, including location and hours; the names and specialties of physicians and other staff; and scheduling, insurance, payment, and other office policies and procedures. Informational brochures help patients maximize the potential of the medical practice to meet their needs in an efficient, professional manner that enhances therapeutic communication between patients and health care providers. Keeping patients fully informed of the medical practice's scheduling policies and procedures creates empowered health care consumers who are more likely to carry a positive image of the physician and the overall quality of care received.

List three different types of medical practices and facilities that would benefit from publishing informational brochures. Some examples include a physical therapy clinic, an OB/GYN practice, a radiology center, and a center for geriatric care.

(1) ____________________

(2) ____________________

(3) ____________________

As a class, compile a complete list of facilities that could benefit from promotional brochures. Choose ten types of facilities and assign one student volunteer for each. The student volunteers will then perform research to find local facilities for each category. The volunteers will contact each facility to obtain any informational brochure materials the practice may have and will bring those materials to class.

Inner City Health Care

Meeting Families' Total Health Care Needs

Commitment to Patient Care
Our staff is committed to providing our patients with the best in medical care. We view your medical care as a team effort—providing you with qualified medical staff while encouraging you to be active participants in your total care. This brochure is designed to help you understand how our practice can best serve you. You are a very important part of our practice and we welcome your questions and comments.

Professional Staff
We are pleased to service the metropolitan area with a well-trained staff of physicians and support staff. Our team of physicians is available to meet your medical needs, assisted by our registered nurses, and certified medical assistants, lab technicians, and radiology technicians. Our urgent care clinic is an alternative to expensive emergency room visits and is open Monday through Saturday.

Services
We provide your family with complete medical facilities through our on-site diagnostic services, including X rays and clinical laboratory. In addition, we are located within five minutes of the local hospital should more extensive services be required. Our **triage line** is available 24 hours a day to assist in assessing problems.

Scheduling
To better serve you we utilize different methods of scheduling your visits.

In our **Urgent Care Center** no appointments are necessary. Patients will be seen on a first-come first-served basis but patients with an urgent need for care will be attended to first. We do, however, request that you call the office first to let us know you are coming. This clinic is best suited for problems that arise (fevers, flus, fractures, etc.).

Our **Clinics** require scheduled appointments. General medical appointments are made every day during regular hours. We make every attempt to see you as close to your scheduled appointment time as possible. Our **specialty clinics** utilize a clustering system so that we reserve certain days and times for particular types of appointments. These are as follows.

Orthopedics—Cast removals,
Mon/Wed 9 AM - 3 PM
Tues/Fri 11 AM - 7 PM
Obstetrics
Mon/Wed 9 AM - 2 PM Friday 1 - 7 PM
Gynecology—Tues and Thurs, 9-7
Pre-Surgery—Mon-Fri, 9 AM - noon
Vascular Lab—Tues and Thurs, 1-7 PM

Cancellations
We request you provide 24 hours notice of an appointment cancellation. You will be billed $20 if you fail to show without notifying our office at least one hour in advance.

Payment Plans
To assist you in obtaining proper medical care and minimizing your concerns for cost, we have established several methods of payment. We directly bill Blue Cross/Blue Shield, HMO Michigan, Shield Care, Care Michigan, and Medicare/Medicaid. Our **billing coordinator**, Karen Ritter, CMA, will be happy to assist you in setting up payment plans if you do not have insurance coverage. In addition, we accept pre-approved credit card payments.

For More Information
Our staff is here to assist you with questions and concerns you may have. Please refer to the following phone numbers for quicker service with specific needs:

Billing
Karen Ritter, CMA, 555-7155, ext. 4

Insurance Preauthorization
Jane O'Hara, CMA, 555-7155, ext. 12

Lab Results
555-7155, ext. 22

Appointment Scheduling
555-7158

Triage Line
555-7159

Clinic #1
Office Hours: Monday-Thursday, 9-7
Closed Friday

Clinic #2
Office Hours: Monday, Wednesday, and Friday, 10-7, Saturday, 10-3
Closed Tuesday and Thursday

Dr. Brown's Hours:
Clinic #1—Monday-Thursday, 9-2
Clinic #2—Monday & Wednesday, 2-7
Friday, noon-7, Saturday, 9-4

Dr. Rice's Hours:
Clinic #1—Monday-Thursday, 2-7
Clinic #2—Monday & Wednesday, 10-2,
Friday, 10-12

Urgent Care Center
Office Hours: Monday-Friday, 9-8
Saturday, 9-2

Dr. George's Hours:
Monday & Wednesday, 9-5
Friday & Saturday, 9-2 every other week

Dr. Woo's Hours:
Monday and Wednesday, 1-8
Friday & Saturday, 9-2 every other week

Dr. Reynolds' Hours:
Tuesday, 1-8, Wednesday, 9-1, Thursday, 9-2,
Friday, 9-2

Dr. Esposito's Hours:
Monday, 9-8, Tuesday, noon-8, Wednesday, 4-8,
Thursday, 11-8, Friday, 3-8, Saturday, 9-2

Dr. Whitney's Hours:
Tuesday, 9-8. Thursday & Friday, 11-8,
Saturday, 9-2

Using the Inner City Health Care brochure and the brochures researched by the class, analyze each brochure and discuss the following.

1. How complete is the information in the brochure? Is the information well organized and easy to access?
2. Does the design and layout of the brochure give patients a sense of order and professionalism? Does the brochure inspire confidence in a potential patient or health care consumer?
3. Are scheduling policies and procedures clearly stated in the brochure? Are there policies concerning cancellations, no-shows, and walk-ins?
4. What is the role of the medical assistant in educating patients about the scheduling policies and procedures of the ambulatory care setting? In addition to distributing informational brochures, what can medical assistants do to aid in the smooth flow of patients through a medical facility?

CASE STUDY

When patient Lenore McDonell falls from the examination table and lacerates her arm while attempting an independent transfer from the table to her wheelchair, clinical medical assistant Joe Guerrero alerts Dr. Winston Lewis, and the two begin to implement emergency procedures to control Lenore's bleeding and assess damage to the arm. Lenore's fall occurred at the end of her appointment, a routine check-up with Dr. Lewis.

Administrative medical assistant Ellen Armstrong must adjust Dr. Lewis's schedule to accommodate the emergency situation. Martin Gordon, a man in his mid-sixties diagnosed with prostate cancer, waits in the reception area for Dr. Lewis's next appointment. Martin's appointment, a six-month follow-up, is expected to take 30 minutes. Martin is also being treated for depression related to his cancer diagnosis. Hope Smith, a new patient in good general health, is scheduled for a complete examination; Hope is due to arrive at the offices of Drs. Lewis & King at the Northborough Family Medical Group within 20 minutes. Jim Marshall, an impatient and aggressive businessman, is scheduled for the first afternoon appointment after Dr. Lewis's lunch commitment. Jim's appointment, for a physical examination and ECG to investigate chest pains he has suffered recently, is expected to take 45 minutes. Dr. Lewis's schedule is completely booked for the rest of the day.

Discuss the following:

1. What scheduling alternatives will Ellen offer to Martin, who is already waiting in the reception area? What special considerations regarding Martin should Ellen take into account and why?
2. What is Ellen's first action regarding Hope, Dr. Lewis's next patient due to arrive at the office? What scheduling alternatives should Ellen offer to Hope?
3. What scheduling alternatives, if any, should Ellen present to Jim? Explain your logic.
4. How is patient triage important to Ellen's rescheduling of Dr. Lewis's patients? What important administrative and communication skills will Ellen use to handle this emergency situation efficiently and professionally?

SUPPLEMENTARY RESOURCES

Study Guide Disk: Additional practice exercises for this chapter are available on the Study Guide disk found in the back of the textbook.

Medical Assisting Videos: Appropriate content is available on Delmar's Medical Assisting Videos, 2nd ed., Tape 3, for the following topics:

Perform Administrative Duties
- Manage Physician's Professional and Hospital Schedule
- Triage Skills

SKILLS COMPETENCY ASSESSMENT

Procedure 14–1: Establishing the Appointment Matrix

Student's Name: ______________________________ Date: ____________

Objective: To have a current and accurate record of appointment times available for scheduling patient visits.

Conditions: The student demonstrates the ability to establish a current and accurate record of appointment times available for scheduling patient visits using the following equipment and supplies: appointment book, physician's schedule, staff schedule, and office calendar.

Time Requirements and Accuracy Standards: 30 minutes. Points assigned reflect importance of step to meeting objective: Important = (5) Essential = (10) Critical = (15). Automatic failure results if any of the **critical** tasks are omitted or performed incorrectly.

SKILLS ASSESSMENT CHECKLIST

Task Performed	Possible Points	TASKS
❑	15	Blocks off times in the appointment book when patients are *not* to be scheduled by marking a large *X* through these time slots.
❑	10	Writes in all vacations, holidays, and other office closures as soon as they are known.
❑	15	Notes staff absences that might affect patient scheduling.
❑	10	Writes in all physician meetings, hospital rounds, appointments, conferences, vacations, and other prescheduled physician commitments.
❑	5	Color-codes with highlighters if the office has a scheduling system for certain examinations or procedures.
❑	5	Completed the tasks within 30 minutes.
❑	15	Results obtained were accurate.

________	Earned	ADD POINTS OF TASKS CHECKED
75	Points	TOTAL POINTS POSSIBLE
________	SCORE	DETERMINE SCORE (divide points earned by total points possible, multiply results by 100)

Actual Student Time Needed to Complete Procedure: ____________

Student's Initials: ____________ Instructor's Initials: ____________ Grade: ____________

Suggestions for Improvement: ______________________________

____

Evaluator's Name (print) ______________________________

Evaluator's Signature ______________________________

Comments ______________________________

SKILLS COMPETENCY ASSESSMENT

Procedure 14–2: Checking in Patients

Student's Name: ______________________________ Date: ____________

Objective: To ensure the patient is given prompt and proper care; to meet legal safeguards for documentation.

Conditions: The student demonstrates the ability to ensure the patient is given prompt and proper care and meets legal safeguards for documentation using the following equipment and supplies: patient chart, required forms, and check-in list and/or appointment book.

Time Requirements and Accuracy Standards: 30 minutes. Points assigned reflect importance of step to meeting objective: Important = (5) Essential = (10) Critical = (15). Automatic failure results if any of the **critical** tasks are omitted or performed incorrectly.

SKILLS ASSESSMENT CHECKLIST

Task Performed	Possible Points	TASKS
❑	15	Prepares a list of patients to be seen and assembles the charts the previous evening or in the morning before opening the ambulatory care setting.
❑	15	Checks charts to see that all information is up to date.
❑	10	Acknowledges patient immediately when she or he arrives.
❑	10	Checks the patient in and reviews vital information.
❑	5	Checks the patient's name off in appointment book and/or day sheet with an ink pen.
❑	5	Asks politely for the patient to be seated and indicates the appropriate wait time.
❑	15	Places the chart where it will be used to route the patient to an appropriate location for the visit.
❑	5	Completed the tasks within 30 minutes.
❑	15	Results obtained were accurate.
	________	Earned ADD POINTS OF TASKS CHECKED
	95	Points TOTAL POINTS POSSIBLE
	________	SCORE DETERMINE SCORE (divide points earned by total points possible, multiply results by 100)

Actual Student Time Needed to Complete Procedure: ____________

Student's Initials: ____________ Instructor's Initials: ____________ Grade: ____________

Suggestions for Improvement: ____

____

____

____

Evaluator's Name (print) ____

Evaluator's Signature ____

Comments ____

DOCUMENTATION

Chart the procedure for the patient's medical record.

Date: ________________

Charting: ____

____

____

____

Student's Initials: __________

SKILLS COMPETENCY ASSESSMENT

Procedure 14–3: Cancellation Procedures

Student's Name: ______________________________ Date: ____________

Objective: To protect the physician from legal complications; to free up care time for other patients; to ensure quality patient care.

Conditions: The student demonstrates the ability to implement cancellation procedures using the following equipment and supplies: appointment sheet, pen (red), and patient chart.

Time Requirements and Accuracy Standards: 10 minutes. Points assigned reflect importance of step to meeting objective: Important = (5) Essential = (10) Critical = (15). Automatic failure results if any of the **critical** tasks are omitted or performed incorrectly.

SKILLS ASSESSMENT CHECKLIST

Task Performed	Possible Points	TASKS
❑	15	Develops a system so it is evident to staff making appointments that, due to cancellations, time is now open to schedule other appointments.
❑	10	*Changes:* Indicates on the appointment sheet all appointments that were changed by noting changes in the appointment sheet margin and directly in the patient's chart, then indicating the new appointment time.
❑	10	*Cancellations:* Indicates cancellations on the appointment sheet and the patient chart. Draws a single red line through canceled appointments. Dates and initials notations in patient chart.
❑	10	*No-shows:* Indicates in the appointment book with a red *X*; notes in patient chart; dates and initials notation.
❑	5	Completed the tasks within 10 minutes.
❑	15	Results obtained were accurate.

_______	Earned	ADD POINTS OF TASKS CHECKED
65	Points	TOTAL POINTS POSSIBLE
_______	SCORE	DETERMINE SCORE (divide points earned by total points possible, multiply results by 100)

Actual Student Time Needed to Complete Procedure: ____________

Student's Initials: ____________ Instructor's Initials: ____________ Grade: ____________

Suggestions for Improvement: ____

____

____

____

Evaluator's Name (print) ____

Evaluator's Signature ____

Comments ____

DOCUMENTATION

Chart the procedure for a no-show, a cancellation, and/or an appointment change in the patient's medical record.

Date: ________________

Charting: ____

____

____

____

Student's Initials: __________

EVALUATION OF CHAPTER KNOWLEDGE

How has your instructor evaluated the knowledge you have gained?

	Instructor Evaluation		
Knowledge	*Good*	*Average*	*Poor*
Chooses appropriate scheduling tools and can describe advantages	_____	_____	_____
Able to establish an appointment matrix	_____	_____	_____
Prepares daily appointment sheet	_____	_____	_____
Prepares daily worksheet	_____	_____	_____
Understands importance of triage in scheduling patient appointments	_____	_____	_____
Understands basic considerations in scheduling appointments	_____	_____	_____
Reviews procedures for cancellations, no-shows, and appointment changes	_____	_____	_____
Reviews procedures for patient check-in	_____	_____	_____
Recalls three types of reminder systems	_____	_____	_____
Reviews six major scheduling systems	_____	_____	_____
Understands purpose and content of patient informational brochure	_____	_____	_____
Recognizes the importance of communication skills in the scheduling process	_____	_____	_____

Student's Initials: ______ Instructor's Initials: ______

Grade: _______

CHAPTER 15

Medical Records Management

PERFORMANCE OBJECTIVES

Accurate filing of patient medical records is an essential administrative task in the ambulatory care setting. To provide the highest quality care, patient medical records and other important files must be easily and promptly accessed by the physician and other members of the health care team. The contents of all medical charts and other files must be kept complete and up-to-date. Medical assisting students can use this workbook chapter to review the filing systems commonly used in the ambulatory care setting and the correct procedures for medical records management.

EXERCISES AND ACTIVITIES

Vocabulary Builder

Fill in the blanks in the following sentences using the words listed below.

accession record	identification label	purging
captions	indexing	release mark
coding	inspection	shingling
color coding	key unit	SOAP
consecutive or serial filing	nonconsecutive filing	Source-Oriented Medical Record (SOMR)
cross-reference	out guide	tickler file
cut	Problem-Oriented Medical Record (POMR)	units
guides		

1. To remember to check with the reference laboratory on Friday to obtain patient Martin Gordon's test results, Ellen Armstrong, CMA places a note in her ______________________.
2. When using the ______________________ approach for all progress notes, Dr. Lewis enters information about a patient's problem in this order: S: subjective impressions; O: objective clinical evidence; A: assessment or diagnosis; P: plans for further studies, treatment, or management.

3. Every six months, Marilyn Johnson, CMA, follows office policy and procedures for ____________________ inactive files to remove and archive those not in active use.
4. The organized method of identifying and separating items to be filed into small subunits is accomplished with the use of ____________________ units.
5. When Liz Corbin, CMA, retrieves Annette Samuels's chart for Dr. Woo she places an ____________________ in the filing cabinet to show that the file has been removed from storage.
6. When filing, Ellen Armstrong, CMA, makes a thorough ____________________ of the item to be filed to identify the key name, business, and subject the information relates to.
7. When returning a patient's chart to the filing cabinet, Walter Seals, CMA, inspects the patient's name to identify the indexing ____________________.
8. When a patient comes into Inner City Health Care for the first time, Karen Ritter, CMA, makes a file for the new patient and then prepares an ____________________, which she adheres along the side of the folder for easy filing in a lateral file cabinet.
9. File folders are available with tabs placed in several positions on the folder. The position of the tab is called the ____________________ of the folder.
10. The ____________________ is a journal (or computer listing) where numbers in a numeric filing system are preassigned. The log sequentially lists numbers to be used to assign to numeric records.
11. The ____________________ filing system uses groups of two, three, or four or more digits, such as the patient's social security number or telephone number, as the filing reference in a numeric filing system.
12. When Dr. King is finished using a patient chart and is ready for it to be returned to the file cabinet, she puts a ____________________ on it.
13. The file for Kent Memorial Hospital contains three indexing ____________________ to be considered when preparing the filing label.
14. If a ____________________ card is required in the alphabetic card file of a numeric filing system, such as when making note of an established patient's married name, a card is prepared that includes an "X" next to the file number to indicate that this card does not designate the primary location card for the file.
15. In the ____________________ system of recordkeeping, patient problems are identified by a number that corresponds to the charting relevant to that problem number: that is, asthma #1; dermatitis #2; and so on.
16. ____________________ are used to separate file folders; they are somewhat larger than folders and are of a heavier stock.
17. When a filing system other than alphabetic is being used, the proper ____________________ must be determined for the chart or file so it can be retrieved.

18. Ellen Armstrong, CMA, uses the ____________________ method for filing laboratory reports; the reports are stacked across the page with the most recent report placed on top of the previous one.
19. Ellen Armstrong, CMA, uses the ____________________ method for handling invoices, sales orders, and requisitions; each record is numbered and filed in ascending order.
20. ____________________ filing systems make retrieval of files more efficient with the use of visible color differences that facilitate easier maintenance of the files.
21. ____________________ are used to identify major sections of file folders by more manageable subunits, such as GA-GE, or Miscellaneous. Captions are marked on the tabs of the guides.
22. Inner City Health Care uses the ____________________ method of recordkeeping, which groups information according to its origin; for example, laboratories, examinations, physician notes, consulting physicians, and other types of information.

Learning Review

1. Assign the correct units to the following items to be filed using the rule for filing patient records that is listed for each.

   A. Names that are hyphenated are considered one unit.

   1. Jackson Hugh Levine-Dwyer

   unit 1______________ unit 2______________ unit 3______________

   2. Leslie Jane Poole-Petit

   unit 1______________ unit 2______________ unit 3______________

   B. Seniority units are indexed as the last indexing unit.

   1. Keith Wildasin Sr.

   unit 1______________ unit 2______________ unit 3______________

   2. Gerald Maggart III

   unit 1______________ unit 2______________ unit 3______________

   C. Titles are considered as separate indexing units. If the title appears with first and last names, the title is considered the last indexing unit.

   1. Dr. Louise Udolf

   unit 1______________ unit 2______________ unit 3______________

   2. Prof. Valerie Rajah

   unit 1______________ unit 2______________ unit 3______________

D. The names of individuals are assigned indexing units respectively: last name, first name, middle, and succeeding names.

1. Lindsay Adair Martin

unit 1________________ unit 2________________ unit 3________________

2. Abigail Sue Johnson

unit 1________________ unit 2________________ unit 3________________

E. When indexing names of married women, the name is indexed by the legal name.

1. Mary Jane O'Keefe (Mrs. John)

unit 1____________ unit 2____________ unit 3____________ unit 4____________

2. Nora Patrice Fowler (Mrs. Herb)

unit 1____________ unit 2____________ unit 3____________ unit 4____________

F. Foreign language units are indexed as one unit with the unit that follows. Spacing, punctuation, and capitalization are ignored.

1. Joseph Jack de la Hoya

unit 1________________ unit 2________________ unit 3________________

2. Maurice John van de Veer

unit 1________________ unit 2________________ unit 3________________

2. Using the numbers 1, 2, and 3, label the patient names in each group according to the correct filing order of names in an alphabetic filing system.

A. _______ Larry Peter Sanders

_______ Larry Paul Samuels

_______ Lawrence Paul Sanders

B. _______ James Edward Reed Sr.

_______ James Edward Reed

_______ James Edward Reed Jr.

C. _______ Lynn Elaine Brenner

_______ Lynn Ellen Brenner

_______ Lynn Eloise Brenner

D. _______ Patrick Sam Saint

_______ Patrick Sam St. Bartz

_______ Paul Sam Saint

3. Assign units to the following items to be filed, using the rule for business/organization filing that is listed for each.

A. When indexing numbers, the numbers are indexed as written.

Riverview One Locksmith

unit 1______________ unit 2______________ unit 3______________

B. When indexing hyphenated numbers, they are indexed only by the number before the hyphen.

24-7 Office Cleaning

unit 1______________ unit 2______________ unit 3______________

C. The order assignment of units for indexing businesses/organizations is as written.

Target Specimen Laboratory

unit 1______________ unit 2______________ unit 3______________

D. When indexing the $ sign before a number, the first unit is the number.

$10 Filing Cabinets

unit 1__________ unit 2__________ unit 3__________ unit 4__________

E. When indexing numbers, if the number is written with a word, it is indexed as one unit with the word.

Janoff's Office Supplies 2Go

unit 1__________ unit 2__________ unit 3__________ unit 4__________

F. When the (in, at, and other prepositions and articles) is the first unit of a business-organization, it is indexed as the last unit.

The Richmond Therapy Group

unit 1__________ unit 2__________ unit 3__________ unit 4__________

G. When indexing numbers, if the number is written as a single word, it is indexed as a single unit.

Laboratory Kits 4 Analysis

unit 1__________ unit 2__________ unit 3__________ unit 4__________

H. When punctuation marks are included as part of the indexing unit, they are disregarded.

"Ace" Prosthetics Inc.

unit 1______________ unit 2______________ unit 3______________

I. When indexing figures, the numbers are written as figures.

1st Metropolitan Hospital

unit 1______________ unit 2______________ unit 3______________

4. Circle the right answer(s) from the choices below.

   A. Jane O'Hara, CMA, is filing patient records using a nonconsecutive numeric filing system. For the patient file labeled 618 32 6445, what is unit 1?

      1. 6445
      2. 618
      3. 32 6445

   B. Physician coding is:

      1. a filing system in which each physician keeps records in her or his office.
      2. a filing system in which physicians do their own coding.
      3. a filing system in which patients are identified by their primary care physician.

   C. The most important reason for using numeric filing is that:

      1. it preserves patient confidentiality.
      2. a larger number of records can be easily filed.
      3. a computer can more readily read numeric filing labels.

   D. Walter Seals, CMA, is filing using a consecutive numeric filing system. For the patient file labeled 67 843, what is unit 1?

      1. 3
      2. 6
      3. 843

   E. Outgoing correspondence is:

      1. friendly correspondence.
      2. correspondence sent out of the medical office.
      3. correspondence to be thrown away.

   F. Karen Ritter, CMA, is filing patient files using a numeric filing system. She comes across a file for a patient who has not yet been assigned a number. Karen should:

      1. put the file in the miscellaneous numeric file section.
      2. put the file in a pending filing bin until the physician can assign a number.
      3. put the file directly behind the rest of the files.

   G. An out guide should contain:

      1. a record of when the chart was removed.
      2. the signature of the patient's physician.
      3. a record of when the file is expected to be returned.

Investigation Activity

Filing skills are mastered through memorization and practice. By memorizing the basic rules of filing, medical assistants will be more confident about filing records and documents accurately. Filing becomes less of a mystery and filing duties can be performed with efficiency, speed, and ease.

Memorization

Create index cards with a basic filing rule written on each one. Consult your textbook for the twenty basic filing rules (see textbook pages 238–241). Also create cards for the filing rules associated with numeric filing (see textbook page 245), cross-references (see textbook pages 248–249), and the filing procedure examples for correspondence (see textbook page 254).

Now, divide the class into small groups of students seated in a circle of no more than five people. Each group has a complete set of filing rule index cards. Shuffle the cards, face down, so the information cannot be read. The first student, designated by the group, takes a card from the shuffled deck of filing rule cards and reads the rule out loud to the group. The first person in the group to give a correct example of the rule "wins" the round. The student's correct answer is written on the index card and initialed. Then, the deck is passed to this student who chooses another card and begins a new round. The game continues until all index cards have been used. The complete deck, now annotated with student answers and initials, is given to the instructor.

As a class, discuss the process of memorizing filing rules and how easy or hard it is to apply filing rules.

Practice

Each student in the class agrees to volunteer to perform two hours of filing for a campus organization, department, administrative office, or library within one designated school week. The following week, discuss in class the different filing systems used on campus. Assess the general experience. For example, how organized was the filing system? Was the system up to date? Was the filing process efficient, confusing, streamlined, disorderly, a no-brainer? Did the office staff exhibit a high knowledge of the inner workings of their filing system? Discuss the impact of effective records management on the smooth operation of any workplace environment, including the ambulatory care setting.

CASE STUDY

At the offices of Drs. Lewis & King, co-office managers Marilyn Johnson and Shirley Brooks stress the importance of maintaining accurate, up-to-date, and complete documentation in all patient medical records. The practice uses the POMR method of recordkeeping for patient files within an alphabetical color-coded filing system. Drs. Lewis & King use the SOAP approach in charting patient progress notes. Twice each year, the office managers hold a special staff meeting devoted solely to a discussion of the filing system. The meeting is used to answer staff questions and consider ideas for streamlining the filing system to increase efficiency and ease of use.

Discuss the following:

1. Why is accurate, up-to-date, and complete documentation in patient medical records essential in the ambulatory care setting?
2. Why is the POMR system commonly used by family practice offices?
3. Why is a color-coding system effective in the ambulatory care setting?
4. How important is an effective, easy to use, and easy to access filing system to the efficiency of the ambulatory care setting?

SUPPLEMENTARY RESOURCES

Study Guide Disk: Additional practice exercises for this chapter are available on the study guide disk found in the back of the textbook.

Medical Assisting Videos: Appropriate content is available on Delmar's Medical Assisting Videos, 2nd ed., for the following topics:

Tape 2: Legal Aspects and Confidentiality of Medical Records
- Access to Medical Records
- Control of and Access to the Computerized Medical Record
- Use Appropriate Guidelines When Releasing Medical Records
- Document Accurately
- Complete Medical Records

Tape 3: Perform Administrative Duties
- Use Basic Office Equipment
- Prepare and Maintain Medical Records
- Apply Computer Concepts for Office Procedures

SKILLS COMPETENCY ASSESSMENT

Procedure 15–1: Steps for Manual Filing with a Numeric System

Student's Name: ______________________________ Date: __________

Objective: To demonstrate an understanding of the principles of the numeric filing system.

Conditions: The student demonstrates the ability to perform manual filing with a numeric filing system using the following equipment and supplies: documents to be filed, dividers with guides, miscellaneous numeric file section, alphabetic card file and cards, accession journal, if needed.

Time Requirements and Accuracy Standards: 10 minutes. Points assigned reflect importance of step to meeting objective: Important = (5) Essential = (10) Critical = (15). Automatic failure results if any of the **critical** tasks are omitted or performed incorrectly.

SKILLS ASSESSMENT CHECKLIST

Task Performed	Possible Points	TASKS
		Inspects and indexes.
❑	10	Codes for filing units. Checks alphabetic card file to see if card already exists.
❑	10	Writes the number in the upper right-hand corner, if the piece is assigned a number.
❑	10	Checks the miscellaneous file, if no number is assigned. If miscellaneous item is ready to be assigned a number, makes a card and notes number in the right-hand corner of card file, crosses out the "M," and makes a chart file.
❑	10	If there is no card, makes up an alphabetic card including a complete name and address, and then writes either "M" or assigns a number.
❑	15	Cross-references if necessary and files the card properly.
❑	15	Files documents in appropriate file folders/charts in ascending order.
❑	5	Completed the tasks within 10 minutes.
❑	15	Results obtained were accurate.

________	Earned	ADD POINTS OF TASKS CHECKED
90	Points	TOTAL POINTS POSSIBLE
________	SCORE	DETERMINE SCORE (divide points earned by total points possible, multiply results by 100)

Actual Student Time Needed to Complete Procedure: __________

Student's Initials: __________ Instructor's Initials: __________ Grade: __________

Suggestions for Improvement: ______________________________

Evaluator's Name (print) ______________________________

Evaluator's Signature ______________________________

Comments ______________________________

SKILLS COMPETENCY ASSESSMENT

Procedure 15–2: Steps for Manual Filing with a Subject Filing System

Student's Name: ______________________________ Date: ____________

Objective: To demonstrate an understanding of the principles of the subject filing system.

Conditions: The student demonstrates the ability to understand the principles of a subject filing system using the following equipment and supplies: documents to be filed by subject, subject index list or index card file listing subjects, alphabetic card file and cards.

Time Requirements and Accuracy Standards: 10 minutes. Points assigned reflect importance of step to meeting objective: Important = (5) Essential = (10) Critical = (15). Automatic failure results if any of the **critical** tasks are omitted or performed incorrectly.

SKILLS ASSESSMENT CHECKLIST

Task Performed	Possible Points	TASKS
❑	10	Reviews the item to find the subject.
❑	15	Matches the subject of the item with an appropriate category on the subject index list.
❑	5	Decides on the proper cross-reference if the item contains information that may pertain to more than one subject.
❑	10	Underlines the subject title, if it appears on the material.
❑	5	If subject title is not on the material, writes the subject title clearly in the upper right-hand corner and underlines it.
❑	10	Uses a wavy line for cross-referencing and an *X*, as with alphabetic and numeric filing.
❑	15	Underlines the first indexing unit of the coded units.
❑	5	Completed the tasks within 10 minutes.
❑	15	Results obtained were accurate.

______	Earned	ADD POINTS OF TASKS CHECKED
90	Points	TOTAL POINTS POSSIBLE
______	SCORE	DETERMINE SCORE (divide points earned by total points possible, multiply results by 100)

Actual Student Time Needed to Complete Procedure: ____________

Student's Initials: ____________ Instructor's Initials: ____________ Grade: ____________

Suggestions for Improvement: ______________________________

Evaluator's Name (print) ______________________________

Evaluator's Signature ______________________________

Comments ______________________________

EVALUATION OF CHAPTER KNOWLEDGE

How has your instructor evaluated the knowledge you have achieved?

Knowledge	Instructor Evaluation *Good*	*Average*	*Poor*
States the reasons for accurately maintaining ambulatory care office files	_____	_____	_____
Recalls common supplies used in medical records management	_____	_____	_____
Names and describes basic rules for filing	_____	_____	_____
Recalls steps for filing medical documentation in patient files	_____	_____	_____
Recalls filing procedures for correspondence	_____	_____	_____
States advantages and disadvantages of the alphabetic filing system	_____	_____	_____
Distinguishes between filing systems, such as alphabetic, numeric, and subject filing	_____	_____	_____
Understands color-coded filing systems	_____	_____	_____
Analyzes the purposes of cross-referencing			
Recalls four common documents filed in the patient's medical record	_____	_____	_____
Describes computer databases and their usefulness to the ambulatory care setting	_____	_____	_____
Understand rules of confidentiality when handling patients' medical records	_____	_____	_____

Student's Initials: ______ Instructor's Initials: ______

Grade: _______

CHAPTER 16

Written Communications

PERFORMANCE OBJECTIVES

Written correspondence in the ambulatory care setting has three important functions: it conveys necessary information to patients, other physicians, and health care organizations; it reflects on the professional standards of the office; and it provides permanent legal documentation in the event of any type of litigation. It is essential that medical assisting students understand the importance of written communication skills. Valuable skills include being able to distinguish between and compose the four major letter styles used in the ambulatory care setting; being able to proofread for spelling, grammar, and content; and being able to describe the significance of accuracy in, and the basic rules of, medical transcription.

EXERCISES AND ACTIVITIES

Vocabulary Builder

Fill in the blanks in the passage below with the appropriate vocabulary terms.

bond paper	optical character reader (OCR)
full block letter	simplified letter
keyed	voice recognition technology (VRT)
medical transcription	watermark
indented modified block letter	ZIP+4
standard modified block letter	

There are four major types of letters that medical assistants commonly write. Of these, the ________________ is the most time-efficient, as it does not use excessive tab indentations for the address, complimentary close, or keyed signature. In the ________________, all lines begin at the left margin with the exception of the date line, complimentary closure, and keyed signature. In the ________________, paragraphs may be indented five spaces. Medical assistants may choose to use the ________________, the style of letter recommended by the Administrative Management Society. In this style, all lines are ________________, or input by keystroke, flush with the left margin. When selecting paper supplies the medical assistant should choose ________________ with a ________________, or image imprinted during the paper-making process that is visible when a sheet is held up to the light. When preparing letters for outgoing shipments, it is important for the medical assistant to pay attention to several factors, including addressing. Medical assistants should machine print addresses (including the ________________ code) with a uniform left hand margin so that the addresses can be read by the U. S. Postal Service's ________________.

One of the most important aspects of written communication in the ambulatory setting is the management of ________________, the process by which medical data is documented. One of the latest tools in this process is ________________, by which physicians speak into a microphone that translates spoken words into a typed report via the computer. This new method can cut down on errors and aid medical assistants in maintaining confidentiality and protecting the privacy of patients in the process of medical documentation.

Learning Review

A. Identify the letter style of workbook Figure 16–1. ________________________

B. Proofread the letter in workbook Figure 16–1, correcting all errors by inserting the proper proofreader's marks. Make your marks directly on to the text. Consult your textbook (page 263) for a list of common proofreader's marks. Refer to a medical dictionary, if necessary.

C. To practice your skills of medical transcription, record the content of the letter in workbook Figure 16–1 by speaking into a tape recorder. Play back the tape and transcribe the letter accurately on a sheet of stationery using the standard modified block style.

JAMES CARTER, MD, NEUROLOGY

Metropolitan University Medical Center, 8280 Wright Avenue, Northborough, OH 12382

February 2, xxxx

Elizabeth Kind, M.D
Northborough Medical Family Group
The Offices of Lewis & King, MD
2501 Center Street
Nrothborough, OH 12345

RE: MARGARET THOMAS

Dear Dr. King:

Thank you for refering Margaret Thomas to my neurological practice. Margaret come to you recently as a new patient for a comprehensive physical examination to evaluate troubling symptoms she had been experiencing for several months. Margaret notices symtoms of tremor, difficulty walking, defective judgement, and hot flushes; she is not able to poinpoint the exac ttime symptoms began. Your physical examination suggested the possible diagnoisis of parkingson's Disease. Margaret presented today for a complete nuerological evaluation.

MEDICAL/SURGICAL HISTORY. The patient is posiitive for the usual childhood diseases and the births of three children, following normal pregnancies. Her surgical history includes an Appendectomy performed 10 years ago. She has a food allergy to shellfish, but no known allergies to medications. She takes Pepto-Bismol and Metamusil for frequent stomach upset and constipation. She is a widow with two children, ages twenty three, twenty-five, and 29, and is a retired homemaker. She does not smoke and has an occassional glass of wine. Her family history is positive for colon cancer in her mother and parenteral grandfather and for lung cancer in her father.

PYHSICALEXAMINATION. VITAL SIGNS: The patient has normal vital signs for a 52-year old Caucasian female. HEENT: The patient had a normacephalic and atraumatic exam. There is mild bobing of the head and facial expressions appear fixed. Pupils equal, round, regular, react to light and acommodation. The fundi were benign. There was normal cup to disc ratio of 0.3. Tympanic Membranes were both clear and mobile. Her nose was clear. the oropharynz ws clear without any evidence of lezions. There was not cervical adenopathy, no thyromegely, or other masses. NECK: Musles of the neck are quite rigid and stiff. CHEST: Cear to percussion and auscultation. HEART: Regular rate and rhythm without murmurs or gallops. there was no jugular venous distention, no peripheral edema, no carotid buits. Pulses were 2+ and symetrical. Abdomen. Some what obese, but benigh. There was not organomegaly or masses. Bowel tones were normal. There was no rebound tenderness. BACK: Examination reveals loss of posturalreflexe and patient stands with head bent forward and wals as if in danger of falling forward. There is difficulty in pivoting and loss of balance. GENITOURINARY: Normal. EXTREMITIES: Thre is moderate bradykinesia. Chracteristic slow, turning motion (pronation-supination) of, the forearm and the hand and a motion of the thumb against the fingers as if rolling a pill between the fingers is noted. This condition seems to worsen when the patient is concentrating or feeling anxious.

```
NEUROLOGICAL. The patient was cooperative and answered all questions. There is
no history past of mental disorders or cardiovascular disease. There is muscle
weakness and rigidity in all four extremities. Intellect remains intact;

LABORATORY DATA: Urinanalysis reveals low levels of dopamin. Cat scan reveals
degeneration of nerve cells occuring in the basel ganglia.

ASSESSMENT. Based on the patient history and neurologic examination, it appears
most likely that the patient has mild to moderate Parkinsons Disease.

PLAN. 1. Recommend physical therapy focussed on learning how to manage difficult
movements such as descneding stairs safely.
2. Exercises to maintain flexibility, motility, and mental well-being.
3. Levadopa to increase dopamine levels in the brain to control symptoms. Please
advise the patient that alchohol consumption shoudl be limited because it acts
antegonistically to levodopa.
4. Relaxation and stress management counseling.

PROGNOSIS. Parkinson's disease progresses slowly. Patient should be follow on a
regular basis and observed for any signs of damentia which may result in about
1-third of cases.

Sincerely,


James Carter, MD

DD: February 2, xxxx
DT: February 3, xxxx

JC/bl
```

Investigation Activity

Written Communications Self-Test

In your written communications, are you able to express yourself accurately and concisely? Able to communicate ideas effectively? Capable of proofreading and editing for content? Use this simple self-test to gauge your comfort and proficiency in written communications by identifying strengths and pinpointing any weak areas that could use improvement. For each statement below, circle the corresponding letter to the response that best describes you.

1. When writing a letter, I generally feel
   A. confident. I communicate effectively on the page and enjoy writing letters.
   B. at ease. My written communication skills are acceptable.
   C. uncomfortable. I would rather communicate verbally than through writing.

2. As far as content goes, when I am given the required information and asked to compose a letter, I
   A. almost always understand exactly what I am being asked to communicate and am able to convey it precisely in letter form.
   B. generally understand what I am being asked to communicate, but sometimes have to fine-tune my letters.

C. often have trouble understanding what I am being asked to communicate and usually have to go back and ask questions about the letter's content.

3. In general, when choosing words for written correspondence, I feel
   A. secure about my ability to select appropriate language and use medical terminology accurately.
   B. pretty confident, although my general vocabulary and knowledge of medical terminology could use some improvement.
   C. frustrated; I always seem to confuse words and medical terms no matter how hard I try not to.

4. As far as spelling goes, I am
   A. a top-notch speller; I always keep both a standard and medical dictionary on hand for the words I am not sure of.
   B. an adequate speller; sometimes I confuse a word here or there. I always have to proofread carefully for spelling errors.
   C. a below-par speller; my letters are always littered with misspellings and someone else has to proofread my work.

5. Grammatically speaking, I am
   A. above average; I routinely find mistakes in my colleagues' work.
   B. passable; I make minor mistakes but usually catch them while proofreading.
   C. hopeless; people find mistakes in my work even after I have checked it twice!

6. Regarding proofreader's marks, I am
   A. highly capable of proofreading my work; if colleagues need someone to proof their work, I am first on their list.
   B. an okay proofreader; I occasionally overlook a mistake, but nobody's perfect.
   C. frightened; proofreading marks are just a bunch of meaningless squiggles to me.

7. How would you describe your formatting skills?
   A. Exemplary. I understand all basic letter forms, and all of my letters are rigorously formatted according to correct specifications.
   B. Satisfactory. Every so often, I confuse styles or forget an annotation, but in general, all my letters are formatted correctly.
   C. Fair to nonexistent. I have trouble understanding why every letter has to be so formally constructed.

8. When adhering to office style guidelines, I
   A. always follow the guidelines.
   B. usually have no problem sticking to style guidelines; when I make a mistake, it is a rare event.
   C. need improvement. My letters are frequently littered with style inconsistencies. I do not understand the need for an office style as long as each letter is written with accurate information.

9. If you had to rate your transcription skills, you would describe them as:
   A. Impeccable. I make very few errors and use critical thinking skills to problem-solve trouble spots before giving up and asking for help.
   B. Sufficient. What I do not understand I automatically flag and ask for clarification.

C. Not as good as they should be. I hate trying to enter data from a taped voice; it is a frustrating experience.

10. Overall, I think of writing letters in the health care environment as
    A. one of my strong suits.
    B. a task that I am able to accomplish, just not one I particularly enjoy.
    C. a necessary evil.

Scoring: If your answers were mostly "A" responses, you have strong written communications skills and enjoy writing letters. If your responses were mostly "B"s, your written communications skills are good but could stand some improvement. Try reviewing pertinent information in this chapter to strengthen areas that need it. If your answers were mostly "C"s, you need to work on your written communication skills. Volunteer to take on as many written correspondence assignments as you can—practice may help you overcome your apprehension about writing letters and will almost certainly raise the quality of your work.

CASE STUDY

Ellen Armstrong, CMA, enjoys working on correspondence for Drs. Lewis & King and takes pride in her written communications skills. As an ongoing project, office manager Marilyn Johnson, CMA, asks Ellen to make suggestions for updating and revising the style manual used in the medical office for written communications guidelines. Ellen suggests the addition of a section in the style manual to discuss bias in language. Bias-free language is sensitive in applying labels to individuals or groups and uses gender-specific words and pronouns appropriately. For example, dementia is used instead of crazy or senile. Instead of using layman, consider using lay person. Apply he or she only in gender-specific usage. Marilyn and the physician-employers ask Ellen to implement the addition to the style manual.

Discuss the following:

1. Why is bias-free language an important consideration in written communications for the ambulatory care setting?
2. List other examples of biased language and give suggestions for bias-free alternatives.

SUPPLEMENTARY RESOURCES

Study Guide Disk: Additional practice exercises for this chapter are available on the study guide disk found in the back of the textbook.

Medical Assisting Videos: Appropriate content is available on Delmar's Medical Assisting Videos, 2nd ed., for the following topics:

Tape 1:	Communication Skills
Tape 2:	Legal Aspects and Confidentiality of Medical Records
	Access to Medical Records
	Use Appropriate Guidelines When Releasing Records
Tape 3:	Perform Administrative Duties
	Use Basic Office Equipment
	Prepare and Maintain Medical Records
	Triage Skills

SKILLS COMPETENCY ASSESSMENT

Procedure 16–1: Preparing and Composing Business Correspondence Using All Components

Student's Name: ______________________________ Date: ____________

Objective: To prepare and compose a rough draft and final-copy business letter.

Conditions: The student demonstrates the ability to prepare and compose a rough draft and final-copy letter using appropriate language and letter style to convey a clear and accurate message to the recipient using the following equipment and supplies: computer or word processor and printer, or typewriter; printed letterhead and plain second sheet; dictionary; thesaurus; medical dictionary; style manual; index cards.

Time Requirements and Accuracy Standards: 15 minutes. Points assigned reflect importance of step to meeting objective: Important = (5) Essential = (10) Critical = (15). Automatic failure results if any of the **critical** tasks are omitted or performed incorrectly.

SKILLS ASSESSMENT CHECKLIST

Task Performed	Possible Points	TASKS
❑	5	Writes information to be included in the letter on index cards.
❑	5	Organizes the index cards in a logical sequence, then composes a rough draft of the letter.
❑	5	Uses language that is easily understood.
❑	10	States the reason for the letter in the first paragraph and encourages action in the last paragraph.
❑	15	Proofreads the draft for grammar, spelling, and punctuation. Uses the appropriate reference material to check any inaccuracies.
❑	5	Chooses the letter format customary to the ambulatory care setting.
❑	10	Begins keying the letter referring to the chosen format. Enters complete date on line 15 or two to three lines below the letterhead.
❑	5	Keys the recipient's name and address flush with the left margin beginning on line 20.
❑	5	Keys the salutation flush with the left margin on the second line below the recipient's address. Follows salutation with a colon, unless using open punctuation.
❑	5	Keys the subject of the letter on the second line below the salutation flush with the left margin.
❑	10	Begins the body of the letter on the second line below the salutation or subject line. Uses correct letter style.

SKILLS COMPETENCY ASSESSMENT — continued

Procedure 16–1: Preparing and Composing Business Correspondence Using All Components

Task Performed	Possible Points	TASKS
☐	5	Keys the complimentary closure on the second line below the body of the letter, capitalizing only the first word.
☐	5	Keys the signature four to six lines below the complimentary closing.
☐	5	Keys reference initials, if used, two lines below the keyed signature.
☐	5	Keys the enclosure or carbon copy notation one or two lines below the reference initials.
☐	15	Proofreads the document and makes corrections as necessary.
☐	10	Prepares the envelope and attaches to the letter.
☐	15	Places the letter on the physician's desk for review and signature.
☐	5	Completed the tasks within 15 minutes.
☐	15	Results obtained were accurate.

______	Earned	ADD POINTS OF TASKS CHECKED
160	Points	TOTAL POINTS POSSIBLE
______	SCORE	DETERMINE SCORE (divide points earned by total points possible, multiply results by 100)

Actual Student Time Needed to Complete Procedure: ____________

Student's Initials: ____________ Instructor's Initials: ____________ Grade: ____________

Suggestions for Improvement: ______________________________

____

____

____

Evaluator's Name (print) ______________________________

Evaluator's Signature ______________________________

Comments ______________________________

SKILLS COMPETENCY ASSESSMENT

Procedure 16–2: Addressing Envelopes According to United States Postal Regulations

Student's Name: ______________________________ Date: __________

Objective: To address envelopes correctly.

Conditions: The student demonstrates the ability to address envelopes according to U.S. postal regulations using the following equipment and supplies: computer or word processor and printer with envelope tray, or typewriter; envelopes; U.S. Postal Service Publication 25; U.S. Postal Service Notice 221.

Time Requirements and Accuracy Standards: 10 minutes. Points assigned reflect importance of step to meeting objective: Important = (5) Essential = (10) Critical = (15). Automatic failure results if any of the **critical** tasks are omitted or performed incorrectly.

SKILLS ASSESSMENT CHECKLIST

Task Performed	Possible Points	TASKS
☐	5	Inserts the envelope in the typewriter or selects the envelope format from the software program.
☐	10	Visualizes an imaginary rectangle on the envelope, extending ⅝ inch to 2¼ inches from the bottom of the envelope, with 1 inch on each side.
☐	15	Accurately keys the address in uppercase letters within the rectangle using uniform left margin. Keys address and ZIP+4 code according to U. S. postal regulations.
☐	15	Accurately keys the return address in uppercase letters in the upper left corner of the envelope.
☐	10	Proofreads the envelope, makes corrections as necessary.
☐	5	Completed the tasks within 10 minutes.
☐	15	Results obtained were accurate.
______	Earned	ADD POINTS OF TASKS CHECKED
75	Points	TOTAL POINTS POSSIBLE
______	SCORE	DETERMINE SCORE (divide points earned by total points possible, multiply results by 100)

Actual Student Time Needed to Complete Procedure: __________

Student's Initials: __________ Instructor's Initials: __________ Grade: __________

Suggestions for Improvement: ______________________________

Evaluator's Name (print) ______________________________

Evaluator's Signature ______________________________

Comments ______________________________

SKILLS COMPETENCY ASSESSMENT

Procedure 16–3: Folding Letters for Standard Envelopes

Student's Name: ______________________________ Date: __________

Objective: To fold and insert letters into envelopes.

Conditions: The student demonstrates the ability to fold and insert letters into envelopes so the letters fit properly using the following equipment and supplies: letters, number 6¾ envelope, number 10 envelope, window envelope.

Time Requirements and Accuracy Standards: 10 minutes. Points assigned reflect importance of step to meeting objective: Important = (5) Essential = (10) Critical = (15). Automatic failure results if any of the **critical** tasks are omitted or performed incorrectly.

SKILLS ASSESSMENT CHECKLIST

Task Performed	Possible Points	TASKS
		Number 6¾ Envelope
❑	5	Folds the letter up from bottom, leaving ¼ inch to ½ inch at the top and creases.
❑	5	Folds the letter from the right edge about one-third the width of the letter and creases.
❑	5	Folds left edge over to within ¼ inch to ½ inch of the right-edge crease.
❑	10	Inserts the left creased edge first into the envelope.
		Number 10 Envelope
❑	5	Folds the letter up about one-third the length of the sheet and creases.
❑	5	Folds the top of the letter down to within ¼ inch to ½ inch of the bottom crease; creases top.
❑	10	Inserts the top creased edge first into the envelope.
		Window Envelope
❑	15	Turns the letter over and folds the top up about one-third the length of the page so the address is facing up and creases.
❑	5	Folds the bottom of the letter back to the first crease.
❑	15	Inserts the letter into the envelope bottom first to reveal entire address through the window.
❑	5	Prepares envelopes in shingled pattern for moistening prior to sealing.

Task Performed	Possible Points	TASKS
☐	5	Completed the tasks within 10 minutes.
☐	15	Results obtained were accurate.

________	Earned	ADD POINTS OF TASKS CHECKED
75	Points	TOTAL POINTS POSSIBLE
________	SCORE	DETERMINE SCORE (divide points earned by total points possible, multiply results by 100)

Actual Student Time Needed to Complete Procedure: ____________

Student's Initials: ____________ Instructor's Initials: ____________ Grade: ____________

Suggestions for Improvement: ____

____

____

____

Evaluator's Name (print) ____

Evaluator's Signature ____

Comments ____

SKILLS COMPETENCY ASSESSMENT

Procedure 16–4: Preparing Outgoing Mail According to United States Postal Regulations

Student's Name: ______________________________ Date: ____________

Objective: To prepare outgoing mail for expeditious delivery.

Conditions: The student demonstrates the ability to prepare outgoing mail according to U.S. postal regulations using the following equipment and supplies: manual or electronic scale, postage meter or stamps, envelope or package to be mailed.

Time Requirements and Accuracy Standards: 10 minutes. Points assigned reflect importance of step to meeting objective: Important = (5) Essential = (10) Critical = (15). Automatic failure results if any of the **critical** tasks are omitted or performed incorrectly.

SKILLS ASSESSMENT CHECKLIST

Task Performed	Possible Points	TASKS
❑	10	Sorts the mail according to postal class.
❑	15	Uses the manual or electronic scale to weigh the item to be mailed. Calculates postage from weight, or reads correct postage on electronic display.
❑	15	Uses a postal meter or stamps to affix the appropriate postage to the piece to be mailed.
❑	10	Places the prepared mail in the area of the office designated for outgoing mail or delivers the mail to the post office according to office policy.
❑	5	Completed the tasks within 10 minutes.
❑	15	Results obtained were accurate.

________	Earned	ADD POINTS OF TASKS CHECKED
70	Points	TOTAL POINTS POSSIBLE
________	SCORE	DETERMINE SCORE (divide points earned by total points possible, multiply results by 100)

Actual Student Time Needed to Complete Procedure: ____________

Student's Initials: ____________ Instructor's Initials: ____________ Grade: ____________

Suggestions for Improvement: ______________________________

____

Evaluator's Name (print) ______________________________

Evaluator's Signature ______________________________

Comments ______________________________

SKILLS COMPETENCY ASSESSMENT

Procedure 16–5: Preparing, Sending, and Receiving a Fax

Student's Name: ______________________________ Date: ____________

Objective: To send and receive information quickly and accurately by fax (facsimile).

Conditions: The student demonstrates the ability to send and receive information quickly and accurately by fax using the following equipment and supplies: fax machine, telephone, correspondence, fax cover sheet.

Time Requirements and Accuracy Standards: 10 minutes. Points assigned reflect importance of step to meeting objective: Important = (5) Essential = (10) Critical = (15). Automatic failure results if any of the **critical** tasks are omitted or performed incorrectly.

SKILLS ASSESSMENT CHECKLIST

Task Performed	Possible Points	TASKS
		To Send a Fax
❑	10	Prepares a cover sheet or uses a preprinted cover sheet for the document to be faxed. Includes on cover sheet the addresses of sender and receiver, total number of faxed pages (including cover sheet), and short message.
❑	15	*Rationale:* Understands that confidential information must be faxed only with the advance permission of the receiver. The cover sheet must include a notice on confidentiality.
❑	10	Places the document face down in the fax machine.
❑	15	Dials the telephone or dedicated fax number of the receiver. Checks accuracy of number dialed.
❑	10	Requests a receipt or report after the document passes through the fax machine.
❑	10	Removes the document from the machine; calls recipient to ensure that fax was received.
		To Receive a Fax
❑	15	Ensures that the fax machine is turned on and that the telephone line to the machine is not being used.
❑	10	Removes the document from the machine after it is received.
❑	15	Immediately delivers the faxed document to the addressee.
❑	5	Completed the tasks within 10 minutes.
❑	15	Results obtained were accurate.

________		Earned	ADD POINTS OF TASKS CHECKED
	130	Points	TOTAL POINTS POSSIBLE
________		SCORE	DETERMINE SCORE (divide points earned by total points possible, multiply results by 100)

SKILLS COMPETENCY ASSESSMENT — continued

Procedure 16–5: Preparing, Sending, and Receiving a Fax

Actual Student Time Needed to Complete Procedure: ____________

Student's Initials: ____________ Instructor's Initials: ____________ Grade: _____________

Suggestions for Improvement: ____

____

____

____

Evaluator's Name (print) ____

Evaluator's Signature ____

Comments ____

EVALUATION OF CHAPTER KNOWLEDGE

How has your instructor evaluated the knowledge you have achieved?

Knowledge	Instructor Evaluation *Good*	*Average*	*Poor*
Understands the importance of written correspondence in the professional health care setting	_____	_____	_____
Understands the four basic types of letters medical assistants usually write and how to compose them	_____	_____	_____
Correctly spells difficult and commonly misspelled and misused words	_____	_____	_____
Uses medical terminology appropriately	_____	_____	_____
Frequently consults standard and medical dictionaries and references when writing	_____	_____	_____
Understands and can apply proofreader's marks	_____	_____	_____
Understands the components of business letters, (e.g., date line, salutation, body of letter, reference initials, postscripts, etc.)	_____	_____	_____
Can identify and use supplies for written communications	_____	_____	_____
Can accurately process incoming and outgoing mail and packages according to U.S. postal regulations	_____	_____	_____
Understands how to use new technologies designed for written communications (i.e., facsimile machines, modems)	_____	_____	_____
Comprehends the importance of medical transcription	_____	_____	_____
Is able to recall the basic tools of medical transcription	_____	_____	_____
Is sensitive to bias in language and can develop strategies for bias-free writing	_____	_____	_____
Applies computer concepts to office procedures	_____	_____	_____
Adapts communication to individuals' abilities to understand	_____	_____	_____

Student's Initials: ______ Instructor's Initials: ______

Grade: _______

CHAPTER 17

Daily Financial Practices

PERFORMANCE OBJECTIVES

Ambulatory care settings depend on sound financial practices to thrive, grow, and continue to provide good patient care. To that end, medical assistants should strive to understand basic accounting and bookkeeping terms, forms, principles, and both manual and computerized systems related to these financial activities. Medical assistants should be prepared to handle a variety of financial tasks, including procedures related to accounts receivable, accounts payable, patient billing, banking, checkbook, purchasing, and petty cash systems.

EXERCISES AND ACTIVITIES

Vocabulary Builder

Complete the vocabulary exercises by identifying the correct key term for each from the list that follows.

Accounts payable	Credit	Petty cash
Accounts receivable	Currency	Petty cash voucher
Adjustment	Day sheet	Posting
Balance	Disbursement	ROA
Charge	Ledger card	Superbill
Charge slip	Pegboard system	Write-it-once system

A. Identify the following financial forms used in the ambulatory care setting.

________________________ (1) Records individual cash transactions for minor or unexpected expenses.

________________________ (2) Records charges, payments, and adjustments for individual patients and/or family members.

______________________ (3) A form that records daily patient transactions, used in conjunction with pegboard systems.

______________________ (4) Records services supplied and the charges and payments for those services; functions as a billing form for insurance reimbursement.

B. Identify the correct financial term or function for each definition.

______________________ (1) The most commonly used manual medical accounts receivable system.

______________________ (2) Small cash sum kept on hand in the office for minor or unexpected expenses.

______________________ (3) Abbreviation for received on account.

______________________ (4) Decreases the balance due.

______________________ (5) The fee for services recorded; it increases the balance due.

______________________ (6) A term for paper money.

______________________ (7) A synonym for *charge slip.*

______________________ (8) This accounting function assigns general ledger account information to a financial transaction.

______________________ (9) As a noun, this term denotes "the amount owed"; as a verb, the term means "to verify posting accuracy."

______________________ (10) This accounting function describes the act of recording financial transactions into bookkeeping or accounting systems.

______________________ (11) An increase or decrease to a patient account not due to charges incurred or payments received.

______________________ (12) This accounting system consists of day sheets, ledger cards, charge slips, and receipt forms. All forms have matching columns that align and are held in place when the system is in use.

______________________ (13) This is the sum owed by a business for services or goods received.

______________________ (14) This is the sum owed to a business for services or goods supplied.

Learning Review

1. A. The checking account is the account most often used by medical assistants in the ambulatory care setting. Checking accounts are accounts that allow depositors to write checks against money placed in the account. What are seven features that may be offered to checking account holders?

(1) ______________________ (3) ______________________

(2) ______________________ (4) ______________________

(5) ______________________ (7) ______________________

(6) ______________________

B. Administrative medical assistant Karen Ritter is responsible for assisting the office manager and accountant in performing accounts payable activities for Inner City Health Care. On September 4, she receives a $323.45 bill from RJ Medical Supply Company for blood pressure equipment the office received on August 30. Noting that the company demands payment within 30 days of billing, Karen writes a check disbursing funds to the company on September 15. The balance in the office's checking account before this check is written equals $2,610.00. Using this information, write out the check and stub below. Karen will submit the check to Susan Rice, M. D., for her signature.

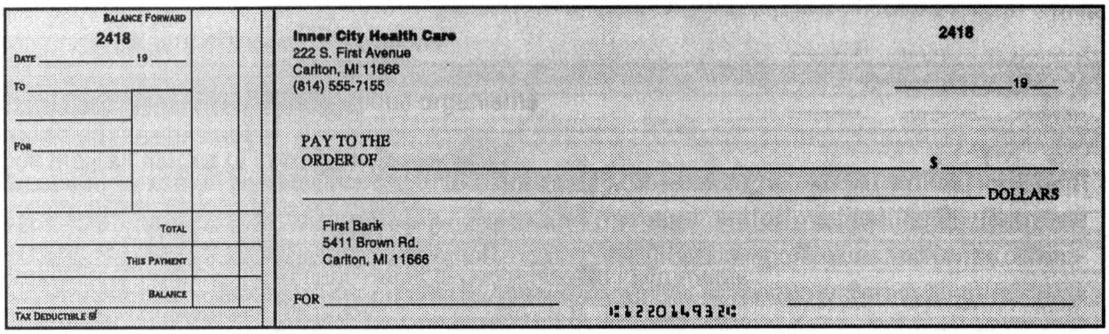
BALANCE FORWARD
2418
DATE ______ 19 ____
TO ______
FOR ______
TOTAL
THIS PAYMENT
BALANCE
TAX DEDUCTIBLE ☐

Inner City Health Care
222 S. First Avenue
Carlton, MI 11666
(814) 555-7155

2418

______ 19 ____

PAY TO THE ORDER OF ______ $ ______

______ DOLLARS

First Bank
5411 Brown Rd.
Carlton, MI 11666

FOR ______

⑆1220114932⑆

C. What are five rules to ensure that checks are properly written and recorded?

(1) ______________________

(2) ______________________

(3) ______________________

(4) ______________________

(5) ______________________

2. A. The first rule of purchasing: Nothing is ordered or paid for without a purchase order or purchase order number. Give four reasons why it is important to ensure proper control over purchasing supplies and equipment.

(1) ______________________

(2) ______________________

(3) ______________________

(4) ______________________

B. Office manager Walter Seals, CMA, is responsible for purchasing office supplies for Inner City Health Care. On September 10, Walter completes purchase order #1743 for supplies ordered from Mayflower Supply, requested by administrative medical assistant Karen Ritter. The items are taxed at 8 percent, and the shipping fee is prepaid. The items are billed and shipped to Inner City Health Care; the terms are net due 30 days. Complete the purchase order form.

Inner City Health Care
222 S. First Avenue
Carlton, MI 11666
(814) 555-7155

Mayflower Supply, Inc.
642 East 65th Street
Carlton, MI 11623
(814) 555-9999

2 boxes of fax paper, #62145, at $8.99 a box
5 day-view desk calendars, #24598, at $4.25 each
4 cases of copier paper, #72148, at $20.00 a box
5 boxes of highlighter pens, 12 to a box, #26773, at $3.98 a box
4 computer printer cartridges, #96187, at $49.99 each

PURCHASE ORDER

NO. ____

Bill To:	Ship To:	Vendor:

REQ BY	BUYER	TERMS

QTY	ITEM	UNITS	DESCRIPTION	UNIT PR	TOTAL
				SUBTOTAL	
				TAX	
				FREIGHT	
				BAL DUE	

C. When the office supplies ordered from Mayflower Supply arrive, what should be done to verify that the correct items and quantities are received? What should be done to prepare the invoice from Mayflower Supply for payment?

____

____

____

____

____

____

3. Describe the following types of checks, which are different from checks issued from a standard business checking account.
   (1) Cashier's check ______________________________

   ____

   (2) Certified check ______________________________

   ____

   (3) Money order ______________________________

   ____

   (4) Voucher check ______________________________

   ____

   (5) Traveler's check ______________________________

   ____

4. A. Ledger cards maintain a permanent record of services provided and charges, adjustments, and payments made for each patient who is seen by the medical practice. Ledger cards may be prepared manually or on a computerized system. Consult the computerized patient ledger card for Mary O'Keefe, reproduced below. Transfer all relevant information to the manual ledger card, correctly entering all charges, adjustments, payments, and other information for Mary O'Keefe.

PATIENT LEDGER

Patient #218 | O'KEEFE, MARY | 43 KINGSBORO AVENUE | NORTHBOROUGH, OH 12345 | Date: 06/24/-- | PHONE: (404) 555-6123

Insured #1: SAME

Insured #2: O'KEEFE, JOHN | 43 KINGSBORO AVENUE | NORTHBOROUGH, OH 12345

Insurance #1: PRUDENTIAL | Policy #: 987654321 | Group #: 987700

Insurance #2: BLUE CROSS | Policy #: 321654907 | Group #: 123456987

01/26/--	59400	TOTAL OBSTETRICAL CARE	2000.00
01/26/--	99202	INTERMEDIATE EXAM, NEW PT.	75.00
01/26/--	88150	PAPANICOLAOU SMEAR	25.00
01/26/--	PMT	DEPOSIT OB CARE	-250.00
02/18/--	PMT	Insur. Pmt. 01/26/-- 90015	-20.00
02/18/--	ADJ	Adj. Cat. #1 01/26/-- 90015	-10.00
02/25/--	85022	CBC	12.50
02/25/--	99212	LIMITED EXAM, ESTAB. PT.	42.00
02/25/--	PMT	Cash Pmt. 01/26/-- 94000	-75.00
04/26/--	85022	CBC	12.50
04/26/--	99212	LIMITED EXAM, ESTAB. PT.	42.00
04/26/--	76805	DIAGNOSTIC ULTRASOUND	82.00
04/26/--	88150	PAPANICOLAOU SMEAR	25.00
		Balance for MARY O'KEEFE	$1,961.00

STATEMENT

L&K LEWIS & KING, MD
2501 CENTER STREET
NORTHBOROUGH, OH 12345

DATE	REFERENCE	DESCRIPTION	CHARGES	CREDITS	BALANCE
	BALANCE FORWARD →				

RB40BC-2

PLEASE PAY LAST AMOUNT IN BALANCE COLUMN

THIS IS A COPY OF YOUR ACCOUNT AS IT APPEARS ON OUR RECORDS

B. Adjustments are entries made to a patient's account that do not represent charges or payment. Name three reasons why adjustments may sometimes be made to a patient's account.

(1) ______________________________

(2) ______________________________

(3) ______________________________

5. Identify two work guidelines and six habits essential to creating and maintaining accurate financial records:

A. Guidelines:

(1) ______________________________

(2) ______________________________

B. Good work habits:

(1) ______________________________

(2) ______________________________

(3) ______________________________

(4) ______________________________

(5) ______________________________

(6) ______________________________

6. Examine the sample bank statement that follows and answer the following questions.

______________ A. How many checks are not listed on the bank statement?

______________ B. What is the total amount of these outstanding checks?

______________ C. According to the bank statement, when was the last deposit made?

______________ D. What was the amount of the last deposit?

______________ E. According to the worksheet, what is the total of the deposits not listed on the bank statement?

______________ F. What are the fees the bank charged this month?

Summary of Account Balance — Closing Date 1/15/95

Account # 1257-164013 — Ending Balance $8,347.62

Beginning Balance	$7,152.18
Total Deposits and Additions	$8,643.86
Total Withdrawals	$7,433.21
Service Charge	$ 15.24

Number	Date	Amount	Number	Date	Amount
201	12/18/94	173.82	234	1/4/95	96.31
223*	12/18/94	44.12	235	1/4/95	73.48
224	12/20/94	586.00	236	1/6/95	325.40
225	12/21/94	24.15	237	1/7/95	40.00
226	12/22/94	33.90	238	1/8/95	66.77
228*	12/23/94	1250.00	241*	1/9/95	15.55
229	12/24/94	11.75	242	1/10/95	12.45
230	12/24/94	19.02	243	1/10/95	4441.64
231	1/2/95	43.80	244	1/10/95	64.55
232	1/3/95	39.00			
233	1/4/95	71.50			

*Denotes gap in check sequence

Date	Deposit Amount	Date	Deposit Amount
18-Dec	361.75	4-Jan	825.00
19-Dec	586.00	5-Jan	1286.71
20-Dec	918.21	7-Jan	608.00
21-Dec	201.00	8-Jan	811.15
2-Jan	475.00	9-Jan	1092.68
3-Jan	1478.36		

Front

1. Enter Ending Balance from the front of this statement
$ 8,347.62

2. Enter deposits not shown on this statement
$ 3,162.50

3. Subtotal (add 1 & 2)
$ 11,510.12

4. List outstanding checks or other withdrawals here

Check #	Amount
222	37.89
227	161.15
239	11.50
240	92.12
245	835.17
246	21.75
247	586.00

5. Total outstanding checks
$ 1,745.58

Balance (subtract #5 from #3)
$ 9,764.54

This should equal your checkbook balance

Back

7. A. Deposits are generally made daily. All checks to be deposited must be endorsed. Define *endorsement*. Identify three methods of endorsing checks and give the benefits or potential disadvantages of each.

____

____

____

B. Checks received from patients and others must be inspected before preparing the checks for deposit. What guidelines should medical assistants follow in accepting and inspecting checks?

____

____

If a check is returned to the ambulatory care setting for insufficient funds, what procedures should be followed?

____

____

8. It is crucial to balance all financial information for each day and for the month's end. Month-end figures on the day sheet must agree with the patient ledgers. Why is it important to go through this time-consuming accounting process?

____

____

____

9. Office manager Marilyn Johnson, CMA, is responsible for managing a variety of accounts payable and accounts receivable duties for the offices of Drs. Lewis and King. Consider the following financial tasks Marilyn performs in the course of a typical week and indicate which ones are accounts payable (AP) functions and which ones are accounts receivable (AR) functions.

_____ A. Prepares a purchase order for pharmaceutical supplies.

_____ B. Lists the check numbers, patient names, and check amounts on a bank deposit slip.

_____ C. Writes a check to the American Medical Association to renew the office's subscription to its journal.

_____ D. Generates a petty cash voucher to document the purchase of coffee and pastry for an office open house.

_____ E. Completes a charge slip detailing procedures and fees for patient Martin Gordon's follow-up examination to check on his treatment progress with chemotherapy for prostate cancer.

_____ F. Completes a registration form and writes a check to Harvard University for Dr. King to attend a weekend medical seminar.

Investigation Activity

Medical assistants are often responsible for performing many financial duties within the ambulatory care setting. Also, medical assistants often interface with the medical practice's bank and banking personnel. To better understand the various services and policies available, choose three student volunteers to visit three different banking establishments in your community. With the financial needs of an ambulatory care setting in mind, the student volunteers will investigate these banks' checking and savings account features, policies, fees, and any special services that might be helpful in managing a medical facility's financial activities. Student volunteers will gather relevant literature and brochures about policies provided by each bank and will bring those materials to class. If possible, the student volunteers may set up an appointment with a bank representative, explaining in advance that the appointment is for the purpose of class research. Student volunteers will then report their findings to the class.

As a class, compare the services and features offered by each bank, citing specific advantages and/or disadvantages. Consider the following questions as well. How convenient is each bank? What are the banking hours and locations? Can depositors establish personal banking representatives to manage their accounts within the bank? Compile a class list of the banking services and features considered most important for the needs of the ambulatory care setting.

CASE STUDY

Suzanne Berry is a new patient at the offices of Drs. Lewis & King in the Northborough Family Medical Group. Suzanne is a single mother of two small children. Suzanne and her children are covered by medical insurance through her employer. The policy covers 80 percent of the usual, reasonable, and customary fees for the family's medical expenses after a $100 per person deductible, which the Berrys have already reached from expenses incurred with the family's previous health care provider. Northborough Family Medical Group requires that patients pay for services not covered by insurance at the time of treatment. The office also charges for all scheduled office visits, unless the patient provides a 24-hour notice of cancellation. The practice accepts personal checks, major credit cards, and under special circumstances, installment payments.

Discuss the following:

1. Take the role of office manager Marilyn Johnson, who meets with Suzanne during her first office visit and explain the practice's policies regarding patient fees and financial obligations.
2. Suzanne asks Marilyn to clarify what she means by "usual, reasonable, and customary fees." Explain.
3. Suzanne tells Marilyn she is interested in the option of charging some larger medical fees to her credit card. What should Marilyn explain to Suzanne about the use of credit cards in the ambulatory care setting?

SUPPLEMENTARY RESOURCES

Study Guide Disk: Additional practice exercises for this chapter are available on the study guide disk found in the back of the textbook.

Medical Assisting Videos: Appropriate content is available on Delmar's Medical Assisting Videos, 2nd ed., for the following topics:

Tape 3	Use Manual Bookkeeping System
	Billing Cycle and Collections
	Electronic Banking
Tape 4	Charge Slip

SKILLS COMPETENCY ASSESSMENT

Procedure 17–1: Preparation for Posting a Day Sheet

Student's Name: ______________________________ Date: __________

Objective: To ensure that the individual in charge of recording patient transactions is organized and prepared *before* patients arrive.

Conditions: The student demonstrates the ability to record patient transactions using the following equipment and supplies: pegboard, new charge slips and receipt forms, new day sheet, and ledger cards of patients scheduled for the day.

Time Requirements and Accuracy Standards: 30 minutes. Points assigned reflect importance of step to meeting objective: Important = (5) Essential = (10) Critical = (15). Automatic failure results if any of the **critical** tasks are omitted or performed incorrectly.

SKILLS ASSESSMENT CHECKLIST

Task Performed	Possible Points	TASKS
❑	10	Places a new day sheet and strip of charge slips on the pegboard.
❑	10	Fills in information at the top of the day sheet (date and page number).
❑	15	Carefully enters forwarded balances in Section 4, "Previous Page" columns A–D, and the "Previous Day's Total" and "Accts. Rec. 1st of Month" in the Accounts Receivable Control and Accounts Receivable Proof boxes.
❑	15	Pulls ledger cards from the storage file for all scheduled patients and keeps them available in the order in which the patients will be seen.
❑	5	Keeps a strip of receipt forms on hand in case someone comes into the office to make payment on account.
❑	5	Completed the tasks within 30 minutes.
❑	15	Results obtained were accurate.

______	Earned	ADD POINTS OF TASKS CHECKED
75	Points	TOTAL POINTS POSSIBLE
______	SCORE	DETERMINE SCORE (divide points earned by total points possible, multiply results by 100)

Actual Student Time Needed to Complete Procedure: __________

Student's Initials: __________ Instructor's Initials: __________ Grade: __________

Suggestions for Improvement: ______________________________

Evaluator's Name (print) ______________________________

Evaluator's Signature ______________________________

Comments ______________________________

SKILLS COMPETENCY ASSESSMENT

Procedure 17–2: Recording Charges and Payments Requiring a Charge Slip (Patient Visits)

Student's Name: ______________________________ Date: __________

Objective: To record information pertaining to a patient's visit to the physician on the patient's ledger and the day sheet and to provide a charge slip for insurance billing.

Conditions: The student demonstrates the ability to record patient information using a patient ledger card and day sheet and to generate an insurance bill using a charge slip.

Time Requirements and Accuracy Standards: 10 minutes. Points assigned reflect importance of step to meeting objective: Important = (5) Essential = (10) Critical = (15). Automatic failure results if any of the **critical** tasks are omitted or performed incorrectly.

SKILLS ASSESSMENT CHECKLIST

Task Performed	Possible Points	TASKS
		When a patient comes in for an appointment
❑	10	Lines up the patient's ledger under the next charge slip and turns back the first two pages of the slip.
❑	10	Writes the date, name of patient, and name of responsible party.
❑	10	Writes any previous balance on the charge slip.
❑	15	Removes the charge slip from the pegboard and clips it to the front of the patient's chart to be given to the physician.
		When the patient returns the form to the front desk
❑	15	Enters the charge next to each procedure and writes in the total on the front of the slip.
❑	15	Replaces the charge slip on the pegboard, carefully lining it up with the patient's name on the day sheet, and correctly inserts the ledger card under the last page of the charge slip.
❑	15	Turns back the first two pages for the charge slip and enters the total charge and any patient payments in the correct columns.
❑	15	Arrives at the final balance by looking at the column on the day sheet that shows the previous balance, adding the day's charges and subtracting payments made.
		If the day sheet has additional columns to the right of the charge slip
❑	5	Records receipt number, if appropriate.
❑	5	Records method of payment.

Task Performed	Possible Points	TASKS
❑	15	Applies business analysis as outlined by office procedures.
		To complete the procedure
❑	15	Completes the posting of each transaction all the way to the far right and on the same line of the day sheet as instructed by office procedure.
❑	10	Keeps first copy of charge slip for filing in patient's chart and gives other copies to patient: one for the patient's personal records and one for submission for insurance reimbursement.
❑	5	Completed the tasks within 10 minutes.
❑	15	Results obtained were accurate.
	______	Earned ADD POINTS OF TASKS CHECKED
	175	Points TOTAL POINTS POSSIBLE
	______	SCORE DETERMINE SCORE (divide points earned by total points possible, multiply results by 100)

Actual Student Time Needed to Complete Procedure: ____________

Student's Initials: ____________ Instructor's Initials: ____________ Grade: ____________

Suggestions for Improvement: ______________________________

____

____

____

Evaluator's Name (print) ______________________________

Evaluator's Signature ______________________________

Comments ______________________________

SKILLS COMPETENCY ASSESSMENT

Procedure 17–3: Receiving a Payment on Account Requiring a Receipt

Student's Name: ______________________________ Date: __________

Objective: To record a payment on the day sheet and patient's ledger card and to provide a receipt to the patient.

Conditions: Student demonstrates the ability to record a payment and provide receipts to patients using a day sheet, patient ledger card, and new receipt form.

Time Requirements and Accuracy Standards: 5 minutes. Points assigned reflect importance of step to meeting objective: Important = (5) Essential = (10) Critical = (15). Automatic failure results if any of the **critical** tasks are omitted or performed incorrectly.

SKILLS ASSESSMENT CHECKLIST

Task Performed	Possible Points	TASKS
		When someone comes into the office to make a payment
❑	5	Places receipt forms on the pegboard in place of the charge slips.
❑	10	Pulls the patient's ledger and places it under the receipt form with the first blank line of the ledger under the carbon strip.
❑	15	Enters the following information on the top of the receipt: date, reference, description, payment, amount, and previous balance.
❑	10	Calculates the new balance by subtracting the payment amount from the previous balance.
❑	5	Gives the receipt to the person making the payment.
❑	5	*Rationale:* Can state reason why no copy of the receipt is needed for the office.
❑	5	Completed the tasks within 5 minutes.
❑	15	Results obtained were accurate.

_______	Earned	ADD POINTS OF TASKS CHECKED
70	Points	TOTAL POINTS POSSIBLE
_______	SCORE	DETERMINE SCORE (divide points earned by total points possible, multiply results by 100)

Actual Student Time Needed to Complete Procedure: __________

Student's Initials: __________ Instructor's Initials: __________ Grade: __________

Suggestions for Improvement: ______________________________

Evaluator's Name (print) ______________________________

Evaluator's Signature ______________________________

Comments ______________________________

SKILLS COMPETENCY ASSESSMENT

Procedure 17–4: Recording Payments Received Through the Mail

Student's Name: ______________________________ Date: ____________

Objective: To record payments received in the mail on the day sheet and patient ledger card, including payments received from patients and from insurance companies on patients' behalf.

Conditions: The student demonstrates the ability to record patient and insurance payments received in the mail using the day sheet and patient ledger cards.

Time requirements and accuracy standards: 5 minutes. Points assigned reflect importance of step to meeting objective: Important = (5) Essential = (10) Critical = (15). Automatic failure results if any of the **critical** tasks are omitted or performed incorrectly.

SKILLS ASSESSMENT CHECKLIST

Task Performed	Possible Points	TASKS
		If a patient mails in a payment or if a payment is sent by an insurance company
☐	15	Pulls the appropriate ledger card and places it directly on the day sheet.
☐	10	Temporarily removes the strip of charge slips from the pegboard.
☐	10	Enters the patient's previous balance on the day sheet (ledger card does not extend to this column).
☐	15	Posts directly onto the ledger card the date, reference (patient name), description (ROA or ROA ins), and payment amount.
☐	10	Calculates the new balance by subtracting the payment amount from the previous balance.
☐	5	Completed the tasks within 5 minutes.
☐	15	Results obtained were accurate.

________	Earned	ADD POINTS OF TASKS CHECKED
80	Points	TOTAL POINTS POSSIBLE
________	SCORE	DETERMINE SCORE (divide points earned by total points possible, multiply results by 100)

Actual Student Time Needed to Complete Procedure: ____________

Student's Initials: ____________ Instructor's Initials: ____________ Grade: ____________

Suggestions for Improvement: ______________________________

Evaluator's Name (print) ______________________________

Evaluator's Signature ______________________________

Comments ______________________________

SKILLS COMPETENCY ASSESSMENT

Procedure 17–5: Balancing Day Sheets

Student's Name: ______________________________ Date: __________

Objective: To verify that all entries to the day sheet are correct and that the totals balance.

Conditions: The student demonstrates the ability to verify day sheet entries and confirm that totals are in balance using the following equipment and supplies: day sheet and calculator.

Time Requirements and Accuracy Standards: 30 minutes. Points assigned reflect importance of step to meeting objective: Important = (5) Essential = (10) Critical = (15). Automatic failure results if any of the **critical** tasks are omitted or performed incorrectly.

SKILLS ASSESSMENT CHECKLIST

Task Performed	Possible Points	TASKS
		Column totals
❑	10	Totals columns A, B1, B2, C, and D and enters the total for each column in the boxes marked "Totals This Page."
❑	10	Adds column totals to the figures entered in the "Previous Page" column boxes to arrive at the "Month to Date" totals.
		Proof of posting (all figures are taken from the "Totals This Page" column boxes)
❑	10	Enters today's column D total which shows the sum of all the previous balances entered when the transactions were posted.
❑	15	Enters column A total and adds column A and D totals to arrive at subtotal.
❑	15	Adds columns B1 and B2 to arrive at sum for total credits for the day. Enters total in space provided for "Less Cols. B1 and B2." Subtracts the total of credits from the subtotal listed in the previous box.
❑	15	Verifies that result equals the amount in column C to indicate that transactions are balanced.
❑	5	*Rationale:* Can state the posting process from an individual transaction to achieving a new balance.
		Accounts Receivable (A/R) Control
❑	10	Carries column A and column B totals from the "Proof of Posting" box to the corresponding spaces in the "A/R Control" box.
❑	10	Adds the amount already entered in the "Previous Day's Total" space to the column A amount to arrive at subtotal.
❑	10	Subtracts the amount carried over from the "Less Cols. B1 and B2" box to find the new "Accounts Receivable" amount.
		Accounts Receivable Proof
❑	5	Enters the "Accounts Receivable" amount from the first working day of the month.
❑	5	Enters the column A "Month-to-Date" total where shown.

Task Performed	Possible Points	TASKS
❑	10	Adds the column A amount to the "Accounts Receivable" amount from the first of the month and enters sum in the subtotal space.
❑	10	Enters the sum of column B1 and B2 month-to-date amounts in the space provided and subtracts this sum from the subtotal. Enters amount in the "Total Accounts Receivable" space.
❑	15	Verifies that the total "Accounts Receivable" amounts in the "A/R Control" and "A/R Proof" boxes match to confirm that posting is correct and the day is balanced.
		Deposit verification
❑	15	Totals the columns in Section 2 of the day sheet and enters the sum of the columns in the space marked "Total Deposit."
❑	15	Verifies that the "Total Deposit" and the total of payments received from column B1 are equal.
		Business analysis summary
❑	5	Totals each column in the summary section.
❑	10	If the summary is used to break out charges by type or by physician, verifies that the sum of the column equals the day's column A total.
❑	10	If the summary is used to credit payments to different physicians, verifies that the sum of the columns equals the day's payment column.
		To transfer balances after the day sheet is balanced
❑	5	Takes out a new day sheet for the next day.
❑	10	Transfers the "Month-to-Date" column totals to the "Previous Page" column boxes on the new sheet.
❑	10	Enters the "Total Accounts Receivable" amount from the last day sheet in the "Previous Day's Total" space of the "A/R Control" box on the new day sheet.
❑	10	Enters the "Accounts Receivable 1st of Month" amount in the "A/R Proof" box on the new sheet.
❑	5	Completed the tasks within 30 minutes.
❑	15	Results obtained were accurate.

______	Earned	ADD POINTS OF TASKS CHECKED
265	Points	TOTAL POINTS POSSIBLE
______	SCORE	DETERMINE SCORE (divide points earned by total points possible, multiply results by 100)

Actual Student Time Needed to Complete Procedure: ____________

Student's Initials: ____________ Instructor's Initials: ____________ Grade: ____________

Suggestions for Improvement: ______________________________

Evaluator's Name (print) ______________________________

Evaluator's Signature ______________________________

Comments ______________________________

SKILLS COMPETENCY ASSESSMENT

Procedure 17–6: Preparing a Deposit

Student's Name: ______________________________ Date: __________

Objective: To create a deposit slip for the day's receipts.

Conditions: The student demonstrates the ability to create a deposit slip using a deposit slip, check endorsement stamp, calculator, and the cash and checks received for the day.

Time Requirements and Accuracy Standards: 30 minutes. Points assigned reflect importance of step to meeting objective: Important = (5) Essential = (10) Critical = (15). Automatic failure results if any of the **critical** tasks are omitted or performed incorrectly.

SKILLS ASSESSMENT CHECKLIST

Task Performed	Possible Points	TASKS
❑	5	Separates all checks from currency.
❑	10	Counts all currency to be deposited, gathering the bills in order (i.e., fifties, twenties, tens, fives, ones), and enters the amount in the space provided.
❑	10	Counts all coins to be deposited and enters amount. Wraps coins if required.
❑	5	Lists each check separately on the back of the deposit slip, including patient name in left-hand column and amount of check in right-hand column.
❑	5	Totals checks listed and copies total on front of deposit slip where indicated.
❑	15	Verifies that sum of currency, coins, and checks equals the total in the "Payments" column on that day's day sheet.
❑	10	Attaches the top copy of the deposit slip to the deposit, leaving the carbon on pad.
❑	5	Enters the date and amount of the deposit in the space provided on the checkbook stub.
❑	5	Adds the amount of the deposit to the checkbook balance.
❑	15	Deposits at the bank and receives record of deposit.
❑	5	*Rationale:* Can provide reasoning for safest method of depositing checks and currency.
❑	5	Completed the tasks within 30 minutes.
❑	15	Results obtained were accurate.

______	Earned	ADD POINTS OF TASKS CHECKED
105	Points	TOTAL POINTS POSSIBLE
______	SCORE	DETERMINE SCORE (divide points earned by total points possible, multiply results by 100)

Actual Student Time Needed to Complete Procedure: __________

Student's Initials: __________ Instructor's Initials: __________ Grade: __________

Suggestions for Improvement: ______________________________

Evaluator's Name (print) ______________________________

Evaluator's Signature ______________________________

Comments ______________________________

SKILLS COMPETENCY ASSESSMENT

Procedure 17–7: Reconciling a Bank Statement

Student's Name: ______________________ Date: __________

Objective: To verify that the balance listed in the checkbook agrees with the balance shown by the bank.

Conditions: The student demonstrates the ability to reconcile a bank statement using a checkbook, bank statement, and calculator.

Time Requirements and Accuracy Standards: 30 minutes. Points assigned reflect importance of step to meeting objective: Important = (5) Essential = (10) Critical = (15). Automatic failure results if any of the **critical** tasks are omitted or performed incorrectly.

SKILLS ASSESSMENT CHECKLIST

Task Performed	Possible Points	TASKS
❑	10	Checks that the balance in the checkbook is current.
❑	5	Subtracts any service charge listed on the statement from the last balance listed in the checkbook.
❑	5	In the checkbook, checks off each check listed on the statement and verifies the amount against the check stub.
❑	5	In the checkbook, checks off each deposit listed on the statement.
❑	10	Copies ending balance listed on the front of the bank statement in the space indicated on the worksheet found on the reverse side of the statement.
❑	10	Using the check stubs, finds any checks and deposits not listed on the bank statement and lists them on the bank statement worksheet.
❑	10	Totals the checks not cleared on the bank statement worksheet.
❑	10	Totals the deposits not credited on the worksheet.
❑	10	Adds together the statement balance and the total of deposits not credited.
❑	10	Subtracts the total of checks not cleared.
❑	15	Verifies that this amount agrees with the balance in the checkbook.
❑	5	If checkbook balances, files statement in appropriate place.
❑	5	Completed the tasks within 30 minutes.
❑	15	Results obtained were accurate.

______	Earned	ADD POINTS OF TASKS CHECKED
125	Points	TOTAL POINTS POSSIBLE
______	SCORE	DETERMINE SCORE (divide points earned by total points possible, multiply results by 100)

SKILLS COMPETENCY ASSESSMENT — continued

Procedure 17–7: Reconciling a Bank Statement

Actual Student Time Needed to Complete Procedure: ____________

Student's Initials: ____________ Instructor's Initials: ____________ Grade: ____________

Suggestions for Improvement: ____

____

____

____

Evaluator's Name (print) ____

Evaluator's Signature ____

Comments ____

SKILLS COMPETENCY ASSESSMENT

Procedure 17–8: Balancing Petty Cash

Student's Name: ______________________________ Date: ____________

Objective: To verify that the amount of petty cash is consistent with the beginning amount, less expenditures shown on receipts.

Conditions: The student demonstrates the ability to balance the petty cash amount using petty cash box, vouchers, and calculator.

Time Requirements and Accuracy Standards: 15 minutes. Points assigned reflect importance of step to meeting objective: Important = (5) Essential = (10) Critical = (15). Automatic failure results if any of the **critical** tasks are omitted or performed incorrectly.

SKILLS ASSESSMENT CHECKLIST

Task Performed	Possible Points	TASKS
❑	5	Counts the money remaining in the petty cash box.
❑	5	Totals amounts of all vouchers in the petty cash box.
❑	10	Subtracts the amount of receipts from the original amounts in petty cash. This amount should equal the amount of cash remaining in the box.
❑	15	After balancing, writes check only for the amount that was used, bringing petty cash back up to the original amount.
		For petty cash check disbursement
❑	5	Sorts all vouchers by account.
❑	10	Lists accounts involved on a sheet of paper.
❑	15	Totals vouchers for each account and records individual totals on the list.
❑	10	Copies this list with its totals on the "Memo" portion of the stub for the check written to replenish petty cash.
❑	10	Files the list with the vouchers and receipts attached, after noting the check number on the list.
❑	5	Completed the tasks within 15 minutes.
❑	15	Results obtained were accurate.

________	Earned	ADD POINTS OF TASKS CHECKED
105	Points	TOTAL POINTS POSSIBLE
________	SCORE	DETERMINE SCORE (divide points earned by total points possible, multiply results by 100)

Actual Student Time Needed to Complete Procedure: ____________

Student's Initials: ____________ Instructor's Initials: ____________ Grade: ____________

Suggestions for Improvement: ______________________________

____

Evaluator's Name (print) ____________________ Evaluator's Signature____________________

Comments ______________________________

EVALUATION OF CHAPTER KNOWLEDGE

How has your instructor evaluated the knowledge you have gained?

	Instructor Evaluation		
Knowledge	*Good*	*Average*	*Poor*
Defines key vocabulary terms	_____	_____	_____
Demonstrates understanding of procedures, policies, and services	_____	_____	_____
Understands importance of informing patients of the office's financial policies and procedures	_____	_____	_____
Documents various financial forms correctly	_____	_____	_____
Understands documentation and reporting needs	_____	_____	_____
Able to use manual bookkeeping systems	_____	_____	_____
Applies computer concepts to computerized accounting systems	_____	_____	_____
Demonstrates ability to manage accounts receivable	_____	_____	_____
Demonstrates ability to manage accounts payable	_____	_____	_____
Able to establish, track, balance, and replenish a petty cash fund	_____	_____	_____
Displays ability to write and record checks and reconcile accounts	_____	_____	_____
Demonstrates understanding of purchasing procedures and ability to prepare purchase orders	_____	_____	_____

Student's Initials: ______ Instructor's Initials: ______

Grade: _______

CHAPTER 18

Medical Insurance and Coding

PERFORMANCE OBJECTIVES

With the growing influence of managed care, many traditional insurance carriers, such as Blue Cross and Blue Shield are joining HMOs and other managed care options in transforming the health care insurance industry. While managed care coverage has simplified the patient's responsibility for payment in some ways, medical assistants have the responsibility to be accurate, timely, and conscientious both in filing insurance claim forms and in understanding the conditions of individual insurance policies. Medical assisting students can use this workbook chapter to explore the role of insurance, learn insurance terminology, and apply accurate insurance coding of diagnosis and procedure codes. Students also discover the medical assistant's important role as a patient educator, helping patients understand the terms and conditions of their health insurance policies.

EXERCISES AND ACTIVITIES

Vocabulary Builder

Across

1. The 40-mile radius of a military base where medical care is available to military dependents.
2. Basis for the Medicare Fee Schedule.
4. The use of the number of members enrolled in a plan to determine the salary of the physician.
7. Those procedures not necessary for the health of the patient are considered__________.
8. The person covered under the terms of the policy.
9. The national administrator of Medicare.
11. When children of undivorced parents are covered under both parents' policies, often this method is used to determine which policy is primary.
13. A classification of patients into categories based on primary diagnosis, procedure, and discharge status.
16. That percentage paid by the company or that paid by the insured.
18. Payment made directly to the physician by the insurance company.

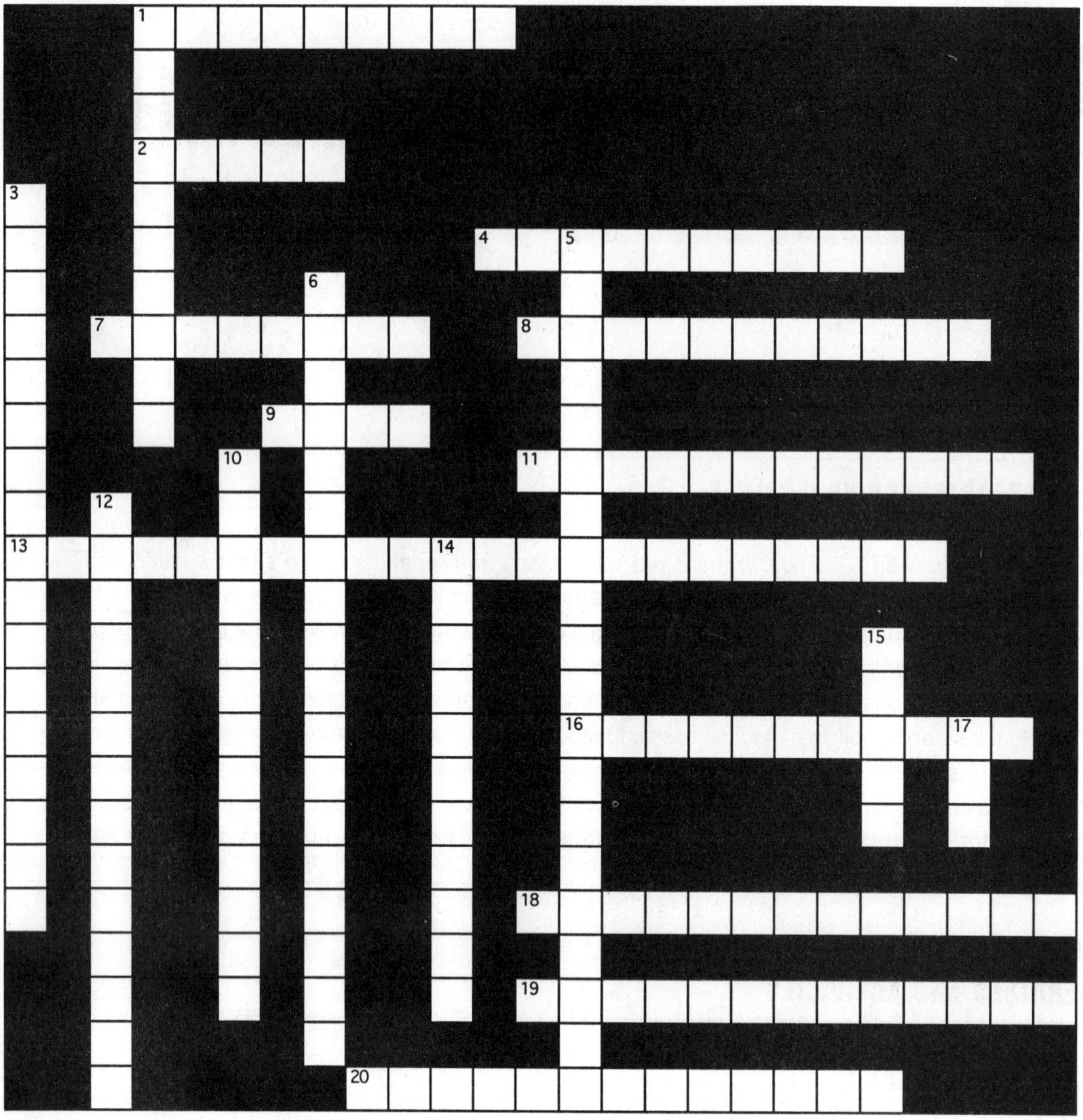

19. The numerical designation for a specific illness, injury, or disease.
20. The length of time defined in the insurance policy before the policy will begin to pay benefits for a pre-existing condition.

Down

1. In some offices, these are referred to as superbills.
3. A physician who has signed a contract with a particular insurance carrier or HMO to provide care for a reduced rate in exchange for direct payment from the insurer.
5. An illness, disease, or injury that occurred before the inception of the policy.
6. The local administrator for Medicare.
10. A numerical code signifying a specific medical procedure.
12. Medical insurance that covers most physician fees, hospital expenses, and surgical fees according to the terms of the policy.

14. An insurance report that is sent with claim payments explaining the reimbursement of the insurance carrier is called an ____________ of benefits.
15. A demand by the beneficiary to the insurance company for payment of medical expenses incurred during the effective dates of the medical policy.
17. This reference lists standard codes for procedures and services.

Learning Review

1. Coding for procedures done and for visits of all kinds—office, hospital, nursing facility, home services—is found in *Current Procedural Terminology* (CPT).

   A. CPT is divided into seven sections. This volume is updated annually and published by the American Medical Association. Name the seven sections.

   (1) ______________________ (5) ______________________
   (2) ______________________ (6) ______________________
   (3) ______________________ (7) ______________________
   (4) ______________________

   B. For each procedure listed, give the correct procedure code and name the CPT section in which the code can be found.

   1. Chemotherapy administration, infusion technique, up to one hour
      code: ____________ section: ______________________
   2. Hepatitis B surface antibody
      code: ____________ section: ______________________
   3. Simple repair of superficial wounds of scalp, neck, axillae, external genitalia, trunk and/or extremities (including hands and feet) 7.6 cm to 12.5 cm
      code: ____________ section: ______________________
   4. Electrocardiogram, routine ECG with at least 12 leads; with interpretation and reports
      code: ____________ section: ______________________
   5. Hepatic venography, wedged or free, with hemodynamic evaluation, radiological supervision, and interpretation
      code: ____________ section: ______________________
   6. Hepatitis Be antigen (HBeAg)
      code: ____________ section: ______________________
   7. Anesthesia for arthroscopic procedures of hip joint
      code: ____________ section: ______________________

2. A. Codes for diagnoses are found in the *International Classification of Diseases, 9th Revision, Clinical Modification* (ICD-9-CM). ICD-9-CM is divided into three volumes. Specify below what information each volume contains.

   Volume I: ____
   ____

Volume II: ____

____

Volume III: ____

____

B. Provide answers to the following questions.
In which volume of the ICD would a CMA first look to find the diagnosis code for osteomyelitis? ____________ What is the diagnosis code for unspecified osteomyelitis of the ankle or foot? ____________ Injury codes cannot stand alone, but must be accompanied by "E" codes. What do "E" codes stand for ? ____________ What is the diagnosis code for obesity? ____________ "V" codes are the last main section of Volumes I and II. What do "V" codes stand for? ____________.

3. Errors in coding insurance claims can have far-reaching effects for both the patient and the physician. Name three effects.
(1) ____

____

(2) ____

____

(3) ____

____

4. For each entry in the following table, check whether the entry represents a diagnosis or procedure. Then, enter the appropriate diagnosis or procedure code, referencing this textbook, the current revision of the ICD, or the current edition of the CPT. In the explanation column, identify whether the procedures are laboratory procedures (LAB), part of the physician's physical examination process (PE), diagnostic procedures (DP), examples of medication administration (MA), preventive measures (PM), procedures related to litigation (LEG), or rehabilitative medicine procedures (RP). For each diagnosis, give a brief definition of the patient condition or illness, consulting a medical encyclopedia if necessary.

Diag.	Proced.	Entry	Code	Explanation
❑	❑	1. Services requested after hours in addition to basic services	____	____________
❑	❑	2. Medicine given or taken in error	____	____________
❑	❑	3. Anorexia nervosa	____	____________
❑	❑	4. Pneumonocentesis, puncture of lung for aspiration	____	____________
❑	❑	5. Diabetic Ketoacidosis	____	____________
❑	❑	6. Urinalysis; qualitative or semi-quantitative, except immunoassays, microscopic only	____	____________

Diag.	Proced.	Entry	Code	Explanation
❑	❑	7. Bruxism	_____	_____
❑	❑	8. Pneumocystis carinii pneumonia	_____	_____
❑	❑	9. Amniocentesis	_____	_____
❑	❑	10. Epstein-Barr virus infection	_____	_____
❑	❑	11. Gait training (includes stair climbing)	_____	_____
❑	❑	12. Medical testimony	_____	_____
❑	❑	13. DTP (diphtheria-tetanus-pertussis) vaccination	_____	_____
❑	❑	14. Therapeutic or diagnostic injection (specify material injected); subcutaneous or intramuscular	_____	_____
❑	❑	15. Narcotics affecting fetus via placenta or breast milk	_____	_____

Investigation Activity

Most people do not think about their health insurance policy or the extent of the coverage it allows until they are faced with a serious illness or condition necessitating immediate medical treatment and/or surgery. The issues involved extend not only to the amount of money an insurance carrier will pay for treatment or surgery, but to whether the procedure, treatment, or surgery is allowed under the policy. In addition to helping patients understand their responsibility in filing claims for traditional insurance carriers or providing proper referral forms when required by HMOs or managed care providers, medical assistants should also encourage patients to learn more about their health insurance policies, including the extent and nature of benefits and specific coverage.

A. Research your own health insurance coverage. What type of coverage is provided: traditional, PPO network, managed care organization or HMO? What deductibles are allowed? How much will the insurer pay after deductibles are met? Are you responsible for the amounts charged that are more than the insurance company's assessment of usual, reasonable, and customary charges? If so, how can you find out how much your carrier will pay for a specific procedure before the procedure is done and the physician's charge is incurred? Is there an out-of-pocket maximum? Is there a lifetime maximum benefit allowed?

If you are covered by a managed care organization or an HMO, are you able to choose your own primary care physician from the organization's network? Must all care from a specialist or other health care professional be preauthorized and referred by the primary care physician? What can you do if your primary care physician will not approve a referral you request? What can you do if a treatment you want is not approved by the HMO? What kinds of alternative medicine are covered (biofeedback, chiropractic, etc.)? What kinds of preventive care are covered (well-baby visits, gynecological exams and Pap tests for women, participation in cardiovascular exercise programs, etc.)?

B. Choose three student volunteers to contact three health insurance carriers: one traditional insurance carrier, one PPO network, and one managed care organization or HMO. Request information about the different types of insurance policies and coverage offered by each. Bring the information to class for discussion and comparison.

CASE STUDY

Lourdes Austen, a one-year survivor of breast cancer, is covered by an HMO. Lourdes's primary care physician, Dr. King, recommends that Lourdes receive a colonoscopy as she has a family history that is positive for colon cancer; medical studies have demonstrated a link between colon and breast cancers in families. Lourdes's HMO requires preauthorization before a specialist's care can be provided. Dr. King supplies the referral to a gastroenterologist who will perform the colon screening test and gives Lourdes the necessary completed referral form to take with her to her scheduled appointment.

During the colonoscopy procedure, one benign polyp is removed and the gastroenterologist requests that Lourdes return for a follow-up examination in one week. Lourdes makes an appointment with the specialist's administrative medical assistant. When she returns one week later, the medical assistant informs Lourdes that she must have a new referral form for the office visit or the HMO will not approve payment; Lourdes will have to pay for the examination herself. "But we drove 40 minutes to get here, and no one ever told me I'd need another form for this. I thought it was all covered under the colonoscopy," Lourdes says.

Discuss the following:

1. Lourdes's HMO policy requires preauthorization. Is there anything that can be done to secure a proper referral without having to schedule another appointment for the patient or force the patient to pay for the office visit?
2. What is the role of the specialist's administrative medical assistant in this situation? Could the situation have been prevented?
3. Lourdes's colonoscopy required the following diagnoses and procedures. Give the correct coding for processing the insurance claim for this patient.

   colonoscopy with biopsy, single or multiple ____________________

   flex sig (colon) ____________________

   family history, malignant neoplasm GI tract ____________________

   personal history, malignant neoplasm, breast ____________________

   low complexity office visit ____________________

SUPPLEMENTARY RESOURCES

Study Guide Disk: Additional practice exercises for this chapter are available on the study guide disk found in the back of the textbook.

Medical Assisting Videos: Appropriate content is available on Delmar's Medical Assisting Videos, 2nd edition, for the following topics:

Tape 4: Types of Reimbursement
- Charge Slip
- Implement Current Procedural Terminology
- Analyze and Use Third Party Guidelines
- Common Problems in the Use of ICD-9 and CPT Manuals
- Responses from Insurers
- Computerized Management of Reimbursement Systems
- Dealing With Frequently Asked Questions from Patients

EVALUATION OF CHAPTER KNOWLEDGE

How has your instructor evaluated the knowledge you have achieved?

Knowledge	**Instructor Evaluation** *Good*	*Average*	*Poor*
Describes the history of medical insurance in this country and its evolution in recent years	_____	_____	_____
Defines the terminology necessary to understand and submit medical insurance claims	_____	_____	_____
Knows at least five examples of medical insurance coverage	_____	_____	_____
Explains the significance of diagnosis-related groups	_____	_____	_____
Understands the process of procedure and diagnosis coding	_____	_____	_____
Codes a sample claim form	_____	_____	_____
Documents accurately	_____	_____	_____
Explains the difference between the HCFA-1500 and the UB92 forms	_____	_____	_____
Describes the way in which computers have altered the claims process	_____	_____	_____
Discusses why claims follow-up is important to the ambulatory care setting	_____	_____	_____
Discusses the legal and ethical issues associated with insurance coding	_____	_____	_____
Is comfortable as a patient educator about insurance issues	_____	_____	_____

Student's Initials: ______ Instructor's Initials: ______

Grade: _______

CHAPTER 19

Billing and Collections

PERFORMANCE OBJECTIVES

Accurate and timely patient billing is essential to maintaining the financial health of an ambulatory care facility. Medical assistants play a vital role in managing accounts receivables. Establishing and monitoring patient billing, using either a manual or computerized system, requires attention to detail, accurate documentation, and excellent communications skills when performing duties related to the collection of outstanding debt. When performing billing and collection tasks, it is important to remember that patients have the right to choose their health care providers and should be respected as consumers.

EXERCISES AND ACTIVITIES

Vocabulary Builder

Match each key vocabulary term to its correct definition.

A. Aging accounts
B. Statute of limitations
C. Monthly billing
D. Truth-in-Lending Act
E. Cycle billing
F. Collection agency
G. Credit bureau

____ **1.** A method that sends all bills at the same time each month, usually on or about the 25th day of each month.

____ **2.** A process by which accounts are determined to be overdue.

____ **3.** Also known as the Consumer Credit Protection Act of 1968; an act requiring providers of installment credits to state the charges in writing and to express the interest as an annual rate.

____ **4.** An outside agency that provides information about an individual's credit history.

____ **5.** An outside establishment that collects outstanding debt.

____ **6.** Statute that defines the period of time in which legal action can take place.

____ **7.** A method of spreading billing over the whole month instead of sending bills at the end of the month.

Learning Review

1. A billing efficiency report allows for careful monitoring of follow-up bills: whether they were paid, if the insurance was paid, and assessing the patient's responsibility for payment. What five pieces of data are included in these reports, from which production efficiency is calculated?

   1. ____________________ 4. ____________________

   2. ____________________ 5. ____________________

   3. ____________________

2. Identify and explain the three most common reasons some patient accounts become past due.

   (1) ____

   ____

   (2) ____

   ____

   (3) ____

   ____

3. A. In the pegboard system, what method is used to identify the age of accounts?

   ____

   ____

   B. A written code "OD2/ 4/1" is entered on a patient ledger card. What does the code mean?

   C. Name five criteria according to which computer programs can age accounts.

   1. ____________________ 4. ____________________

   2. ____________________ 5. ____________________

   3. ____________________

   D. The computer can also generate accounts receivable reports. Name three pieces of information included on a computer-generated accounts receivable report.

   1. ______________ 2. ______________ 3. ______________

4. Credit bureaus, or collection agencies, generally provide two services to an ambulatory care facility. Name and describe each type of service.

   (1) ____

   ____

   (2) ____

   ____

5. Collection of fees when a patient has died are directed to the executor of the estate. Place a checkmark next to each action below that represents a responsible action in collecting past due accounts from deceased patients' estates.

____ A. Address the statement to "Estate of (insert patient's name)" and mail to the patient's last known address.

____ B. Send an invoice with a complete breakdown of all monies owed to the deceased patient's spouse or closest relative, noting that the survivor is responsible for making payment in full.

____ C. Wait a minimum of ten days after the death to send a statement to the estate, out of respect for the family of the deceased.

____ D. When no executor or representative of the deceased has been appointed, contact the office's attorney or the probate court for advice on how to proceed.

____ E. Write off unpaid amounts as uncollectible.

6. A statement is returned to the office marked "no forwarding address." What three actions can medical assistants take to track down the "skip" without the risk of violating laws, such as the Fair Debt Collection Practices Act?

(1) ______________________________

(2) ______________________________

(3) ______________________________

7. With regard to collections, the statute of limitations is usually defined by the class of the overdue account. Name the three classes of accounts.

1. ____________ 2. ____________ 3. ____________

Investigation Activity

Communication skills are essential to performing collections duties in the ambulatory care setting. A compassionate tone and diplomatic manner are required. However, while displaying empathy, medical assistants also must be firm in requesting payment or making arrangements with patients for payment schedules. When dealing with the general public, it is always wise to expect the unexpected. Medical assistants may encounter avoidance, anger, guilt, or embarrassment from patients when attempting telephone collections. What is the best way of handling each of the patient responses below? Role-play the conversations with a partner. To simulate a telephone conversation, make sure you cannot see you partner during the spoken exchange. The partner who is role-playing the patient should use a variety of moods and tones to convey his or her responses.

1. "I've been a patient here for ten years and always paid my bills on time. And now when I've got a serious illness and I'm overwhelmed with medical bills and I need your understanding, all you care about is getting your money."
2. "The physician makes me wait two hours every time I have an appointment. So, the physician can wait to be paid."
3. "Bill? What bill? I never got a bill."
4. "I may be getting a little older and more forgetful, but I always look for my bills and pay them on time. My children come and help me. Your records must be wrong."
5. "The insurance was supposed to cover that charge. I'm just not paying. Call them."
6. "The check is in the mail." (in response to a third collection notice)

CASE STUDY

Charles Williams, 62 years old, is a new patient of Dr. Winston Lewis's at the offices of Drs. Lewis & King. On July 1, xxxx, five days before the patient's birthday, Charles comes to see Dr. Lewis for a 1:00 P.M. appointment with a chief complaint of intermittent, irregular heartbeats or palpitations, dizziness, and chest pain. Dr. Lewis performs a comprehensive physical examination and orders several tests, including an EKG, CBC, and urinalysis with microscopy. The total fee for the office visit and tests is $345: $200 for the physical examination, $75 for the EKG, $25 for the urinalysis, $25 for routine venipuncture, and $20 for a complete blood count, which Charles pays for by check at the time of service. Charles is insured by a private carrier, All American Insurance Company, group #333210, ID number 112-45-9980, which he receives through his employer, HighTech Computer Group. Dr. Lewis asks Ellen Armstrong, CMA, to schedule a return appointment in exactly one week to go over the results of Charles's tests. Ellen schedules the appointment and prepares a charge slip for Charles's visit. She refers to his patient information sheet for the correct personal information. Charles Williams lives at 123 Greenside Street, Northborough, OH, 12346.

Complete the charge slip for Charles Williams's office visit.

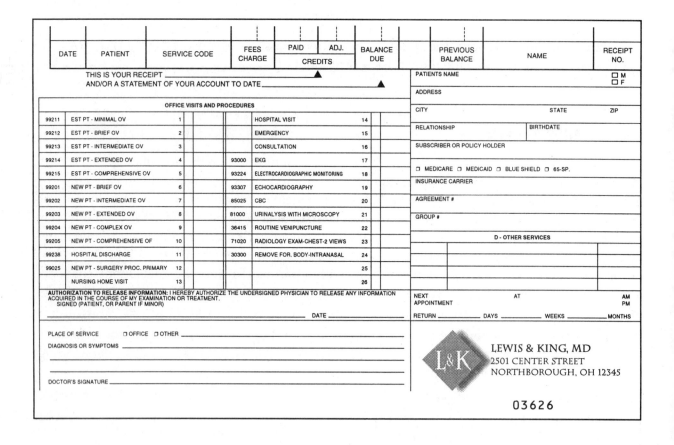

DATE	PATIENT	SERVICE CODE	FEES CHARGE	CREDITS: PAID	CREDITS: ADJ.	BALANCE DUE		PREVIOUS BALANCE	NAME	RECEIPT NO.

THIS IS YOUR RECEIPT ▲
AND/OR A STATEMENT OF YOUR ACCOUNT TO DATE ▲

PATIENTS NAME ☐ M ☐ F

ADDRESS

CITY STATE ZIP

RELATIONSHIP BIRTHDATE

SUBSCRIBER OR POLICY HOLDER

☐ MEDICARE ☐ MEDICAID ☐ BLUE SHIELD ☐ 65-SP.

INSURANCE CARRIER

AGREEMENT #

GROUP #

OFFICE VISITS AND PROCEDURES

99211	EST PT - MINIMAL OV	1			HOSPITAL VISIT	14	
99212	EST PT - BRIEF OV	2			EMERGENCY	15	
99213	EST PT - INTERMEDIATE OV	3			CONSULTATION	16	
99214	EST PT - EXTENDED OV	4		93000	EKG	17	
99215	EST PT - COMPREHENSIVE OV	5		93224	ELECTROCARDIOGRAPHIC MONITORING	18	
99201	NEW PT - BRIEF OV	6		93307	ECHOCARDIOGRAPHY	19	
99202	NEW PT - INTERMEDIATE OV	7		85025	CBC	20	
99203	NEW PT - EXTENDED OV	8		81000	URINALYSIS WITH MICROSCOPY	21	
99204	NEW PT - COMPLEX OV	9		36415	ROUTINE VENIPUNCTURE	22	
99205	NEW PT - COMPREHENSIVE OF	10		71020	RADIOLOGY EXAM-CHEST-2 VIEWS	23	
99238	HOSPITAL DISCHARGE	11		30300	REMOVE FOR. BODY-INTRANASAL	24	
99025	NEW PT - SURGERY PROC. PRIMARY	12				25	
	NURSING HOME VISIT	13				26	

D - OTHER SERVICES

AUTHORIZATION TO RELEASE INFORMATION: I HEREBY AUTHORIZE THE UNDERSIGNED PHYSICIAN TO RELEASE ANY INFORMATION ACQUIRED IN THE COURSE OF MY EXAMINATION OR TREATMENT.
SIGNED (PATIENT, OR PARENT IF MINOR)

_______________ DATE _______________

NEXT APPOINTMENT AT AM PM

RETURN ________ DAYS ________ WEEKS ________ MONTHS

PLACE OF SERVICE ☐ OFFICE ☐ OTHER ____________

DIAGNOSIS OR SYMPTOMS ____________

DOCTOR'S SIGNATURE ____________

L&K

LEWIS & KING, MD
2501 CENTER STREET
NORTHBOROUGH, OH 12345

03626

SUPPLEMENTARY RESOURCES

Study Guide Disk: Additional practice exercises for this chapter are available on the study guide disk found in the back of the textbook.

Medical Assisting Videos: Appropriate content is available on Delmar's Medical Assisting Videos, 2nd ed., for the following topics:

Tape 3: Billing Cycle and Collections
Tape 4: Charge Slip
Computerized Management of Reimbursement Systems
Dealing With Frequently Asked Questions from Patients

EVALUATION OF CHAPTER KNOWLEDGE

How has your instructor evaluated the knowledge you have achieved?

	Instructor Evaluation		
Knowledge	*Good*	*Average*	*Poor*
Understands credit and collection policies and procedures	_____	_____	_____
Understands process of aging accounts	_____	_____	_____
Recognizes components of a complete patient statement	_____	_____	_____
Accurately completes a charge slip	_____	_____	_____
Possesses ability to hold a professional telephone collection call	_____	_____	_____
Identifies collection techniques and describes the use of each	_____	_____	_____
Possesses ability to compose collection letters	_____	_____	_____
Understands importance of accounts receivables to the financial health of the ambulatory care setting	_____	_____	_____
Knows the function of credit bureaus and collection agencies	_____	_____	_____
Identifies special collection situations and strategies for handling them	_____	_____	_____
Considers legal ramifications of billing and collection procedures, including the Truth-in Lending Act, Fair Debt Collection Practices Act, small claims court, and the statute of limitations	_____	_____	_____

Student's Initials: ______ Instructor's Initials: ______

Grade: _______

CHAPTER 20

Accounting Practices

PERFORMANCE OBJECTIVES

The management of practice finances in the ambulatory care setting is one of the most important aspects in the operation of the facility. The proper management of medical facility finances includes daily financial practices, the accurate coding and processing of insurance forms, collection of accounts, and accounting practices. Accounting in the ambulatory care setting includes the collection of data on all aspects of the financial operation. If done properly, accounting can monitor the profitability of a facility and ensure that any new activities, such as computerization, result in optimum financial health. The administrative duties of medical assistants will require them to become involved in the financial operations of the ambulatory care setting. A working knowledge of accounting processes will also help medical assistants become aware of the manner in which financial realities influence workplace decisions in the ambulatory care setting, such as purchasing new equipment, hiring new employees, or implementing a facility newsletter for community outreach and patient education.

EXERCISES AND ACTIVITIES

Vocabulary Builder

_____ 1. Accounting
_____ 2. Accounts payable
_____ 3. Accounts receivable ratio
_____ 4. Assets
_____ 5. Balance sheet
_____ 6. Collection ratio
_____ 7. Cost accounting
_____ 8. Cost analysis
_____ 9. Cost ratio
_____ **10.** Financial accounting
_____ **11.** Fixed costs
_____ **12.** Income statement
_____ **13.** Liabilities
_____ **14.** Managerial Accounting
_____ **15.** Owner's equity
_____ **16.** Utilization review
_____ **17.** Variable costs

A. The financial statement showing net profit or loss.

B. These vary in direct proportion to patient volume.

C. Provides information for entities external to the practice, for example, the federal government.

D. The outstanding accounts receivable divided by the average monthly gross income for the past twelve months.

E. A procedure that determines the cost of each service.

F. An itemized statement of assets, liabilities, financial condition, and equity.

G. Generates information to enable more efficient internal management.

H. These do not vary in total as the number of patients varies.

I. System of monitoring the financial status of a facility and the financial results of its activities, providing information for decision making.

J. Debts, financial obligations, for which one is responsible.

K. The gross income divided by the amount that could have been collected, less disallowances.

L. Properties of value that are owned by a business entity.

M. An unwritten promise to pay a supplier for property or merchandise purchased on credit or for a service rendered.

N. The amount by which business assets exceed business liabilities.

O. A formula that shows the cost of a procedure or service and helps determine the financial value of maintaining certain services.

P. Determines what it costs for a practice to perform particular services.

Q. A review of medical services before they can be performed.

Learning Review

1. There are a variety of methods used for financial management in the ambulatory care setting. Name three bookkeeping systems that are appropriate for use in an noncomputerized, or manual, environment.

(1) ______________________________

(2) ______________________________

(3) ______________________________

Match the appropriate bookkeeping system to the following duties performed by the medical assistant.

______________________ A. Office manager Walter Seals, CMA, was responsible for implementing a computer system at Inner City Health Care. Before the computerized accounting program was put into effect, the urgent care center relied on a manual system of checks and balances that allowed the physician-employers to keep a firm hold on the relationship between the facility's assets and the sum of liabilities and net worth.

____________________ B. During a temporary one-week down period in the computer system at the offices of Drs. Lewis & King while a system upgrade is installed, administrative medical assistant Ellen Armstrong completes each day's financial transactions in a daily journal, then transfers this information to the ledger through the posting process. The information will be entered into the computer once the system is up and running again.

____________________ C. When the patient returns the charge slip to the reception desk after an examination, Karen Ritter, CMA, carefully replaces and lines up the charge slip with the patient's name on the day sheet, then correctly inserts the ledger card under the last page of the charge slip. She proceeds to enter the total charges due and any patient payments.

2. A. Medical software packages have the ability to code information obtained in the ambulatory care setting for use in a database. When completing insurance claim forms or generating reports, the software has the capability to include the most common ________________ and ____________________ codes. What other kinds of codes can a computerized accounting system generate that will facilitate the billing functions?

____

____

____

B. The computer can also be used in the preparation of these four financial documents:

(1) ____

(2) ____

(3) ____

(4) ____

3. Name three ways computer service bureaus handle accounts from medical facilities.

(1) ____

____

(2) ____

____

(3) ____

____

4. What five points are important to consider when an ambulatory care setting makes the decision to move from a manual to a computerized accounting system—whether through a computer service bureau or an on-site system?

(1) ____

(2) ____

(3) ____

(4) ____

(5) ____

5. Fixed costs are expenses that do not vary in total as the number of patients seen by the medical practice grows or shrinks. Variable costs are expenses that are directly affected by patient volume.

   A. From the list below, identify expenses that qualify as fixed costs (FC) and those that are variable costs (VC).

   ____ 1. Interpreting laboratory test results

   ____ 2. Annual depreciation of the cost of an automatic electrocardiograph (ECG) machine

   ____ 3. Medical benefits for the office staff

   ____ 4. Purchase of reagent test strips for urinalysis

   ____ 5. Magazine subscriptions for the facility reception area

   ____ 6. Monthly telephone expenses

   ____ 7. Medical journal subscriptions for the physician-owners

   ____ 8 Purchase of a HemoCue blood glucose system

   ____ 9. Printing cost of a patient education brochure

   ____ 10. Purchase of open-shelf lateral files

   ____ 11. Adding a new position, such as a clinical medical assistant, to the office staff

   ____ 12. Property taxes on the medical facility building and grounds

   ____ 13. The monthly cost of janitorial services

   ____ 14. Purchase of disposable needle-syringe units

   ____ 15. Disposable paper gowns for patient examinations

   B. Calculating and reviewing fixed and variable costs provides data that allow what four functions to be performed in the ambulatory care setting?

   (1) ______________________ (3) ______________________

   (2) ______________________ (4) ______________________

6. A balance sheet, or statement of financial position, itemizes the credits and debits incurred by the ambulatory care setting. The balance sheet is prepared from an analysis of the double-entry bookkeeping records. What four items should be included when making a debit or credit entry in a ledger or journal?

   (1) ____

   (2) ____

   (3) ____

   (4) ____

7. At the offices of Drs. Lewis & King, the total accounts receivable at the end of May is $100,000 and the monthly receipts total is $75,000; the total accounts receivable at the end of June is $82,000 and the monthly receipts total is $31,000; the total accounts receivable at the end of July is $86,000 and the monthly receipts total is $20,000; the total accounts receivable at the end of August is $93,000 and the monthly receipts total is $45,000. What is the accounts receivable ratio for each month? Show your calculations in the space provided.

May	July
June	August

Which month has the healthiest accounts receivable ratio and why?

____

8. A. For the month of September, receipts at the offices of Drs. Lewis & King totaled $35,000. The Medicare/Medicaid adjustment for the month was $1,750 and the managed care adjustment was $4,500. Total charges for the month of September equaled $53,000. What is the collection ratio for the month of September? Show your calculation in the space provided.

____

____

B. For the month of October, receipts at the offices of Drs. Lewis & King totaled $41,000. The Medicare/Medicaid adjustment for the month was $2,000, the Worker's Compensation adjustment was $750, and the managed care adjustment was $4,700. Total charges for October equaled $55,000. What is the collection ratio for the month of October? Show your calculation in the space provided.

____

____

C. Which month has the more desirable collection ratio and why?

9. A. A group practice of radiologists charges $185 for a routine mammogram. Total expenses related to the mammogram procedure equal $30,000 per month, and the practice performs a monthly average of 200 mammograms. What is the average cost ratio for the mammogram procedure? Show your calculations in the space provided.

____

____

B. Given the cost to patients for the mammogram procedure, is the group practice making a profit or loss on performing mammograms? What amount is the profit or loss per procedure? What amount is the profit or loss for the entire month?

____

____

10. A. Income statements reveal the cumulative profit and total expenses for each month. Monthly income and expenses are then added to arrive at year-to-date totals, which are compared to the annual budget for particular income and expense categories. Use the following information to complete the expense analysis for the first quarter office expense costs of the offices of Drs. Lewis and King. The total office expense budget for the year is $20,000 divided evenly per quarter.

Telephone expenses for January = $323.46, February = $425.93, March = $393.87.
Postage and mail expenses for January = $725.45, February = $550.90, March = $601.33.
Office supply expenses for January = $1,200.62, February = $325.45, March = $446.26.
Yearly budget for telephone expenses = $4,000, postage and mail expenses = $8,000, office supply expenses = $8,000.

Office Expenses	January	February	March	Year-to-Date	Budget for Year
Office supplies	$	$	$	$	$
Postage	$	$	$	$	$
Telephone	$	$	$	$	$
TOTALS	$	$	$	$	$

B. How much are the offices of Drs. Lewis and King over or under budget for quarterly office expenses? ____________________ How might the office manager use data from the budget sheet?

____

____

Why is it important to implement and track budgets for specific categories of income and expense in the ambulatory care setting?

____

____

____

Investigation Activity: Business Sense and Savvy Self-test

Personal finances as well as the finances of businesses such as ambulatory care settings require careful planning, management, and budgeting. You can use the systems of business financial management to gain insights into your personal spending patterns and to help develop and fine-tune smart financial habits and attitudes.

For each statement, circle the response that best describes you.

1. I think saving money is
   A. Important; I make effort every to put away a sum of money as savings on a regular basis.
   B. Great if you can find a way; I'd like to save but I have trouble finding ways to do it.
   C. Not important right now; I have too many expenses—what I really need is a loan!

2. When planning a large purchase, such as a computer or a car, I
   A. Set a limit for spending and affordable installment payments and stick to it.
   B. Have a rough idea of what I can afford, but don't do any advance planning.
   C. Try to buy what I want and think about paying for it later.

3. When considering monthly personal income and expenses, I
   A. Know exactly how much money is coming in and how much is going out to pay bills.
   B. Know I can cover my bills but don't keep track of exactly how much I make or spend.
   C. Hope for the best and if I fall short—charge it!
4. When I have extra money, I
   A. Save one-third, use one-third to pay off debts, and use the last third on a special purchase.
   B. Save half or use it to pay off debts and spend the other half on a special purchase.
   C. Spend it all on a special purchase.
5. My checkbook is
   A. Always balanced.
   B. Sometimes balanced.
   C. Rarely balanced.
6. When choosing a bank for my savings and/or checking, I
   A. Research interest rates, features, funds, and services carefully to find the best deal.
   B. Choose the bank that pays the highest interest rate.
   C. Just pick whatever's most convenient; banks are all the same.
7. I think planning for retirement is
   A. A priority now; the sooner you start saving the more your money grows!
   B. Important but not the most essential financial responsibility I have right now.
   C. Not something I think about now—that's too far away; who can predict the future?
8. People think of me as
   A. Someone who pays attention to detail and is neat and organized.
   B. Someone who always manages to get the job done at the last minute.
   C. Someone who struggles to keep up with routine or repetitive tasks.
9. I think analyzing financial data is
   A. A smart way to assess current spending patterns and guide future spending.
   B. A great thing to do if you have enough time and willpower.
   C. A waste of time; besides, I just don't want to know.
10. I am the kind of person who
    A. Sets short- and long-term financial goals for income and spending and works toward implementing them in a responsible way.
    B. Has short- and long-term financial goals but can't get around to planning for them.
    C. Makes financial decisions on a day-to-day basis; it's enough to deal with one day at a time.

Scoring

If your answers were mostly A responses, congratulations! You have developed a financially responsible outlook and good record-keeping habits. If your responses were mostly Bs, you are thinking about financial realities and recognize the importance of a strong financial awareness. Focus on specific areas where you can improve your financial skills. If your responses were mostly Cs, you need to work on achieving good personal financial habits. Start working on your record-keeping skills by taking the plunge and keeping a weekly journal of expenses to see where your money goes!

In personal matters and in business, responsible accounting practices create organized, successful platforms for financial health, well-being, and potential growth.

CASE STUDY

When the offices of Drs. Lewis and King agreed to accept individuals covered by a large managed care organization, the decision of the physician-owners was based on a complete financial analysis and projection of the expected effects the new patient load would have on the medical practice. As a result, the group practice added a second office manager and a new clinical medical assistant to the existing staff.

Discuss the following:

1. As Drs. Lewis and King absorb the new managed care patients into the practice, what can the physician-owners do to determine whether their financial analysis and projection was accurate?
2. Once the practice has assembled financial data on the effects of the new patient load, how will these data be used?
3. What beneficial effects might the addition of a clinical medical assistant have on the medical practice?

SUPPLEMENTARY RESOURCES

Study Guide Disk: Additional practice exercises for this chapter are available on the study guide disk found in the back of the textbook.

Medical Assisting Videos: Appropriate content is available on Delmar's Medical Assisting Videos, 2nd ed., Tape 3, for the following topics:

Perform Administrative Duties
- Use Manual Bookkeeping System
- Billing Cycle and Collection
- Electronic Banking

EVALUATION OF CHAPTER KNOWLEDGE

How has your instructor evaluated the knowledge you have achieved?

	Instructor Evaluation		
Knowledge	*Good*	*Average*	*Poor*
Possesses a knowledge of the importance of medical financial management in the ambulatory care setting	_____	_____	_____
Understands and can define basic accounting terms	_____	_____	_____
Identifies and has a working knowledge of the various accounting and bookkeeping systems	_____	_____	_____
Understands the role computerized systems can play in the medical office	_____	_____	_____
Recognizes the challenges of converting from a manual to a computerized accounting system	_____	_____	_____
Possesses a working knowledge of cost analysis, financial records, and financial ratios	_____	_____	_____
Understands utilization review and the importance it has in the ambulatory care setting	_____	_____	_____
Recognizes the importance of good personal and professional financial practices and habits	_____	_____	_____

Student's Initials: ______ Instructor's Initials: ______

Grade: _______

CHAPTER 21

Medical Asepsis, Disease, and Infection Control

PERFORMANCE OBJECTIVES

During the last century, medical science, an improved standard of living, and public health measures have combined to reduce the incidence and mortality rates of infectious disease in the United States. Antibiotics and vaccines now protect much of the world from numerous ancient, deadly infectious diseases, including smallpox, measles, and tuberculosis. Because the world we live in, however, is teeming with pathogens, microorganisms that can cause disease, humankind is not, and indeed may never be, free from the threat of infectious diseases. Medical assistants who care for patients in an ambulatory care setting can help reduce the risk of infection to themselves, other health care professionals, patients, and visitors by adhering to the principles of infection control. Through the practice of medical and surgical asepsis as well as the observance of the Centers for Disease Control and Prevention's universal and standard precautions and transmission-based precautions, medical assistants will limit the presence of infectious agents, create barriers against transmission, and decrease their own and others' risks of contracting or transmitting infectious diseases.

EXERCISES AND ACTIVITY

Vocabulary Builder

A. *Fill in the blanks with the correct key vocabulary terms listed below.*

Infection control	Excoriated	Medical asepsis
Transmission	Microorganisms	Sanitization
Surgical asepsis	Epidemiology	Contaminated

____________________ is the study of the history, cause, and patterns of infectious diseases. Microscopic living creatures, also known as ____________________, that are capable of causing disease are called pathogens. The spread of infectious diseases can occur through direct contact, indirect contact, inhalation, ingestion, or blood-borne contact.

____________________ refers to various methods, including the CDC's standard precautions, health care professionals use to eliminate or reduce the risk of ____________________ of infectious microorganisms from one person to another. ____________________ involves specific techniques used in the ambulatory care setting that are designed to destroy pathogens after they leave the body and to decrease the risk of spreading infection to others. ____________________ is also performed in the ambulatory care setting and involves techniques designed to maintain sterile conditions during procedures to prevent pathogens from entering a patient's body during an invasive procedure.

To reduce the risk that any item, including equipment, trays, and clothing, could be ____________________ or exposed to microorganisms or infectious material, various sterilization techniques are employed. Medically aseptic hand-washing techniques should be performed on a regular basis to ensure the reduction of pathogens spread by the hands. To reduce the risk of chapped, ____________________ skin, medical assistants can apply water-based antibacterial lotion to the hands after washing. Before instruments or other fomites are disinfected or sterilized, they must be scrubbed or cleaned to remove tissue, debris, or other impurities that may harbor pathogens, a process called ____________________.

B. *Match the following terms with the correct definitions.*

Amebic dysentery	Infectious agent	Pathogen
Blood-borne pathogen	Malaria	Scabies
Fomites	Palliative	Trichomoniasis

____________________ 1. Infestation with a Trichomonas parasite, which may be transmitted through sexual intercourse.

____________________ 2. Infectious skin disease caused by the itch mite, Sarcoptes scabiei, which is transmitted by direct contact with infected persons.

____________________ 3. A pharmacological treatment agent for a viral infection is an example of an agent that relieves only symptoms of the disease instead of curing the infection.

____________________ 4. A pathogen responsible for a specific infectious disease.

____________________ 5. Infectious intestinal disease characterized by inflammation of the mucous membrane of the colon.

____________________ 6. Any microorganism capable of causing disease found in blood or components of blood.

____________________ 7. Infectious disease caused by protozoan parasites within red blood cells; transmitted to humans by female mosquitoes.

____________________ 8. Substances that absorb and transmit infectious material, that is, contaminated items such as equipment.

____________________ 9. Any disease-producing microorganism.

C. Write a brief definition for each key vocabulary term.

1. Resistance ____

2. Vaccine ____

3. Antibody ____

4. Immunoglobulins ____

5. Immunity ____

6. Disinfection ____

7. Antigen ____

Learning Review

1. The following are the common five stages of many infectious diseases. Place the stages in the proper order, starting with initial infection with a pathogen, and describe the identifying characteristics and symptoms associated with each.

Acute	Prodromal
Declining	Convalescent
Incubation	

Stage	Description
(1) ____________	______________________________
(2) ____________	______________________________
(3) ____________	______________________________
(4) ____________	______________________________
(5) ____________	______________________________

2. For each vaccine, identify the disease for which the vaccine provides immunity and the route of vaccine administration.

Vaccine	Disease	Route of Administration
DTP	______	____________________
HBV	______	____________________
MMR	______	____________________
Hib	______	____________________
OPV	______	____________________

3. Health care professionals use many interventions to break the chain of infection transmission. For each intervention below, identify one of the five links of infection it is intended to break.

____________________ A. Hand washing.
____________________ B. Universal and standard precautions.
____________________ C. Rapid accurate identification of organisms.
____________________ D. Aseptic technique.
____________________ E. Recognition of high-risk patients.
____________________ F. Isolation.
____________________ G. Control of excretions and secretions.
____________________ H. Environmental sanitation.
____________________ I. Treatment of underlying disease.
____________________ J. Air flow control.
____________________ K. Trash and waste disposal.
____________________ L. Food handling.

4. A susceptible host is a person who is not resistant or immune to a pathogenic organism and is, therefore, able to contract the pathogenic organism and develop an infection.

A. List the five causes of susceptibility:

(1) ____________________
(2) ____________________
(3) ____________________
(4) ____________________
(5) ____________________

B. Susceptibility of a person depends upon several factors. For each example given, identify the correct factor of susceptibility.

____________________ (1) Dr. Angie Esposito is physically worn down by working double shifts at Inner City Health Care. While she loves the excitement of working intensely with patients in an urgent care setting, flu season is coming and Dr. Esposito is worried that she will succumb.

____________________ (2) Significantly overweight and a heavy smoker, Herb Fowler is prone to colds that just will not go away; Dr. Winston Lewis is treating Herb for a case of chronic bronchitis.

_______________ (3) Mary O'Keefe's three-year-old son, Chris, and several other members of his play group come down with chicken pox after playing with a child infected with the disease, caused by the varicella-zoster virus.

_______________ (4) Pneumocystis pneumonia is an infection common to patients who have a full-blown case of AIDS.

_______________ (5) Jim Marshall, stressed out by the pressure to complete an architectural design ahead of schedule and on a tight budget, is depressed and angry when he gets laid up with the flu and misses two days of work.

_______________ (6) Margaret Thomas's college-age niece is caught in an epidemic of scabies that sweeps through her dorm floor and places the students in temporary isolation until the outbreak is controlled.

_______________ (7) While vacationing at a remote spot in Mexico, Bill Schwartz eats almost a pound of shrimp at a local restaurant and the next day experiences severe diarrhea and vomiting. He is diagnosed with cholera, caused by the Vibrio cholerae bacterium harbored in the shellfish he had eaten.

5. Immunity is defined as the ability of the body to resist disease. Identify the correct terms or the specific form of immunity that may occur in response to specific antigens.

A. The immune response that involves T cells and B cells to attack viruses, fungi, organ transplants, or cancer cells is called _______________.

B. The immune response that produces antibodies to kill pathogens and recognize them in the future is called _______________.

C. The immunity that follows the administration of vaccines is called _______________.

D. The short-term immunity provided to a newborn that occurs when antibodies pass to a fetus from the mother is called _______________.

E. The immunity that results from contracting an infectious agent and experiencing either an acute or a subclinical infectious disease is called _______________.

F. The immunity achieved through administration of ready-made antibodies, such as gamma-globulin is called _______________.

6. For each infectious disease listed below, identify the agent of transmission (virus, bacteria, fungus, etc.), at least one route of transmission, and common symptoms.

A. AIDS

Agent: _______________

Transmission: _______________

Symptoms: _______________

____

____

____

B. TB

Agent:____

Transmission: ____

Symptoms: ____

C. Gastroenteritis

Agent:____

Transmission: ____

Symptoms: ____

D. Hepatitis B

Agent:____

Transmission: ____

Symptoms: ____

E. Chicken pox

Agent:____

Transmission: ____

Symptoms: ____

F. Influenza

Agent:____

Transmission: ____

Symptoms: ____

7. A. Describe three methods of medical asepsis used to reduce the presence of pathogens in an ambulatory care setting.

(1) ______________________________

____

(2) ______________________________

____

(3) ______________________________

____

B. Place a checkmark next to each statement below that represents the appropriate use of medical asepsis in the ambulatory care setting.

_____ (1) Joe Guerrero, CMA, washes his hands before performing the transfer of patient Lenore McDonell from the wheelchair to the examination table.

_____ (2) Wanda Slawson, CMA, runs a clean sheet of disposable paper over the examination table to prepare the room for the next patient. She picks up the cloth gown patient Lydia Renzi leaves unused, still in its plastic protective covering, on a chair in the examination room and places it on the examination table for the next patient to use.

_____ (3) After performing a venipuncture procedure on patient Leo McKay, Bruce Goldman, CMA, tells Leo he can just throw the gauze pad he has been holding on the venipuncture site in the trash can.

_____ (4) Anna Preciado, CMA, moving quickly to assist a patient who may be about to faint, accidentally bumps into a sterile tray of instruments, knocking a scalpel and clamp onto the floor. The patient, who is bent over in front of Anna, picks the instruments up off the floor and places them back on the tray in the sterile field. "You dropped these," he says.

_____ (5) After assisting in the removal of an infected sebaceous cyst from a patient, clinical medical assistant Audrey Jones cleans, dresses, and bandages the wound as directed by Dr. Winston Lewis. She then disposes of all contaminated items per OSHA guidelines, properly removes PPE, removes her gloves, and washes her hands.

C. For each item in part B (above) that does not reflect proper techniques of medical asepsis, explain what went wrong and how the error should be corrected.

____

____

____

____

8. ______________________ is a term used interchangeably for surgical asepsis. Living tissue surfaces, such as skin, cannot be sterilized. Name two examples of ways that skin can be rid of as many pathogens as possible before the use of a sterile covering.

(1) ______________________________

____

(2) ____

____

9. A. For each instrument or item below, identify the method used for proper asepsis: chemical disinfection (CD), chemical sterilization (CS), or steam sterilization (SS) in an autoclave.

Match the following equipment with the correct aseptic method.

_____ (1) Glass thermometers

_____ (2) Wrapped surgical instruments

_____ (3) Stethoscopes

_____ (4) Fiber-optic endoscopes

_____ (5) Countertops

_____ (6) Wheelchairs

_____ (7) Gynecological instruments

_____ (8) Examination tables

B. Why are gynecological instruments sanitized separately from other external physical examination instruments before sterilization?

____

____

10. Identify and describe the most widely used method of sterilization in the ambulatory care setting.

____

____

____

____

11. A. List six general rules that ensure proper sterilization when using an autoclave.

(1) ____

(2) ____

(3) ____

(4) ____

(5) ____

(6) ____

B. Identify the recommended requirements for effective sterilization in an autoclave.

Temperature: ______________________________

Time for sterilization of unwrapped items: ______________________________

Time for sterilization of loosely wrapped items: ______________________________

Time for sterilization of tightly wrapped items: ______________________________

Frequency of draining of water and cleaning of autoclave: ______________________________

Investigation Activity

Physicians are required to report cases of certain infectious diseases to the state Department of Public Health, which in turn sends these data to the Centers for Disease Control and Prevention. In the space provided below, list the five infectious diseases you believe physicians encountered most during the previous year in the state in which you live. Then elect one student volunteer to write, call, or visit your state's Department of Public Health to find out the five infectious diseases that actually were most prevalent that year in your state; obtain statistics regarding the outbreaks as well.

Suspected Five Most Common Infectious Diseases in Your State	*Actual Five Most Common Infectious Disease in Your State*
Year: ______________	Year: ______________
1. ______________________	1. ______________________
2. ______________________	2. ______________________
3. ______________________	3. ______________________
4. ______________________	4. ______________________
5. ______________________	5. ______________________

Discuss the following:

1. Are you surprised at the specific diseases and the number of cases reported in your state? Why or why not? What populations are contracting the infectious diseases? Think about how infectious diseases are spread and if there are social or economic factors that might explain the presence or spread of disease.
2. What steps can people take at home, work, school, and other everyday settings to reduce their chance of exposure to infectious diseases?
3. What details of daily activity (general health, living or workplace conditions, attention to sanitation and cleanliness, exposure to populations at high risk for infection, etc.) might affect your personal risk of infection?

CASE STUDIES

Case 1

Michelle Richards, a medical assisting intern at the Northborough Family Medical Group of Drs. Winston Lewis and Elizabeth King, attends to patient procedures and examinations under the supervision of office manager Marilyn Johnson, CMA. Although Michelle is careful to follow all infection control methods during her observations, she has developed severe dermatitis on her hands. She is concerned that this condition, which has not responded to creams and lotions, is related to the latex gloves she wears during required procedures.

1. Discuss the possible causes of Michelle's symptoms.
2. Suggest a course of action that both addresses Michelle's condition and maintains the proper degree of asepsis.

Case 2

Liz Corbin, CMA, is responsible for maintaining and cleaning the autoclave at Inner City Health Care. Because this equipment is used every day to sterilize instruments used during procedures performed at the clinic, Liz cleans the inner chamber of the autoclave daily. Once a week, she gives the autoclave a thorough cleansing.

1. Describe Liz's daily cleaning procedure.
2. Describe the weekly cleaning procedure for the autoclave.
3. How important is proper maintenance and cleaning of the autoclave in the ambulatory care setting?

Case 3

One-year-old Marissa O'Keefe is a patient at the practice of Drs. Lewis and King. During her well-baby visit, Joe Guerrero, CMA, gives Marissa an MMR vaccine and is about to administer the scheduled fourth DTP immunization when her mother, Mary O'Keefe, voices concern about this vaccination. "I've read that the DPT shot can be dangerous and sometimes causes brain damage. Marissa had a fever after her last DPT, so I don't want to take any risks with this one. I don't think she should have this shot."

1. Should Joe administer the DPT shot to Marissa? How safe is the DPT shot? What is the ICD-9-CM diagnosis code for the DTP vaccination?
2. What is Joe's best therapeutic response to Mary?

SUPPLEMENTARY RESOURCES

Study Guide Disk: Additional practice exercises for this chapter are available on the study guide disk found in the back of the textbook.

Medical Assisting Videos: Appropriate content is available on Delmar's Medical Assisting Videos, 2nd ed., Tape 5, for the following topics:

Standard Precautions
Perform Medical Aseptic Procedure of Handwashing
Use Disposable Single-Contact Gloves (Putting On and Removing)
Personal Protective Equipment
Perform Medical Aseptic Procedures
Ultrasound Cleaners
Wrap and Autoclave an Article
Perform Surgical Aseptic Procedures

SKILLS COMPETENCY ASSESSMENT

Procedure 21–1: Medically Aseptic Handwash

Student's Name: ______________________________ Date: __________

Objective: To reduce pathogens on the hands and wrist, decreasing direct and indirect transmission of infectious microorganisms.

Conditions: The student demonstrates the ability to reduce pathogens on the hands and wrists using the following equipment: sink, soap (bar soap discouraged), water-based antibacterial lotion, disposable paper towels, nail stick or brush.

Time Requirements and Accuracy Standards: 5 minutes. Points assigned reflect importance of step to meeting objective: Important = (5) Essential = (10) Critical = (15). Automatic failure results if any of the **critical** tasks are omitted or performed incorrectly.

STANDARD PRECAUTIONS: 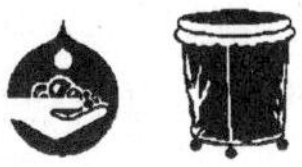

SKILLS ASSESSMENT CHECKLIST

Task Performed	Possible Points	TASKS
☐	5	Removes all jewelry (except plain wedding band).
☐	5	*Rationale:* Jewelry can harbor microorganisms.
☐	5	Prepares disposable paper towel.
☐	5	Does not allow clothing or hands to touch sink.
☐	5	*Rationale:* Remembers sink is contaminated and touching sink with clothes or hands will contaminate them.
☐	10	Turns on faucet with a dry paper towel and adjusts water temperature to lukewarm.
☐	10	*Rationale:* Warm water makes better suds than cold water. Hot water may scald the skin.
☐	15	Wets hands and applies soap, rubbing into a lather.
☐	15	Washes all surfaces of the hands, interlacing the fingers and scrubbing between each finger.
☐	10	*Rationale:* Friction loosens debris and microorganisms.
☐	10	Rinses well, keeping hands and forearms pointed downward.
☐	5	*Rationale:* Prevents water from running down to the elbows, which are less contaminated than the hands.

SKILLS COMPETENCY ASSESSMENT — continued

Procedure 21–1: Medically Aseptic Handwash

Task Performed	Possible Points	TASKS
❑	10	Rinses hands and forearms, keeping them pointed downward.
❑	5	Washes wrists and forearms to height of possible contamination.
❑	5	Rinses hands, wrists, and forearms.
❑	10	Uses orange wood stick or brush for the first handwashing of the day.
❑	10	For the first handwashing of the day, or if hands are contaminated or excessively soiled, repeats hand-washing technique, rewetting hands and applying soap and following all other procedural steps.
❑	5	Dries hands, wrists, and forearms with disposable paper towels; does not touch towel dispenser; blots hands with towel instead of rubbing.
❑	10	If sink is not foot-operated, uses a clean disposable towel to turn off the water faucet.
❑	5	*Rationale:* Clean hands will become contaminated from the dirty sink.
❑	5	Discards paper towel in biohazard waste container.
❑	10	Repeats hand-washing procedure prior to and following each patient contact, procedure, or meal.
❑	5	Applies water-based antibacterial lotion to prevent chapped, excoriated skin.
❑	5	*Rationale:* Cracked skin allows microorganisms to gain entrance and cause infection.
❑	5	Completed the tasks within 5 minutes.
❑	15	Results obtained were accurate.

________	Earned	ADD POINTS OF TASKS CHECKED
205	Points	TOTAL POINTS POSSIBLE
________	SCORE	DETERMINE SCORE (divide points earned by total points possible, multiply results by 100)

Actual Student Time Needed to Complete Procedure: ____________

Student's Initials: ____________ Instructor's Initials: ____________ Grade: ____________

Suggestions for Improvement: ________________________________

Evaluator's Name (print) ________________________________

Evaluator's Signature ________________________________

Comments ________________________________

SKILLS COMPETENCY ASSESSMENT

Procedure 21–2: Instrument Sanitization

Student's Name: ______________________________ Date: ____________

Objective: To properly clean contaminated instruments to remove tissue or debris.

Conditions: The student demonstrates the ability to properly clean contaminated instruments using a sink (or ultrasonic cleaner), sanitizing agent, brush, disposable paper towels, disposable gloves, and biohazard waste container.

Time Requirements and Accuracy Standards: 5 minutes. Points assigned reflect importance of step to meeting objective: Important = (5) Essential = (10) Critical = (15). Automatic failure results if any of the **critical** tasks are omitted or performed incorrectly.

STANDARD PRECAUTIONS:

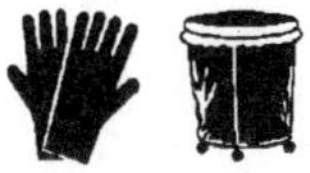

SKILLS ASSESSMENT CHECKLIST

Task Performed	Possible Points	TASKS
☐	5	Wears disposable gloves in accordance with OSHA standards.
☐	10	Rinses contaminated instrument immediately in water and disinfectant solution; rinses instrument again under running water.
☐	5	*Rationale:* Understands importance of rinsing instrument as quickly as possible after a procedure to help prevent debris from adhering to it.
☐	5	To carry contaminated instrument from one place to another to sanitize it, places instrument in a basin labeled "Biohazard."
☐	15	Scrubs each instrument well with detergent and water; scrubs under running water and scrubs any inside edges and all surfaces.
☐	10	Rinses well under hot water.
☐	5	*Rationale:* Understands that rinsing with hot water will remove residue and aid in the drying process while eliminating rust and water spots.
☐	5	After rinsing, places instruments on muslin or disposable paper towel until all instruments are scrubbed.
☐	10	*Rationale:* Understands danger of recontamination of instruments.

SKILLS COMPETENCY ASSESSMENT — continued

Procedure 21–2: Instrument Sanitization

Task Performed	Possible Points	TASKS
❑	10	Dries instruments with muslin or disposable paper towels.
❑	5	*Rationale:* Understands that wet instruments may rust or corrode.
❑	5	Completed the tasks within 5 minutes.
❑	15	Results obtained were accurate.

________	Earned	ADD POINTS OF TASKS CHECKED
105	Points	TOTAL POINTS POSSIBLE
________	SCORE	DETERMINE SCORE (divide points earned by total points possible, multiply results by 100)

Actual Student Time Needed to Complete Procedure: ____________

Student's Initials: ____________ Instructor's Initials: ____________ Grade: ____________

Suggestions for Improvement: ____

____

____

____

Evaluator's Name (print) ____

Evaluator's Signature ____

Comments ____

SKILLS COMPETENCY ASSESSMENT

Procedure 21–3: Removing Contaminated Gloves

Student's Name: ______________________________ Date: __________

Objective: To remove and dispose of contaminated gloves in order to contain exposure.

Conditions: Student demonstrates the ability to remove and dispose of contaminated gloves using a biohazard waste receptacle.

Time Requirements and Accuracy Standards: 5 minutes. Points assigned reflect importance of step to meeting objective: Important = (5) Essential = (10) Critical = (15). Automatic failure results if any of the **critical** tasks are omitted or performed incorrectly.

STANDARD PRECAUTIONS:

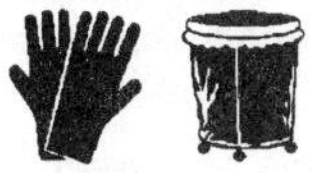

SKILLS ASSESSMENT CHECKLIST

Task Performed	Possible Points	TASKS
☐	10	Grasps the palm of the used left glove with the right hand to begin removing the first glove, holding hands away from the body and pointed downward.
☐	15	Pulls off the used left glove and encases it in the right gloved hand.
☐	10	Holds the left glove that has been removed in the right gloved hand; inserts two fingers of the ungloved left hand between the right arm and the inside of the right glove.
☐	15	Turns the right dirty glove inside out over the other. One glove is now inside the other glove.
☐	15	Disposes of the inverted gloves into a biohazard waste receptacle.
☐	15	*Rationale:* Understands that biological waste should be placed in a red biohazard bag.
☐	10	Immediately washes hands thoroughly.
☐	5	Completed the tasks within 5 minutes.
☐	15	Results obtained were accurate.
______	Earned	ADD POINTS OF TASKS CHECKED
100	Points	TOTAL POINTS POSSIBLE
______	SCORE	DETERMINE SCORE (divide points earned by total points possible, multiply results by 100)

Actual Student Time Needed to Complete Procedure: __________

Student's Initials: __________ Instructor's Initials: __________ Grade: __________

Suggestions for Improvement: ______________________________

Evaluator's Name (print) ______________________________

Evaluator's Signature ______________________________

Comments ______________________________

SKILLS COMPETENCY ASSESSMENT

Procedure 21–4: Instrument/Equipment Chemical Disinfection or Chemical Sterilization

Student's Name: ______________________________ Date: ____________

Objective: To achieve medical asepsis for instruments to be used during external physical examinations or procedures, such as thermometers (chemical disinfection), and to achieve surgical asepsis for instruments and equipment to be used during internal physical examinations or procedures, such as surgical instruments and proctological equipment (chemical sterilization).

Conditions: Student demonstrates the ability to achieve medical and surgical asepsis by appropriately and fully disinfecting or sterilizing instruments or equipment using an airtight container, disinfectant chemical solution, a timer or clock, distilled water for disinfection, sterile water for sterilization, disposable gloves, and a biohazard waste container.

Time Requirements and Accuracy Standards: 5 minutes. Points assigned reflect importance of step to meeting objective: Important = (5) Essential = (10) Critical = (15). Automatic failure results if any of the **critical** tasks are omitted or performed incorrectly.

STANDARD PRECAUTIONS:

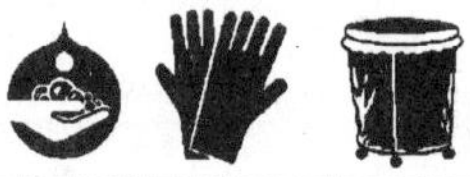

SKILLS ASSESSMENT CHECKLIST

Task Performed	Possible Points	TASKS
		Chemical Disinfection
☐	10	Sanitizes instruments as shown in Procedure 21–2 that require medical aseptic chemical disinfection.
☐	5	*Rationale:* Sanitization must precede disinfection in order to remove debris. Understands that medical asepsis is not sterile and should not be used for instruments employed in invasive procedures requiring sterile technique.
☐	15	Reads the manufacturer's instructions on the original container of chemical disinfectant solution.
☐	5	*Rationale:* Is able to choose the chemical disinfectant solution with the specific preparation instructions and germicidal properties that best suits the needs of the ambulatory care setting.
☐	5	Puts on disposable gloves to prevent burning or irritation to the skin.
☐	15	Prepares solution as indicated by manufacturer.
☐	5	Writes own initials and date of opening or preparation directly on the container.
☐	10	Pours prepared solution into a container with an airtight lid, avoiding splashing.

Task Performed	Possible Points	TASKS
❑	5	*Rationale:* Understands that open containers can cause accidental inhalation of fumes or poisoning; splashing can cause skin, inhalation, or mucous membrane contact.
❑	10	Places sanitized instruments into solution, covering instruments completely; avoids splashing.
❑	5	*Rationale:* Understands that if instruments are not covered with solution, disinfection cannot occur.
❑	5	Closes lid of container.
❑	10	Labels container with name of solution, exposure time, and initials.
❑	15	Does not open or add additional instruments during disinfection period.
❑	5	*Rationale:* Understands that adding instruments during disinfection procedure limits effectiveness of the disinfectant solution.
❑	15	Waits required exposure time and lifts items from the container tray; rinses well under distilled water or tap water, according to the manufacturer's instructions.
❑	5	*Rationale:* Understands that using instruments without rinsing off chemical disinfectant solution can irritate the patient's skin and may corrode instruments over time, as solution is caustic.
❑	10	Removes instruments and places them on muslin or disposable paper towel.
❑	15	Dries instruments with muslin or paper towel.
❑	5	Properly discards used chemical disinfectant.
❑	5	Removes gloves.
❑	5	Stores instruments and/or equipment in a clean, dry area.
❑	5	Documents procedure.
		Chemical Sterilization
❑	10	Follows procedures for chemical disinfection above, beginning with the sanitization of instruments or equipment. Recalls that the difference between chemical disinfection and chemical sterilization is the type of solution used and the exposure time to the chemical solution.
❑	15	Reads the manufacturer's instructions for exposure time to achieve chemical sterilization.
❑	5	*Rationale:* Understands correct exposure time for sterilization is longer than time for disinfection.
❑	15	Following recommended exposure time, removes instruments with sterile transfer forceps to protect sterility. Rinses under sterile water.

SKILLS COMPETENCY ASSESSMENT — continued

Procedure 21–4: Instrument/Equipment Chemical Disinfection or Chemical Sterilization

Task Performed	Possible Points	TASKS
❑	15	Dries instrument with a sterile muslin towel.
❑	5	*Rationale:* Understands that wet instruments will contaminate a sterile field.
❑	15	Places the sterilized dry instrument on the sterile field with the sterile transfer forceps.
❑	5	Changes the solution as recommended by the manufacturer.
❑	5	Removes gloves.
❑	5	Documents the procedure.
❑	5	Completed the tasks within 5 minutes.
❑	15	Results obtained were accurate.

______	Earned	ADD POINTS OF TASKS CHECKED
305	Points	TOTAL POINTS POSSIBLE
______	SCORE	DETERMINE SCORE (divide points earned by total points possible, multiply results by 100)

Actual Student Time Needed to Complete Procedure: ____________

Student's Initials: ____________ Instructor's Initials: ____________ Grade: ____________

Suggestions for Improvement: ____

Evaluator's Name (print) ____

Evaluator's Signature ____

Comments ____

DOCUMENTATION

Record disinfected or sterilized instruments/equipment in the chemical disinfection/sterilization log book.

Date: ____________

Chemical Disinfection Documentation: ____

____

Chemical Sterilization Documentation: ____

____

Student's Initials: ____________

SKILLS COMPETENCY ASSESSMENT

Procedure 21–5: Wrapping Instruments for Sterilization in Autoclave

Student's Name: ______________________________ Date: ____________

Objective: To properly wrap sanitized instruments for sterilization in an autoclave.

Conditions: Student demonstrates the ability to properly wrap sanitized instruments for sterilization in autoclave using the following equipment: sanitized instruments, wrapping material (muslin or disposable wrapping paper), sterilization indicator, 2 × 2 gauze or cotton balls (if instrument has sharp edges), autoclave wrapping tape, and permanent marker or felt-tipped pen.

Time Requirements and Accuracy Standards: 5 minutes. Points assigned reflect importance of step to meeting objective: Important = (5) Essential = (10) Critical = (15). Automatic failure results if any of the **critical** tasks are omitted or performed incorrectly.

SKILLS ASSESSMENT CHECKLIST

Task Performed	Possible Points	TASKS
❑	10	Prepares a clean, dry, flat surface of adequate size to lay wrapping material.
❑	5	*Rationale:* Understands that a clean area reduces the risk of contamination.
❑	5	Selects two wraps of adequate size in which to wrap instruments.
❑	5	Places one square of wrapping material at an angle in front of the body on the dry surface with one corner pointed directly at the torso.
❑	5	Places the sanitized instruments or articles to be placed in the autoclave just below the center of the wrap.
❑	15	Opens instruments with hinges as wide as possible and places a 2 × 2 gauze or cotton ball in the opening.
❑	5	*Rationale:* Understands that instruments with hinged parts that are not spread wide open prior to autoclaving may not be properly sterilized.
❑	10	Places one sterilization indicator with the instrument.
❑	5	Brings corner of the wrap closest to the body up and over the article toward the center.
❑	5	Brings the tip of the same corner back toward the body until it reaches the folded edge, creating a fan-fold effect.
❑	5	Smooths edges of the fold; article remains completely covered.
❑	5	Folds one side edge toward the center line; fan-folds back to side and creases.

SKILLS COMPETENCY ASSESSMENT — continued

Procedure 21–5: Wrapping Instruments for Sterilization in Autoclave

Task Performed	Possible Points	TASKS
❑	15	Repeats previous step for the other side edge.
❑	5	Folds the package up from the bottom.
❑	5	Folds the top edge down and over the entire package.
❑	5	*Rationale:* Understands that if wrap does not cover the entire package, items must be unwrapped and rewrapped with a larger piece of wrapping material.
❑	15	To "wrap twice," places package into the center of a second wrap and repeats correct procedures for wrapping package within the second piece of wrapping material.
❑	5	*Rationale:* Wrap twice allows the outer wrap of a double-wrapped item to be removed so the inside wrapped item can be placed onto a sterile field.
❑	10	Tapes with autoclave tape across the point left exposed.
❑	5	*Rationale:* Understands that autoclave tape is not an indicator of sterilization or quality control, but only that the package has been through the autoclave.
❑	15	Labels the tape with names of instruments or type of pack, date of sterilization, and initials.
❑	5	*Rationale:* Understands that dating package provides a method for assessing its sterility over time.
❑	15	Immediately places wrapped instruments in autoclave after dating. If package is not placed immediately into the autoclave, waits to date package until just before autoclaving.
❑	5	Documents procedure.
❑	5	Completed the tasks within 5 minutes.
❑	15	Results obtained were accurate.

________	Earned	ADD POINTS OF TASKS CHECKED
205	Points	TOTAL POINTS POSSIBLE
________	SCORE	DETERMINE SCORE (divide points earned by total points possible, multiply results by 100)

Actual Student Time Needed to Complete Procedure: ____________

Student's Initials: ____________ Instructor's Initials: ____________ Grade: ____________

Suggestions for Improvement: ____

____

____

____

Evaluator's Name (print) ____

Evaluator's Signature ____

Comments ____

DOCUMENTATION

Record the label information for the instrument or type of pack wrapped.

Date: ______________

Label: ____

____

Student's Initials: __________

SKILLS COMPETENCY ASSESSMENT

Procedure 21–6: Steam Sterilization (Autoclave)

Student's Name: ______________________________ Date: ____________

Objective: To rid instruments for use in invasive procedures of all forms of microbial life.

Conditions: Student demonstrates the ability to rid instruments and other equipment of microorganisms using a steam sterilizer (autoclave), autoclave manufacturer procedure manual, and wrapped sanitized instrument packages with sterilization indicators placed inside (or unwrapped item if removed with sterile transfer forceps).

Time Requirements and Accuracy Standards: 15 minutes. Points assigned reflect importance of step to meeting objective: Important = (5) Essential = (10) Critical = (15). Automatic failure results if any of the **critical** tasks are omitted or performed incorrectly.

SKILLS ASSESSMENT CHECKLIST

Task Performed	Possible Points	TASKS
❑	5	Checks water level in reservoir; adds distilled water to "fill line."
❑	15	Loads packages into autoclave tray; allows three inches between packages; avoids stacking directly on top of other packages.
❑	10	**Jars:** Loads jars of dressings or cups on their sides, with tops ajar or loosely in place.
❑	10	**Packages:** Loads cloth or dressing packages vertically, three inches apart.
❑	15	**Unwrapped items:** Loads unwrapped items vertically, three inches apart, not allowing any item to touch another item.
❑	15	**Unwrapped instruments:** Loads unwrapped instruments flat with handles opened.
❑	5	Closes autoclave door and seals.
❑	15	Turns on autoclave and sets temperature to achieve 250–254° F (121° C) and 15 pounds of pressure according to the manufacturer's guidelines.
❑	10	When the temperature dial indicates that the proper temperature and pressure have been achieved inside the autoclave, begins necessary exposure time by setting timer.
❑	5	*Rationale:* Can identify proper length of exposure time required for wrapped instrument packages or trays, unwrapped items, and unwrapped items covered with cloth.
❑	5	Does not attempt to open the door during the autoclave cycle.
❑	10	Following completion of the autoclave cycle, exhausts steam pressure from the autoclave by following the manufacturer's instructions.
❑	10	Opens the door approximately 1 inch after the pressure gauge indicates zero (0) pressure and the temperature gauge indicates a decrease to at least 212° F. (Some autoclaves have a drying cycle, eliminating the need for opening the autoclave one inch.)

Task Performed	Possible Points	TASKS
☐	5	*Rationale:* Understands that injuries can occur if autoclave door is opened sooner.
☐	15	Allows contents to completely dry, ten to fifteen minutes.
☐	5	*Rationale:* Understands that if wet or damp packages are handled or placed on a countertop while warm, they will become contaminated by microorganisms.
☐	10	Removes wrapped contents with dry, clean hands and stores in clean, dry area reserved for sterilized packages only. If the outer wrapper is required to remain sterile, removes package with sterile transfer forceps and places on a sterile field or in a sterile storage area.
☐	10	Removes unwrapped contents with sterile transfer forceps; resanitizes and resterilizes the transfer forceps following use. (Sterile transfer forceps must have been sterilized immediately prior to or along with the unwrapped item.)
☐	5	Documents the procedure.
☐	10	Performs quality control by monitoring sterilization indicators with each use of sterilized instruments.
☐	15	Documents on a weekly basis sterilization indicator outcome in quality control log; dates and initials log entries.
☐	5	Completed the tasks within 15 minutes.
☐	15	Results obtained were accurate.

_______	Earned	ADD POINTS OF TASKS CHECKED
225	Points	TOTAL POINTS POSSIBLE
_______	SCORE	DETERMINE SCORE (divide points earned by total points possible, multiply results by 100)

Actual Student Time Needed to Complete Procedure: ____________

Student's Initials: ____________ Instructor's Initials: ____________ Grade: ____________

Suggestions for Improvement: ______________________________

Evaluator's Name (print) ______________________________

Evaluator's Signature ______________________________

Comments ______________________________

DOCUMENTATION

Document the procedure in the autoclave quality control log: ______________________________

____

____

____

Student's Initials: __________

EVALUATION OF CHAPTER KNOWLEDGE

How has your instructor evaluated the knowledge you have gained?

	Instructor Evaluation		
Knowledge	*Good*	*Average*	*Poor*
Defines key vocabulary terms correctly	_____	_____	_____
Identifies and understands the importance of infection control in the ambulatory care setting	_____	_____	_____
Observes universal and standard precautions	_____	_____	_____
Defines the five classifications of infectious organisms	_____	_____	_____
Describes the four stages of infectious diseases	_____	_____	_____
States and describes the four phases of immune response	_____	_____	_____
Understands the purpose of rapid sanitization of contaminated instruments	_____	_____	_____
Identifies four methods of sterilization	_____	_____	_____
Defines both surgical and medical asepsis	_____	_____	_____
Demonstrates ability to perform competent wrapping technique and proper operation of the autoclave with sanitized instrument packages	_____	_____	_____
States supplies and equipment used to achieve surgical asepsis when using an autoclave	_____	_____	_____
Performs accurate documentation of procedures	_____	_____	_____

Student's Initials: ______ Instructor's Initials: ______

Grade: _______

CHAPTER 22

Taking a Medical History

PERFORMANCE OBJECTIVES

The patient's medical history is an invaluable tool in helping the physician treat the patient effectively. When taking or updating patient medical histories, medical assistants must be as thorough and accurate in documentation as possible, while remaining respectful of the patient's emotional needs and right to privacy. Therapeutic communication skills, including, but not limited to, active listening, recognizing nonverbal cues, and adapting communication to the patient's ability to understand, are essential to the process of obtaining accurate and complete patient medical histories.

EXERCISES AND ACTIVITIES

Vocabulary Builder

Match each key vocabulary term to the example that best describes it.

A. Allergies
B. Chart
C. Chief complaint
D. Clinical diagnosis
E. Debridement
F. Differential diagnosis
G. Familial
H. Objective sign
I. Problem-Oriented Medical Record (POMR)
J. SOAP
K. Source-Oriented Medical Record (SOMR)
L. Subjective complaint

______ **1.** 3/10/xx CC: NVD × 4 days. T > 100° F × 2 days. Loss of appetite.

Decode this chart note: ____

____

A mistake is made in the chart note on the previous page. Three days should be listed instead of four. Using the proper procedure for notation, enter a correction to the chart note in the space provided below:

3/10/xx CC: NVD × 4 days. T > 100° F × 2 days. Loss of appetite.

______ **2.** Diseases or conditions with genetic links such as breast and colon cancers, coronary artery disease, diabetes mellitus, and hypertension.

______ **3.** Removal of dead or damaged tissue or foreign debris.

______ **4.** Mary O'Keefe calls Dr. King's office to schedule an emergency appointment and tells Ellen Armstrong, CMA, that her 3-year-old son Chris awakened during the night with a high fever and extreme pain in his right ear.

______ **5.** Dr. King examines 3-year-old Chris O'Keefe's right ear with an otoscope and observes that the ear is inflamed; the ear is also draining.

______ **6.** When a 19-year-old young woman comes into Inner City Health Care with extreme abdominal pain localized to the lower right quadrant, vomiting, slight fever, and loss of appetite, Dr. Whitney orders a CBC, a urinalysis, and an abdominal ultrasound to distinguish between possible diagnoses of acute appendicitis or an ovarian cyst that has become twisted.

Include proper insurance coding for each test Dr. Whitney has ordered, to be included on the patient's charge slip.

(1) ______________________________

(2) ______________________________

(3) ______________________________

What are the proper diagnosis codes for the two diagnoses Dr. Whitney is investigating for this emergency patient?

(1) ______________________________

(2) ______________________________

Will the physician code a diagnosis for the patient at this time? If so, what diagnosis will be used? If not, what kind of information will the physician code in place of a diagnosis?

____

____

______ **7.** Dr. Whitney confirms a diagnosis of acute appendicitis for the female emergency patient, based on subjective and objective information accumulated from the patient's history, the findings of the physical examination, and the results of the laboratory tests ordered.

______ **8.** A patient's file of medical history and treatment, kept by the physician.

______ **9.** A traditional form of charting that consists of a chronological set of notes for each visit, beginning with the patient's first visit.

______ **10.** Charting method that lists patient data in the following order: Subjective/Objective/Assessment/Plan.

_____ 11. An acquired sensitivity to a substance (allergen) that does not normally cause a reaction.

_____ 12. The most efficient way of recording chart notes, especially in multi-physician clinics or practices.

Learning Review

1. Every physician/patient interview is a cross-cultural one. List four questions a medical assistant might ask while taking a medical history that will help bridge social and cultural beliefs to obtain accurate information about a patient's condition that the physician will need to give proper care and treatment.

   (1) ______________________________

   (2) ______________________________

   (3) ______________________________

   (4) ______________________________

2. List the nine possible characteristics of patient chief complaints:

   (1) ______________ (6) ______________

   (2) ______________ (7) ______________

   (3) ______________ (8) ______________

   (4) ______________ (9) ______________

   (5) ______________

3. Decode each component of the chart note excerpt listed below.

A.	7/15/xxxx	
B.	CC: lower abdominal pain $\times$ 1 wk $\bar{c}$ $\uparrow$ malaise.	
C.	Wt. 135 Ht. 5'5" T 99.8°F R 19 clear P 78 regular BP 134/82	
D	Pt describes $\uparrow$ urge to urinate $\bar{c}$ burning sensation on urination; pressure in abdomen; lack of energy.	
E.	Past Med Hist	freq. UTIs dx Type II diabetes mellitus 1987; Rx Glynase 3 mg tab qd quit smoking 20 yrs ago weight $\downarrow$ 10lbs in last 2 yrs.
F.	Allergies	no known
G.	Family Hist	no Δ
H.	Habits	< 2 glasses wine per wk no smoking, regular exercise

A. ______________________________

B. ______________________________

C. ______________________________

D. ______________________________

E. ______________________________

F. ______________________________

G. ______________________________

H. ______________________________

4. After the history is taken by the medical assistant, the physician will perform a review of systems (ROS). In addition to the patient's general state of health, list ten body systems the physician will assess during the ROS.

(1) ______________	(6) ______________
(2) ______________	(7) ______________
(3) ______________	(8) ______________
(4) ______________	(9) ______________
(5) ______________	(10) ______________

Investigation Activity

It is important for the medical assistant to be aware of his or her own family medical history. Knowledge of diseases and conditions that occur within one's family can give a health care team invaluable information that may aid in a swift, accurate diagnosis and treatment of health problems. And, a knowledge of diseases and illnesses that "run" in families can give individuals an important head start in pursuing effective preventive measures.

Create your own family medical genogram. This genogram, or "family" tree, can be referenced quickly and easily and will reveal patterns of disease or illness within your family. You'll want to start by including four generations: yourself, your siblings (if any), your children (if any), your parents, and your grandparents. The genogram should only include individuals who are related to you by blood. Create the genogram using the following symbols recommended by the Task Force of the North American Primary Care Research Group:

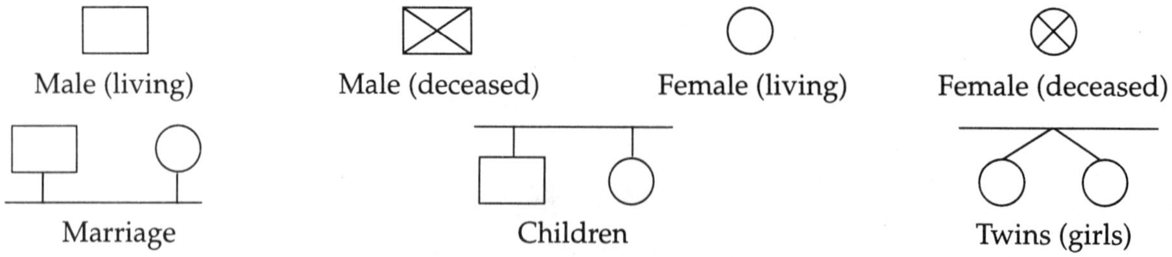

Within each symbol, fill in the relative's name and year of birth. Also include the year of death for those who are deceased. Underneath each symbol, write in as many diseases, conditions, or health care problems specific to that relative of which you are aware. For example, a relative may smoke, be overweight, or have had a heart attack. Use the completed genogram to evaluate your own health priorities and to adopt healthy lifestyle changes accordingly.

Here is a sample completed genogram for Martin Gordon and his sister Margaret.

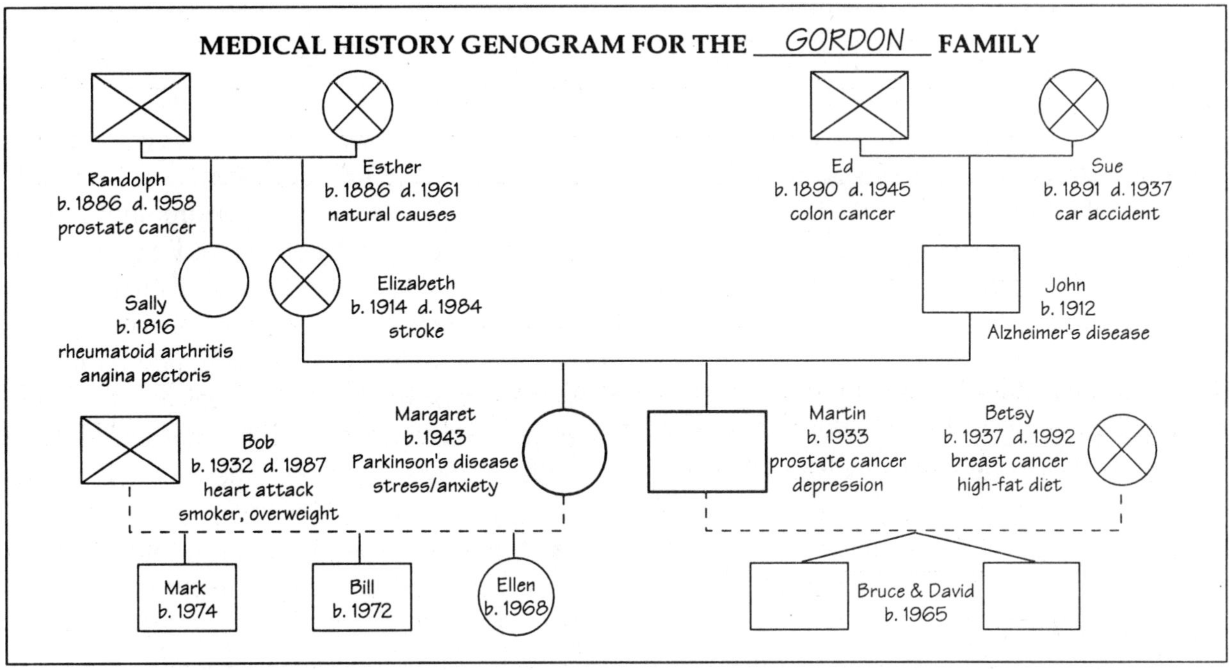

Complete the genogram below, which has been started, by entering symbols to represent your grandparents.

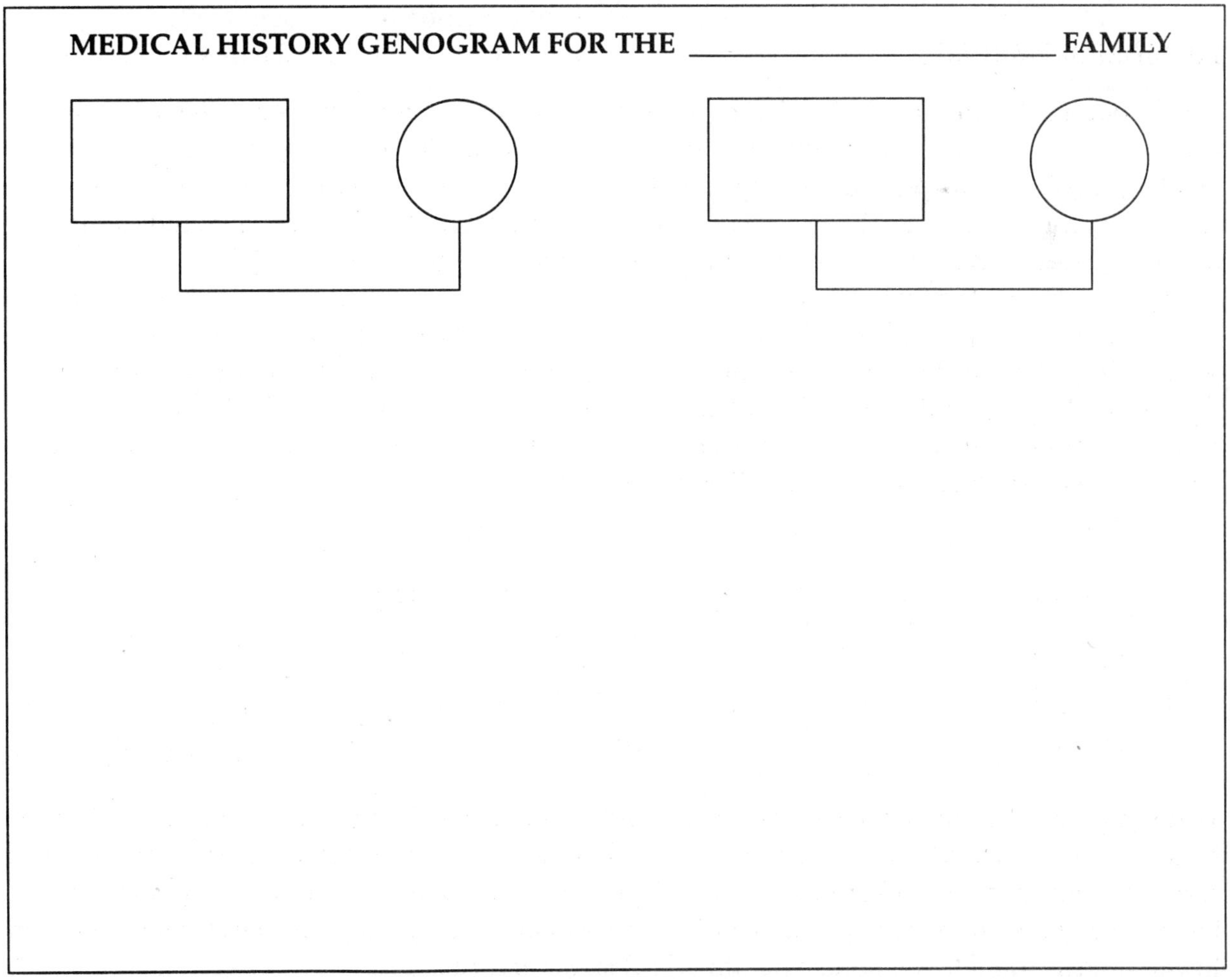

CASE STUDY

Nancy Catalina is a new patient of Dr. Esposito's at Inner City Health Care. Nancy, an 88-year-old Italian-born woman, comes to see Dr. Esposito at the urging of her granddaughter Leslie, who has set up the appointment for her. Nancy's primary care physician of thirty-five years has just retired; her only criteria for a new physician is that the physician must be of Italian descent.

When scheduling the appointment, Leslie notes to Liz Corbin, CMA, her grandmother's past medical history of mild angina pectoris, high blood pressure, hiatal hernia, and rheumatoid arthritis. On the day of the exam, Liz questions Nancy directly about her medical history. Nancy talks extensively about her aches and pains, moving back and forth in time between current problems and problems that took place as distant as forty years ago. In each case, a gentle reminder from her granddaughter brings Nancy back to a discussion of her present physical condition. Upon each reminder, Nancy acknowledges the difference between past and current events and admits she had gotten off track, though this is not readily apparent from her answers to Liz. It is clear that Leslie's knowledge of her grandmother's life and medical history makes it possible for Leslie to distinguish between events in Nancy's past and events in her present, guiding her back to the task at hand: taking a current medical history for the patient's permanent record.

Discuss the following:

1. What communications skills will Liz need to use to get the most accurate information from Nancy?
2. What can the manner in which this patient relates information reveal about her?
3. What effect does Nancy's granddaughter have on the process of taking the medical history? Is the effect beneficial or disruptive?

SUPPLEMENTARY RESOURCES

Study Guide Disk: Additional practice exercises for this chapter are available on the study guide disk found in the back of the textbook.

Medical Assisting Videos: Appropriate content is available on Delmar's Medical Assisting Videos, 2nd ed. Tape 8, for the following topics:

Interview and Take Patient History
Take an In-depth Patient History
Introduction to Health Promotion, Disease Prevention, and Self-Responsibility

SKILLS COMPETENCY ASSESSMENT

Procedure 22–1: Taking a Medical History

Student's Name: ______________________________ Date: ____________

Objective: To obtain a medical history from a patient new to the ambulatory care setting.

Conditions: To obtain a medical history from a new patient using the following equipment and supplies: patient history forms, clipboard, pens.

Time Requirements and Accuracy Standards: 15 minutes. Points assigned reflect importance of step to meeting objective: Important = (5) Essential = (10) Critical = (15). Automatic failure results if any of the **critical** tasks are omitted or performed incorrectly.

SKILLS ASSESSMENT CHECKLIST

Task Performed	Possible Points	TASKS
❑	5	Performs introductions. Confirms identity of new patient and escorts to examination room or private area.
❑	5	Makes eye contact and uses positive body language to put patient at ease.
❑	5	Explains purpose and importance of obtaining patient information. Asks questions on the form, trying to get as much information as possible without letting the patient deviate from the subject.
❑	10	Asks each question clearly. Makes sure patient understands all questions.
❑	15	Repeats the patient's answers when needed to confirm. Is specific in documentation of answers.
❑	10	Writes legibly using dark ink (blue or black).
❑	15	Rechecks the medical history form for completeness. Notes any additional information provided by the patient. Makes sure numbers, dates, spelling, and other information are accurate and legible.
❑	5	Prepares the patient for the review of systems and physical examination, if indicated.
❑	10	Documents the procedure.
❑	5	Completed the tasks within 15 minutes.
❑	15	Results obtained were accurate.
______	Earned	ADD POINTS OF TASKS CHECKED
100	Points	TOTAL POINTS POSSIBLE
______	SCORE	DETERMINE SCORE (divide points earned by total points possible, multiply results by 100)

SKILLS COMPETENCY ASSESSMENT — continued

Procedure 22–1: Taking a Medical History

Actual Student Time Needed to Complete Procedure: ____________

Student's Initials: ____________ Instructor's Initials: ____________ Grade: ____________

Suggestions for Improvement: ____

____

____

____

Evaluator's Name (print) ____

Evaluator's Signature ____

Comments ____

DOCUMENTATION

Chart the procedure in the patient's medical record.

Date: ____________________________

Charting: ____

____

____

____

Student's Initials: ________________

EVALUATION OF CHAPTER KNOWLEDGE

How has your instructor evaluated the knowledge you have achieved?

Knowledge	**Instructor Evaluation** *Good*	*Average*	*Poor*
Understands the necessity and function of the medical history in patient treatment	_____	_____	_____
Defines the parts of the medical history	_____	_____	_____
Identifies and uses effective methods of interacting with patient	_____	_____	_____
Obtains a medical history from patient	_____	_____	_____
Explains different methods of charting/documentation	_____	_____	_____
Defines SOAP and relates the function of this charting approach	_____	_____	_____
Understands issues of cultural sensitivity in taking a medical history	_____	_____	_____
Adapts communication to individuals' abilities to understand	_____	_____	_____
Performs within ethical boundaries	_____	_____	_____
Exhibits therapeutic communications skills	_____	_____	_____
Documents accurately	_____	_____	_____
Serves as liaison between physician and others	_____	_____	_____

Student's Initials: ______ Instructor's Initials: ______

Grade: _______

CHAPTER 23

Vital Signs and Measurements

PERFORMANCE OBJECTIVES

One of the primary tasks of medical assistants is measuring patients' vital signs. The vital or cardinal signs—temperature, pulse, respiration (TPR) and blood pressure (B/P)—are important indicators of general health and must be measured and recorded with care. Because every individual's normal vital signs are different from those of every other person, the initial visit at any medical practice is usually used to record the patient's baseline vital signs. The baseline gives medical professionals an idea of what is normal for that patient and provides a point of comparison for use during future visits. For this reason, accuracy is especially important when recording vital signs at each patient's first visit. Medical assistants need to recognize factors that may influence the results of vital signs. Weight and height measurements may also be taken as further indications of the patient's condition. Aseptic techniques must be observed when taking patients' vital signs.

EXERCISES AND ACTIVITIES

Vocabulary Builder

Insert one of the following key vocabulary terms into each sentence describing a clinical situation.

Apnea
Arrhythmia
Baseline
Bradycardia
Bradypnea
Cheyne-Stokes
Diastole
Dyspnea
Emphysema
Eupnea
Frenulum
Hyperpnea
Hypertension
Hyperventilation
Hypotension
Hypoventilation
Orthopnea
Rales
Rhonchi
Stertorous
Stridor
Systole
Tachycardia
Tachypnea
Wheezes

1. Maria Jover comes to the office of Drs. Lewis and King complaining that she cannot breathe when she lies down. Joe Guerrero, CMA, notes ______________________ on her chart.

(3) After 3 minutes of strong aerobic activity, such as jumping jacks or jogging in place.

____

(4) Note the variations in the characteristics of the pulse and respiration as your body moved from rest to strong activity.

____

____

(5) Calculate the ratio of respiration to pulse for your resting, active, and aerobic rates listed earler. Show your calculations in the spaces provided.

Rest Active Aerobic

____

Investigation Activity

Baseline vital signs can differ widely among healthy people. What is normal for one person may be an indication of illness for another. It is important for medical assistants to appreciate and understand these variations as well as the variations that different measurement methods can cause.

A. Choose one method of temperature measurement and use it to obtain baseline body temperatures for ten different people who are not suffering from any illnesses. Your subjects should be as varied as possible in age and other factors; be sure to include both males and females. Try to take each temperature at the same time of day. Fill in all of the information required in the chart below, using the proper method of recording temperatures.

Baseline Temperature Chart

Measurement Method Used: _______________________

Patient	Age	Gender	Time of Day	Temperature
A				
B				
C				
D				
E				
F				
G				
H				
I				
J				

What conclusions can you draw from this sample? _______________________

____

____

____

What other variables can you think of that might affect baseline body temperature? ________

____

____

____

B. Now take several temperature readings on one patient using each type of measurement equipment. Take the readings in sequence, all at one time. Fill in the chart below, using the proper method of recording temperatures.

Temperature Measurement Methods

Patient Age: __________ **Gender:** ___________ **Time of Day:** __________

Method	Temperature
Mercury thermometer, oral	
Mercury thermometer, rectal	
Mercury thermometer, axillary	
Disposable strip thermometer, oral	
Digital thermometer, oral	
Tympanic thermometer, aural	

What conclusions can you draw from this experiment? ____________________

____

____

____

Why do you think body temperature readings are affected by the methods used to measure them?

____

____

____

CASE STUDIES

As a medical assistant, you can expect to take patients' vital signs as a regular part of your work routine. You will have to make decisions about the equipment and methods used to make these measurements and answer patients' questions about each procedure. For each of the following scenarios, discuss the following.

1. What measurement method and/or site is the medical assistant most likely to use in this case, and why?
2. What is the medical assistant's best therapeutic response to the patient?

Case 1

Wayne Elder lives near Inner City Health Care in a group home for developmentally disabled adults. Wayne has a history of ear infections and colds in both ears. He visits the clinic one morning with dizziness and pain in his right ear. As Wanda Slawson, CMA, prepares to take Wayne's temperature, she learns that he drank a cup of hot coffee just before walking to the clinic. Wayne Elder asks, "How come you need to know what I ate? It's my ear that hurts."

Case 2

Henry Hansen is rushed to Inner City Health Care unconscious. He is bleeding profusely from a cut on his face. "He fell down the stairs," sobs Henry's mother, Juanita. Administrative medical assistant Karen Ritter alerts Dr. James Whitney, one of the clinic physicians, and calls 911 to summon emergency services personnel. The first thing clinical medical assistant Bruce Goldman does, after determining that Henry is breathing, is to take Henry's pulse. "What are you doing?" Juanita who is almost hysterical now, screams. "Why aren't you waking him up?"

Case 3

A. Abigail Johnson, who suffers from many of the problems of advancing age, including diabetes mellitus, is an elderly patient of Elizabeth King, M.D. A friendly woman, Abigail has a good rapport with everyone in the office—all of whom, she says, are "just like family"—and is eager to please the staff. One winter day she comes in with possible flu symptoms. As Audrey Jones, CMA, goes through the usual check of vital signs, Abigail audibly changes her breathing pattern, deepening and regularizing her respiration.

B. When Audrey asks Abigail to prepare for a weight measurement, Abigail says, "Oh, do we have to do that today? I'm just not up to it. Besides, I don't want to know how much I weigh right now. When I feel better, then I'll focus on losing more weight. You understand how I feel, don't you?"

SUPPLEMENTARY RESOURCES

Study Guide Disk: Additional practice exercises for this chapter are available on the study guide disk found in the back of the textbook.

Medical Assisting Videos: Appropriate content is available on Delmar's Medical Assisting Videos, 2nd ed., for the following topics:

Tape 6 Take Vital Signs
- Take and Record Oral Temperature Using a Glass Thermometer
- Take and Record Rectal Temperature
- Take and Record Oral Temperature Using an Electronic Thermometer
- Take and Record An Aural (Ear) Temperature
- Take and Record Axillary (Underarm) Temperature
- Take and Record a Radial Pulse
- Take and Record a Brachial Pulse (Infant)
- Use a Stethoscope to Take an Apical Pulse (Adult)
- Use a Stethoscope to Take an Apical Pulse (Infant)
- Take and Record Respiration

Tape 7 Take and Record Blood Pressure
- Measure Height and Weight Using an Upright Scale

SKILLS COMPETENCY ASSESSMENT

Procedure 23–1: Taking an Oral Temperature Using a Mercury Thermometer

Student's Name: ______________________________ Date: ____________

Objective: To obtain an oral temperature.

Conditions: The student demonstrates the ability to take an oral temperature using the following equipment and supplies: mercury thermometer, disposable thermometer sheaths, gloves, paper towels, biohazard waste container.

Time Requirements and Accuracy Standards: 10 minutes. Points assigned reflect importance of step to meeting objective: Important = (5) Essential = (10) Critical = (15). Automatic failure results if any of the **critical** tasks are omitted or performed incorrectly.

STANDARD PRECAUTIONS:

SKILLS ASSESSMENT CHECKLIST

Task Performed	Possible Points	TASKS
☐	5	Washes hands and follows standard precautions.
☐	5	Assembles equipment.
☐	5	Identifies patient and positions patient comfortably.
☐	10	Determines if patient has ingested hot or cold food or drink, or has smoked, in the previous half hour.
☐	5	*Rationale:* Understands that food ingestion or smoking can arbitrarily affect oral temperature reading.
☐	5	Explains procedure.
☐	10	Shakes thermometer until it reads below 96.0°F.
☐	5	Covers thermometer with sheath.
☐	5	Applies gloves.
☐	5	Inserts thermometer under patient's tongue to the side of the mouth.
☐	5	*Rationale:* Understands the anatomy of the tongue and the need to avoid the patient's frenulum.
☐	10	Instructs patient to close mouth around thermometer but not to place the teeth on it.
☐	5	*Rationale:* Understands the necessity of preventing air leakage and to avoid patient biting.
☐	15	Leaves in place for 3 to 5 minutes.

Task Performed	Possible Points	TASKS
☐	10	Removes thermometer from mouth, removing sheath and disposing it in a biohazard waste container.
☐	5	Holds thermometer at eye level and reads the result.
☐	5	Washes thermometer in cool water, rinses, dries, and places it on clean paper towel.
☐	5	Removes gloves and discards in a biohazard waste container.
☐	5	Washes hands.
☐	5	Places thermometer in disinfectant solution.
☐	5	*Rationale:* Understands that thermometer must remain in disinfectant solution for 30 minutes.
☐	15	Records temperature in patient chart and documents procedure.
☐	5	Completed the tasks within 10 minutes.
☐	15	Results obtained were accurate.

_______	Earned	ADD POINTS OF TASKS CHECKED
170	Points	TOTAL POINTS POSSIBLE
_______	SCORE	DETERMINE SCORE (divide points earned by total points possible, multiply results by 100)

Actual Student Time Needed to Complete Procedure: ___________

Student's Initials: ___________ Instructor's Initials: ___________ Grade: ___________

Suggestions for Improvement: ___________________________

Evaluator's Name (print) ___________________________

Evaluator's Signature ___________________________

Comments ___________________________

DOCUMENTATION

Chart the results in the patient's medical record.

Date: _________

Charting: ___________________________

____

____

____

____

Student's Initials: _________

SKILLS COMPETENCY ASSESSMENT

Procedure 23–2: Taking an Oral Temperature Using a Disposable Oral Strip

Student's Name: ______________________________ Date: ____________

Objective: To obtain an oral temperature.

Conditions: The student demonstrates the ability to measure oral temperature using the following equipment and supplies: oral strip thermometer, gloves, biohazard waste container.

Time Requirements and Accuracy Standards: 5 minutes. Points assigned reflect importance of step to meeting objective: Important = (5) Essential = (10) Critical = (15). Automatic failure results if any of the **critical** tasks are omitted or performed incorrectly.

STANDARD PRECAUTIONS:

SKILLS ASSESSMENT CHECKLIST

Task Performed	Possible Points	TASKS
☐	5	Washes hands and follows standard precautions.
☐	5	Assembles equipment.
☐	5	Identifies patient and positions patient comfortably.
☐	10	Determines if patient has ingested hot or cold food or drink, or has smoked, in previous half hour.
☐	5	*Rationale:* Understands that food ingestion or smoking can arbitrarily affect oral temperature reading.
☐	5	Explains procedure.
☐	5	Applies gloves.
☐	10	Inserts oral strip thermometer under patient's tongue to the side of the mouth.
☐	5	*Rationale:* Understands the anatomy of the tongue and the need to avoid the patient's frenulum.
☐	10	Instructs patient to close mouth around thermometer but not to place the teeth on it.
☐	15	Leaves in place for 60 seconds.
☐	15	Removes thermometer and waits 10 seconds.
☐	5	*Rationale:* Understands that time is needed for strip to stabilize and record accurate temperature.

Task Performed	Possible Points	TASKS
❑	15	Reads temperature by locating the last dot that has changed color.
❑	10	Discards strip in a biohazard waste container.
❑	5	Removes gloves and discards in a biohazard waste container.
❑	5	Washes hands.
❑	10	Records temperature in patient chart and documents procedure.
❑	5	Completed the tasks within 5 minutes.
❑	15	Results obtained were accurate.

________	Earned	ADD POINTS OF TASKS CHECKED
165	Points	TOTAL POINTS POSSIBLE
________	SCORE	DETERMINE SCORE (divide points earned by total points possible, multiply results by 100)

Actual Student Time Needed to Complete Procedure: ____________

Student's Initials: ____________ Instructor's Initials: ____________ Grade: ____________

Suggestions for Improvement: ________________________________

____

____

____

Evaluator's Name (print) ________________________________

Evaluator's Signature ________________________________

Comments ________________________________

DOCUMENTATION

Chart the results in the patient's medical record.

Date: ____________

Charting: ________________________________

____

____

____

Student's Initials: ________

SKILLS COMPETENCY ASSESSMENT

Procedure 23–3: Taking an Oral Temperature Using a Digital Thermometer

Student's Name: ______________________________ Date: ____________

Objective: To obtain an oral temperature.

Conditions: The student demonstrates the ability to measure oral temperature using the following equipment and supplies: digital thermometer, probe covers, biohazard waste container.

Time Requirements and Accuracy Standards: 3 minutes. Points assigned reflect importance of step to meeting objective: Important = (5) Essential = (10) Critical = (15). Automatic failure results if any of the **critical** tasks are omitted or performed incorrectly.

STANDARD PRECAUTIONS:

SKILLS ASSESSMENT CHECKLIST

Task Performed	Possible Points	TASKS
☐	5	Washes hands.
☐	5	Assembles equipment.
☐	5	Identifies patient and positions patient comfortably.
☐	5	Determines if patient has ingested hot or cold food or drink, or has smoked in previous half hour.
☐	5	*Rationale:* Understands that food ingestion or smoking can arbitrarily affect oral temperature reading.
☐	5	Explains procedure.
☐	10	Selects blue probe.
☐	5	*Rationale:* Understands that blue probe is used for oral temperature taking with the digital thermometer.
☐	5	Covers probe with probe cover.
☐	10	Inserts probe under patient's tongue to the side of the mouth.
☐	5	*Rationale:* Understands the anatomy of the tongue and the need to avoid the patient's frenulum.
☐	10	Instructs patient to close mouth around thermometer but not to place the teeth on it.
☐	10	Leaves in place until beep is heard.

Task Performed	Possible Points	TASKS
❑	15	Removes thermometer and reads results on digital display.
❑	10	Discards probe cover in a biohazard waste container.
❑	5	Replaces digital thermometer in base holder.
❑	5	Washes hands.
❑	15	Records temperature in patient chart and documents procedure.
❑	5	Completed the tasks within 3 minutes.
❑	15	Results obtained were accurate.

________	Earned	ADD POINTS OF TASKS CHECKED
155	Points	TOTAL POINTS POSSIBLE
________	SCORE	DETERMINE SCORE (divide points earned by total points possible, multiply results by 100)

Actual Student Time Needed to Complete Procedure: ____________

Student's Initials: ____________ Instructor's Initials: ____________ Grade: ____________

Suggestions for Improvement: ____

Evaluator's Name (print) ____

____

____

____

Evaluator's Signature ____

Comments ____

DOCUMENTATION

Chart the results in the patient's medical record.

Date: ____________

Charting: ____

____

____

____

____

____

Student's Initials: ________

SKILLS COMPETENCY ASSESSMENT

Procedure 23–4: Obtaining an Aural Temperature Using a Tympanic Thermometer

Student's Name: ______________________________ Date: __________

Objective: To obtain an aural temperature using a tympanic thermometer.

Conditions: The student demonstrates the ability to measure aural temperature using the following equipment and supplies: tympanic thermometer, covers or ear speculum, waste container.

Time Requirements and Accuracy Standards: 2 minutes. Points assigned reflect importance of step to meeting objective: Important = (5) Essential = (10) Critical = (15). Automatic failure results if any of the **critical** tasks are omitted or performed incorrectly.

STANDARD PRECAUTIONS:

SKILLS ASSESSMENT CHECKLIST

Task Performed	Possible Points	TASKS
☐	5	Washes hands and follows standard precautions.
☐	5	Assembles equipment.
☐	5	Identifies patient and positions patient comfortably.
☐	5	Explains procedure.
☐	5	Places cover on thermometer.
☐	5	Sets thermometer to start.
☐	10	Gently places probe into ear canal, sealing it.
☐	5	*Rationale:* Understands that air leaks will occur and results will be inaccurate if ear canal is not sealed.
☐	10	Activates system.
☐	15	Waits until results are displayed on screen.
☐	5	Removes probe from ear.
☐	10	Discards cover into waste container by pressing release button.
☐	5	Washes hands.
☐	5	Replaces thermometer.
☐	10	Properly records temperature in patient chart and documents procedure.

Task Performed	Possible Points	TASKS
❑	5	Completed the tasks within 2 minutes.
❑	15	Results obtained were accurate.

________	Earned	ADD POINTS OF TASKS CHECKED
125	Points	TOTAL POINTS POSSIBLE
________	SCORE	DETERMINE SCORE (divide points earned by total points possible, multiply results by 100)

Actual Student Time Needed to Complete Procedure: ____________

Student's Initials: ____________ Instructor's Initials: ____________ Grade: ____________

Suggestions for Improvement: ____

____

____

____

Evaluator's Name (print) ____

Evaluator's Signature ____

Comments ____

DOCUMENTATION

Chart the results in the patient's medical record.

Date: ____________

Charting: ____

____

____

____

____

____

Student's Initials: ________

SKILLS COMPETENCY ASSESSMENT

Procedure 23–5: Taking a Rectal Temperature Using a Mercury Thermometer

Student's Name: ______________________________ Date: __________

Objective: To obtain a rectal temperature using a mercury thermometer.

Conditions: The student demonstrates the ability to measure rectal temperature using the following equipment and supplies: rectal thermometer, sheath, lubricating jelly, gloves, clean paper towels, biohazard waste container.

Time Requirements and Accuracy Standards: 10 minutes. Points assigned reflect importance of step to meeting objective: Important = (5) Essential = (10) Critical = (15). Automatic failure results if any of the **critical** tasks are omitted or performed incorrectly.

STANDARD PRECAUTIONS:

SKILLS ASSESSMENT CHECKLIST

Task Performed	Possible Points	TASKS
☐	5	Washes hands.
☐	5	Assembles equipment.
☐	5	Identifies patient.
☐	5	Explains procedure.
☐	5	Removes patient's clothing from waist down, draping as needed to give patient privacy and warmth.
☐	5	Positions patient in Sims position.
☐	5	Places sheath on thermometer.
☐	10	Applies lubricating jelly to sheath.
☐	5	*Rationale:* Understands that lubrication makes insertion easier and increases patient safety.
☐	15	Spreads patient's buttocks and inserts thermometer into the rectum past the sphincter (1.5 inches in adults).
☐	15	Holds buttocks together, keeping thermometer in place, for 5 minutes.
☐	5	*Rationale:* Understands that patient movement can cause movement of thermometer and injury.
☐	5	Removes thermometer from rectum.
☐	10	Removes sheath and places in a biohazard waste container.

Task Performed	Possible Points	TASKS
❑	10	Reads thermometer.
❑	5	Washes, rinses, and dries thermometer and places it on a clean paper towel.
❑	5	Removes gloves, discarding in a biohazard waste container, and washes hands.
❑	5	Places thermometer in disinfectant solution in a container specifically for rectal thermometers.
❑	5	Offers tissues for patient to wipe anus, assists patient in dressing, and positions comfortably.
❑	15	Properly records temperature in patient chart and documents procedure.
❑	5	Completed the tasks within 10 minutes.
❑	15	Results obtained were accurate.

_______	Earned	ADD POINTS OF TASKS CHECKED
165	Points	TOTAL POINTS POSSIBLE
_______	SCORE	DETERMINE SCORE (divide points earned by total points possible, multiply results by 100)

Actual Student Time Needed to Complete Procedure: __________

Student's Initials: __________ Instructor's Initials: __________ Grade: __________

Suggestions for Improvement: ______________________________

Evaluator's Name (print) ______________________________

Evaluator's Signature ______________________________

Comments ______________________________

DOCUMENTATION

Chart the results in the patient's medical record.

Date: __________

Charting: ______________________________

____

____

____

____

____

Student's Initials: ________

SKILLS COMPETENCY ASSESSMENT

Procedure 23–6: Taking a Rectal Temperature Using a Digital Thermometer

Student's Name: ______________________________ Date: ____________

Objective: To obtain a rectal temperature using a digital thermometer.

Conditions: The student demonstrates the ability to measure rectal temperature using the following equipment and supplies: digital thermometer with red probe, probe cover, lubricating jelly, gloves, biohazard waste container.

Time Requirements and Accuracy Standards: 2 minutes. Points assigned reflect importance of step to meeting objective: Important = (5) Essential = (10) Critical = (15). Automatic failure results if any of the **critical** tasks are omitted or performed incorrectly.

STANDARD PRECAUTIONS:

SKILLS ASSESSMENT CHECKLIST

Task Performed	Possible Points	TASKS
☐	5	Washes hands and applies gloves, following standard precautions.
☐	5	Assembles equipment.
☐	5	Identifies patient.
☐	5	Explains procedure.
☐	5	Removes patient's clothing from waist down, draping as needed to give patient privacy and warmth.
☐	5	Positions patient in Sims position.
☐	5	Places probe cover on red probe.
☐	5	*Rationale:* Understands that red probe is used for rectal temperature measurement.
☐	10	Applies lubricating jelly to probe cover.
☐	5	*Rationale:* Understands that lubrication makes insertion easier and increases patient safety.
☐	15	Spreads patient's buttocks and inserts thermometer into the rectum past the sphincter (1.5 inches in adults).
☐	15	Holds buttocks together, keeping thermometer in place, until beep is heard.
☐	5	*Rationale:* Understands that patient movement can cause movement of thermometer, inaccurate readings, and injury.
☐	10	Reads results on digital display.

Task Performed	Possible Points	TASKS
❑	5	Removes thermometer from rectum.
❑	10	Discards probe cover into a biohazard waste container by pushing release button.
❑	5	Replaces thermometer in base.
❑	5	Removes gloves, discarding in a biohazard waste container, and washes hands.
❑	5	Offers tissues for patient to wipe anus, assists patient in dressing, and positions comfortably.
❑	15	Properly records temperature in patient chart and documents procedure.
❑	5	Completed the tasks within 2 minutes.
❑	15	Results obtained were accurate.

_______	Earned	ADD POINTS OF TASKS CHECKED
165	Points	TOTAL POINTS POSSIBLE
_______	SCORE	DETERMINE SCORE (divide points earned by total points possible, multiply results by 100)

Actual Student Time Needed to Complete Procedure: ____________

Student's Initials: ____________ Instructor's Initials: ____________ Grade: ____________

Suggestions for Improvement: ____________

Evaluator's Name (print) ____________

Evaluator's Signature ____________

Comments ____________

DOCUMENTATION

Chart the results in the patient's medical record.

Date: ____________

Charting: ____________

____

____

____

____

____

Student's Initials: ________

SKILLS COMPETENCY ASSESSMENT

Procedure 23–7: Taking an Axillary Temperature

Student's Name: ______________________________ Date: __________

Objective: To obtain an axillary temperature using a mercury thermometer.

Conditions: The student demonstrates the ability to measure axillary temperature using the following equipment and supplies: mercury thermometer, sheath, Towelettes, paper towels.

Time Requirements and Accuracy Standards: 15 minutes. Points assigned reflect importance of step to meeting objective: Important = (5) Essential = (10) Critical = (15). Automatic failure results if any of the **critical** tasks are omitted or performed incorrectly.

STANDARD PRECAUTIONS:

SKILLS ASSESSMENT CHECKLIST

Task Performed	Possible Points	TASKS
☐	5	Washes hands and follows standard precautions.
☐	5	Assembles equipment.
☐	5	Identifies patient.
☐	5	Explains procedure.
☐	10	Places sheath on thermometer.
☐	5	Asks patient to remove clothing from waist up, gowning as necessary to protect patient's privacy and warmth.
☐	5	Wipes axillary area with dry paper towel.
☐	5	*Rationale:* Understands that moisture in axilla will cause an inaccurate reading.
☐	5	Places thermometer in axilla.
☐	10	Asks patient to fold arm against chest.
☐	5	*Rationale:* Understands that this will keep thermometer in place, prevent air contact, and preserve an accurate reading.
☐	15	Leaves in place 10 minutes.
☐	10	Removes thermometer from axilla and discards sheath into a biohazard waste container.

Task Performed	Possible Points	TASKS
❑	5	Reads thermometer.
❑	5	Washes, rinses, and dries thermometer, placing it on a clean paper towel.
❑	5	Washes hands.
❑	5	Soaks thermometer in disinfectant solution.
❑	10	Properly records temperature in patient chart and documents procedure.
❑	5	Completed the tasks within 15 minutes.
❑	15	Results obtained were accurate.

______	Earned	ADD POINTS OF TASKS CHECKED
140	Points	TOTAL POINTS POSSIBLE
______	SCORE	DETERMINE SCORE (divide points earned by total points possible, multiply results by 100)

Actual Student Time Needed to Complete Procedure: ____________

Student's Initials: ____________ Instructor's Initials: ____________ Grade: ____________

Suggestions for Improvement: ____

____

Evaluator's Name (print) ____

Evaluator's Signature ____

Comments ____

DOCUMENTATION

Chart the results in the patient's medical record.

Date: ____________

Charting: ____

____

____

____

____

____

Student's Initials: _______

SKILLS COMPETENCY ASSESSMENT

Procedure 23–8: Taking a Radial Pulse

Student's Name: ______________________________ Date: ____________

Objective: To obtain a pulse rate.

Conditions: The student demonstrates the ability to measure radial pulse rate using the following equipment and supplies: watch with second hand.

Time Requirements and Accuracy Standards: 2 minutes. Points assigned reflect importance of step to meeting objective: Important = (5) Essential = (10) Critical = (15). Automatic failure results if any of the **critical** tasks are omitted or performed incorrectly.

STANDARD PRECAUTIONS:

SKILLS ASSESSMENT CHECKLIST

Task Performed	Possible Points	TASKS
☐	5	Washes hands.
☐	5	Identifies patient.
☐	5	Explains procedure.
☐	5	Positions patient with wrist resting on his or her lap or on a table.
☐	10	Locates radial pulse with pads of first three fingers.
☐	10	Gently compresses radial artery so pulsations can be clearly felt.
☐	15	Counts pulsations for one full minute.
☐	15	Notes any irregularities in rhythm, volume, and arterial condition.
☐	5	Washes hands.
☐	10	Records pulse rate and any irregularities in patient chart, following the temperature reading, and documents procedure.
☐	5	Completed the tasks within 2 minutes.
☐	15	Results obtained were accurate.

________	Earned	ADD POINTS OF TASKS CHECKED
105	Points	TOTAL POINTS POSSIBLE
________	SCORE	DETERMINE SCORE (divide points earned by total points possible, multiply results by 100)

Actual Student Time Needed to Complete Procedure: ____________

Student's Initials: ____________ Instructor's Initials: ____________ Grade: ____________

Suggestions for Improvement: ____

____

____

____

Evaluator's Name (print) ____

Evaluator's Signature ____

DOCUMENTATION

Chart the results in the patient's medical record. This patient also has an aural temperature of 98.7°F taken with a tympanic thermometer.

Date: __________

Charting: ____

____

____

____

____

____

Student's Initials: ________

SKILLS COMPETENCY ASSESSMENT

Procedure 23–9: Taking an Apical Pulse

Student's Name: ______________________________ Date: __________

Objective: To obtain an apical pulse rate.

Conditions: The student demonstrates the ability to measure apical pulse rate using the following equipment and supplies: stethoscope, watch with second hand.

Time Requirements and Accuracy Standards: 2 minutes. Points assigned reflect importance of step to meeting objective: Important = (5) Essential = (10) Critical = (15). Automatic failure results if any of the **critical** tasks are omitted or performed incorrectly.

STANDARD PRECAUTIONS:

SKILLS ASSESSMENT CHECKLIST

Task Performed	Possible Points	TASKS
☐	5	Washes hands.
☐	5	Assembles equipment.
☐	5	Identifies patient.
☐	5	Explains procedure.
☐	5	Asks patient to remove clothing from waist up, gowning as necessary to protect patient's privacy and warmth.
☐	5	Positions patient in supine position.
☐	5	*Rationale:* Understands that this provides easier access to apex of heart.
☐	10	Locates fifth intercostal space, midclavical, left off sternum.
☐	5	*Rationale:* Understands that this is the location of the apex of the heart.
☐	10	Places stethoscope on site and listens for lub-dub sound of heart.
☐	5	*Rationale:* Understands that each lub-dub pair equals one pulse.
☐	15	Counts pulse for 1 minute.
☐	5	Assists patient to sit up and dress.
☐	5	Washes hands.

Task Performed	Possible Points	TASKS
❑	15	Properly records pulse in patient chart, noting any arrhythmias, and documents the procedure.
❑	5	Completed the tasks within 2 minutes.
❑	15	Results obtained were accurate.
________	Earned	ADD POINTS OF TASKS CHECKED
125	Points	TOTAL POINTS POSSIBLE
________	SCORE	DETERMINE SCORE (divide points earned by total points possible, multiply results by 100)

Actual Student Time Needed to Complete Procedure: ____________

Student's Initials: ____________ Instructor's Initials: ____________ Grade: ____________

Suggestions for Improvement: ____

____

____

____

Evaluator's Name (print) ____

Evaluator's Signature ____

DOCUMENTATION

Chart the results in the patient's medical record. This patient also has an axillary temperature of 98.7°F.

Date: ____________

Charting: ____

____

____

____

____

____

Student's Initials: __________

SKILLS COMPETENCY ASSESSMENT

Procedure 23–10: Measuring the Respiration Rate

Student's Name: ______________________________ Date: ____________

Objective: To obtain an accurate respiration rate.

Conditions: The student demonstrates the ability to measure respiration rate using the following equipment and supplies: watch with second hand.

Time Requirements and Accuracy Standards: 2 minutes. Points assigned reflect importance of step to meeting objective: Important = (5) Essential = (10) Critical = (15). Automatic failure results if any of the **critical** tasks are omitted or performed incorrectly.

STANDARD PRECAUTIONS:

SKILLS ASSESSMENT CHECKLIST

Task Performed	Possible Points	TASKS
☐	5	Washes hands.
☐	5	Identifies patient.
☐	5	Positions the patient comfortably.
☐	15	For 1 minute, monitors and counts the rise and fall of the patient's chest wall: by observation alone, by holding the patient's arm across the chest and feeling for its rises and falls, or by placing a hand on the patient's shoulder and watching chest movements.
☐	15	Notes depth of breathing, rhythm, and breath sounds while counting.
☐	5	Washes hands.
☐	10	Records respiration rate in patient chart, along with any irregularities or sounds, and documents the procedure.
☐	5	Completed the tasks within 2 minutes.
☐	15	Results obtained were accurate.

________	Earned	ADD POINTS OF TASKS CHECKED
80	Points	TOTAL POINTS POSSIBLE
________	SCORE	DETERMINE SCORE (divide points earned by total points possible, multiply results by 100)

Actual Student Time Needed to Complete Procedure: ____________

Student's Initials: ____________ Instructor's Initials: ____________ Grade: ____________

Suggestions for Improvement: ______________________________

____

____

____

Evaluator's Name (print) ______________________________

Evaluator's Signature ______________________________

Comments ______________________________

DOCUMENTATION

Chart the results in the patient's medical record. This patient also has a rectal temperature of 99.4°F and a pulse rate of 72 beats per minute.

Date: __________

Charting: ______________________________

____

____

____

____

____

Student's Initials: ______

SKILLS COMPETENCY ASSESSMENT

Procedure 23–11: Measuring a Blood Pressure

Student's Name: ______________________________ Date: ____________

Objective: To measure blood pressure.

Conditions: The student demonstrates the ability to measure blood pressure using the following equipment and supplies: stethoscope, sphygmomanometer, alcohol wipes.

Time Requirements and Accuracy Standards: 5 minutes. Points assigned reflect importance of step to meeting objective: Important = (5) Essential = (10) Critical = (15). Automatic failure results if any of the **critical** tasks are omitted or performed incorrectly.

STANDARD PRECAUTIONS:

SKILLS ASSESSMENT CHECKLIST

Task Performed	Possible Points	TASKS
☐	5	Washes hands.
☐	10	Assembles equipment, including a cuff of the appropriate size.
☐	5	*Rationale:* Understands that a cuff of the wrong size can give inaccurate results.
☐	5	Cleans stethoscope earpieces with alcohol wipe.
☐	5	Identifies patient.
☐	5	Explains procedure.
☐	10	Positions patient, preferably in a seated position, with feet flat on the floor and arm resting on lap or table.
☐	5	*Rationale:* Understands that crossed legs or an arm above heart level can give inaccurate results.
☐	5	Bares patient's upper arm, asking patient to remove clothing if necessary.
☐	5	Palpates brachial artery.
☐	10	Positions cuff bladder over the brachial artery, about two inches above the elbow.
☐	10	Palpates radial pulse and smoothly inflates cuff until pulse is no longer felt, noting this number.
☐	5	Deflates cuff quickly and allows arm to rest for 1 minute.
☐	5	Calculates peak inflation level.
☐	5	*Rationale:* Understands that this will ensure that an auscultatory gap is not missed.
☐	10	Determines that cuff is completely deflated.
☐	10	Positions stethoscope over brachial artery, holding in position with fingers only.
☐	10	Inflates cuff, smoothly and quickly, to peak inflation level.

Task Performed	Possible Points	TASKS
☐	15	Deflates cuff at 2 to 4 mm Hg per second.
☐	10	Listens for Korotkoff phase I, noting when it appears.
☐	5	Continues deflation, noting each Korotkoff phase.
☐	15	Notes point at which all sounds disappear, Korotkoff phase V.
☐	10	Continues deflating cuff at the same rate for at least 10 more mm Hg after sounds disappear.
☐	5	*Rationale:* Understands this will allow time for an auscultatory gap, should one be present.
☐	5	Deflates cuff quickly and removes it.
☐	5	Cleans stethoscope earpieces with alcohol wipe.
☐	5	Washes hands.
☐	10	Records measurement in patient chart and documents procedure.
☐	5	Completed the tasks within 5 minutes.
☐	15	Results obtained were accurate.

_______	Earned	ADD POINTS OF TASKS CHECKED
230	Points	TOTAL POINTS POSSIBLE
_______	SCORE	DETERMINE SCORE (divide points earned by total points possible, multiply results by 100)

Actual Student Time Needed to Complete Procedure: ____________

Student's Initials: ____________ Instructor's Initials: ____________ Grade: ____________

Suggestions for Improvement: ____

Evaluator's Name (print) ____

Evaluator's Signature ____

Comments ____

DOCUMENTATION

Chart the results in the patient's medical record. This patient also has an oral temperature of 98.6°F taken with an oral strip thermometer, a strong pulse of 62 beats per minute, and a respiratory rate of 15 breaths per minute.

Date: ____________

Charting: ____

____

____

____

Student's Initials: ____________

SKILLS COMPETENCY ASSESSMENT

Procedure 23–12: Measuring Height

Student's Name: ______________________________ Date: __________

Objective: To obtain the height of a patient.

Conditions: The student demonstrates the ability to measure height using the following equipment and supplies: scale with measuring bar; paper towel.

Time Requirements and Accuracy Standards: 5 minutes. Points assigned reflect importance of step to meeting objective: Important = (5) Essential = (10) Critical = (15). Automatic failure results if any of the **critical** tasks are omitted or performed incorrectly.

STANDARD PRECAUTIONS:

SKILLS ASSESSMENT CHECKLIST

Task Performed	Possible Points	TASKS
☐	5	Washes hands.
☐	5	Identifies patient.
☐	5	Explains procedure.
☐	5	Instructs patient to remove shoes.
☐	5	Places paper towel on scale.
☐	10	Instructs patient to stand on the scale platform with back to measuring bar, looking straight ahead.
☐	5	*Rationale:* Understands that facial or eye injuries could result if patient faces the measuring bar, and that a more accurate result is obtained if patient looks straight ahead.
☐	5	Assists patient onto scale platform.
☐	5	*Rationale:* Understands that the movable platform could cause patient to lose balance if unassisted.
☐	10	Lowers measuring bar until headrest is positioned firmly atop patient's head.
☐	10	Assists patient in stepping off the scale, helping him or her to sit and replace shoes if necessary.
☐	15	Reads line where measurement falls.

Task Performed	Possible Points	TASKS
❑	5	Lowers measuring bar to original position.
❑	5	Washes hands.
❑	5	Records height in patient chart.
❑	5	Completed the tasks within 5 minutes.
❑	15	Results obtained were accurate.
_______	Earned	ADD POINTS OF TASKS CHECKED
120	Points	TOTAL POINTS POSSIBLE
_______	SCORE	DETERMINE SCORE (divide points earned by total points possible, multiply results by 100)

Actual Student Time Needed to Complete Procedure: ___________

Student's Initials: ___________ Instructor's Initials: ___________ Grade: ___________

Suggestions for Improvement: ___________________________

____

____

____

Evaluator's Name (print) ___________________________

Evaluator's Signature ___________________________

Comments ___________________________

DOCUMENTATION

Chart the results in the patient's medical record. This patient also has a rectal temperature of 99.9°F, a pulse rate of 75 beats per minute, a respiration rate of 25 breaths per minute, and a blood pressure reading in the left arm, while sitting, of 122/80. Sinus arrhythmia is noted in this patient.

Date: ___________

Charting: ___________________________

____

____

____

____

____

Student's Initials: ___________

SKILLS COMPETENCY ASSESSMENT

Procedure 23–13: Measuring Adult Weight

Student's Name: ______________________________ Date: ____________

Objective: To obtain the weight of the patient.

Conditions: The student demonstrates the ability to measure weight using the following equipment and supplies: balance beam scale; paper towel.

Time Requirements and Accuracy Standards: 5 minutes. Points assigned reflect importance of step to meeting objective: Important = (5) Essential = (10) Critical = (15). Automatic failure results if any of the **critical** tasks are omitted or performed incorrectly.

STANDARD PRECAUTIONS:

SKILLS ASSESSMENT CHECKLIST

Task Performed	Possible Points	TASKS
☐	5	Washes hands.
☐	5	Identifies patient.
☐	5	Explains procedure.
☐	5	Places paper towel on scale.
☐	5	Instructs patient to place any heavy items, including items in pockets, in a safe area provided.
☐	5	Instructs patient to remove shoes, jackets, and other outerwear.
☐	10	Assists patient onto scale platform, positioning patient in platform's center.
☐	5	*Rationale:* Understands that the movable platform could cause patient to lose balance if unassisted.
☐	5	Moves lower weight bar to estimated number (patient may be asked for approximate weight).
☐	5	Slides upper weight bar until balance beam point is centered.
☐	15	Reads weight, adding upper bar measurement to lower bar measurement.
☐	10	Assists patient in stepping off scale, helping him or her to sit and replace shoes if necessary and returning any other items.

Task Performed	Possible Points	TASKS
☐	5	Returns weights to 0.
☐	5	Washes hands.
☐	5	Records measurement in patient chart.
☐	5	Completed the tasks within 5 minutes.
☐	15	Results obtained were accurate.
______	Earned	ADD POINTS OF TASKS CHECKED
115	Points	TOTAL POINTS POSSIBLE
______	SCORE	DETERMINE SCORE (divide points earned by total points possible, multiply results by 100)

Actual Student Time Needed to Complete Procedure: ____________

Student's Initials: ____________ Instructor's Initials: ____________ Grade: ____________

Suggestions for Improvement: ____

____

____

Evaluator's Name (print) ____

Evaluator's Signature ____

Comments ____

DOCUMENTATION

Chart the results in the patient's medical record. This patient also has an oral temperature of 98.3°F; an apical pulse rate of 68 beats per minute; a respiration rate of 19 breaths per minute, with shallow breathing; a blood pressure reading in the right arm, while supine, of 132/78; and a height of 5 feet 7.5 inches.

Date: __________

Charting: ____

____

____

____

____

____

Student's Initials: ________

EVALUATION OF CHAPTER KNOWLEDGE

Evaluate your own strengths and weaknesses in the measurement of vital signs and your understanding of their ramifications. Compare this evaluation to the one provided by your instructor.

	Student Self-evaluation			Instructor Evaluation		
Knowledge	*Good*	*Average*	*Poor*	*Good*	*Average*	*Poor*
Ability to define and describe key terms relating to temperature, pulse, respiration, and blood pressure readings	____	____	____	____	____	____
Understands normal and abnormal body temperatures as well as factors that affect temperature	____	____	____	____	____	____
Identifies various types of thermometers and knows procedures for their care, storage, and use	____	____	____	____	____	____
Knows anatomical locations of pulse sites and procedures for obtaining pulse rate at each one	____	____	____	____	____	____
Identifies normal and abnormal pulse rates, including common arrhythmias	____	____	____	____	____	____
Understands procedure for obtaining respiration rate	____	____	____	____	____	____
Identifies normal and abnormal respiration rates and breath sounds	____	____	____	____	____	____
Ability to use blood pressure equipment and understand measurement procedures	____	____	____	____	____	____
Identifies normal and abnormal blood pressure readings, including factors that affect it	____	____	____	____	____	____
Understands procedures for obtaining height and weight measurements	____	____	____	____	____	____
Ability to accurately record all measurements on patient chart	____	____	____	____	____	____

Student's Initials: ______ Instructor's Initials: ______

Grade: ________

Chief Complaints and Possible Diagnoses

- Vomiting and severe pain in or around one eye, blurred vision (glaucoma)
- Pain on urination with watery mucus discharge (nonspecific urethritis)
- Cough, fever, chest pain, shortness of breath (pneumonia)
- Lethargy, muscle weakness, cramps, slow heart rate, hair loss (hypothyroidism)
- Headache, nausea, dizziness, impaired mental processes; severe breathlessness, cough, and phlegm production (mountain sickness and high-altitude pulmonary edema)
- Abnormal or heavy menstrual bleeding with lower back pain during menstruation (endometriosis)
- Headache with severe pain on one side, nausea, flashing lights create vision disturbance before headache begins (migraine)
- Fever, rash of purple spots, dislike of strong light, pain on bending head forward (meningitis)
- Constipation, regular use of laxatives (overuse of laxatives)
- Inability to concentrate, low sex drive, recurrent headaches (depression)

Patient Characteristics

The patient is

- Aggressive but not rude; asks a lot of questions
- Shy, will not maintain eye contact
- Deaf, communicates by lip-reading and handwritten exchanges
- Unable to concentrate, does not seem to understand or follow directions well
- Complaining constantly
- Confined to a wheelchair
- Making a joke out of everything, but in a nice way
- Distrustful of the medical assistant
- Speaks broken English
- Evasive and does not want to reveal information
- Cooperative and good-natured
- Depressed
- In a great deal of pain
- Fatigued
- Worried
- Trying to self-diagnose and get the medical assistant to confirm the self-diagnosis

CASE STUDY

Rowena Lawrence brings her 5-year-old son Bobby to Inner City Health Care with a suspected case of the mumps contracted from his sister Felicia. As Bruce Goldman, CMA, helps the child remove his clothing, leaving only his underwear, the child becomes increasingly fearful and begins to cry. Rowena's gentle reprimand to "Hush up and do what you're told," makes the boy cry harder. It is obvious that the child is uncomfortable and feverish.

Discuss the following:

1. What can the medical assistant do to calm the child and make him more comfortable? What is Bruce's therapeutic response?

SUPPLEMENTARY RESOURCES

Study Guide Disk: Additional practice exercises for this chapter are available on the study guide disk found in the back of the textbook.

Medical Assisting Videos: Appropriate content is available on Delmar's Medical Assisting Videos, 2nd ed., Tape 8, for the following topics:

Clean Examination Table and Countertop
Assist Physician with Examination and Treatments
Position and Drape the Patient
Role of the Medical Assistant During the Examination
Introduction to Health Promotion, Disease Prevention, and Self-Responsibility

SKILLS COMPETENCY ASSESSMENT

Procedure 24–1: Positioning Patient in the Supine Position

Student's Name: ______________________________ Date: ____________

Objective: To safely and properly assist patient into supine position for examination of anterior surface of the body from head to toe.

Conditions: The student demonstrates the ability to position the patient in the supine position for examination using the following equipment and supplies: examination table, drape, gown.

Time Requirements and Accuracy Standards: 2 minutes. Points assigned reflect importance of step to meeting objective: Important = (5) Essential = (10) Critical = (15). Automatic failure results if any of the **critical** tasks are omitted or performed incorrectly.

STANDARD PRECAUTIONS:

SKILLS ASSESSMENT CHECKLIST

Task Performed	Possible Points	TASKS
❑	5	Washes hands and follows standard precautions.
❑	5	Assembles supplies.
❑	5	Assists patient to sit on the end of the examination table.
❑	10	Assists patient to lie back on table while pulling out the table extension. Supports patient's feet and back while extending foot of table.
❑	5	Covers patient with drape from shoulders to ankles.
❑	5	Places small pillow under patient's head.
❑	10	Upon completion of procedure, assists patient to seated position (allows patient to remain seated to prevent orthostatic hypotension).
❑	5	Pushes table extension back into place while supporting patient's feet.
❑	15	Once patient is stable (checks color or patient's skin, checks pulse), gives further instructions as required.
❑	5	Completed the tasks within 2 minutes.
❑	15	Results obtained were accurate.

_______	Earned	ADD POINTS OF TASKS CHECKED
85	Points	TOTAL POINTS POSSIBLE
_______	SCORE	DETERMINE SCORE (divide points earned by total points possible, multiply results by 100)

Actual Student Time Needed to Complete Procedure: ____________

Student's Initials: ____________ Instructor's Initials: ____________ Grade: ____________

Suggestions for Improvement: ______________________________

Evaluator's Name (print) ______________________________

Evaluator's Signature ______________________________

Comments ______________________________

SKILLS COMPETENCY ASSESSMENT

Procedure 24–2: Positioning Patient in the Dorsal Recumbent Position

Student's Name: ______________________ Date: __________

Objective: To safely and properly assist patient to dorsal recumbent position for pelvic or rectal examination; urinary catheterization; and head, chest, or neck examination.

Conditions: The student demonstrates the ability to position patient in the dorsal recumbent position using the following equipment and supplies: examination table, drape, gown.

Time Requirements and Accuracy Standards: 2 minutes. Points assigned reflect importance of step to meeting objective: Important = (5) Essential = (10) Critical = (15). Automatic failure results if any of the **critical** tasks are omitted or performed incorrectly.

STANDARD PRECAUTIONS:

SKILLS ASSESSMENT CHECKLIST

Task Performed	Possible Points	TASKS
❑	5	Washes hands and follows standard precautions.
❑	5	Assists patient to sit on the end of the examination table.
❑	10	Assists patient to lie back on table; extends the foot of the table while supporting the patient's feet and back.
❑	5	Assists patient to bend knees and place feet flat on the surface of the table.
❑	5	Covers patient with drape (diamond shape) from shoulders to ankles.
❑	5	Places small pillow under patient's head.
❑	5	Upon completion of procedure, assists patient to seated position while pushing table extension back into place and supporting patient's feet.
❑	10	Has patient sit at end of table for a few minutes to prevent dizziness.
❑	15	Once patient is stable (checks color of patient's skin, checks pulse), gives further instructions as required.
❑	5	Completed the tasks within 2 minutes.
❑	15	Results obtained were accurate.

______	Earned	ADD POINTS OF TASKS CHECKED
85	Points	TOTAL POINTS POSSIBLE
______	SCORE	DETERMINE SCORE (divide points earned by total points possible, multiply results by 100)

Actual Student Time Needed to Complete Procedure: __________

Student's Initials: __________ Instructor's Initials: __________ Grade: __________

Suggestions for Improvement: ______________________

Evaluator's Name (print) ______________________

Evaluator's Signature ______________________

Comments ______________________

SKILLS COMPETENCY ASSESSMENT

Procedure 24–3: Positioning Patient in the Lithotomy Position

Student's Name: ______________________________ Date: ____________

Objective: To safely and properly assist patient in lithotomy position for pelvic or rectal examination or for urinary catheterization.

Conditions: The student demonstrates the ability to position patient in the lithotomy position using the following equipment and supplies: examination table, drape, gown.

Time Requirements and Accuracy Standards: 5 minutes. Points assigned reflect importance of step to meeting objective: Important = (5) Essential = (10) Critical = (15). Automatic failure results if any of the **critical** tasks are omitted or performed incorrectly.

STANDARD PRECAUTIONS:

SKILLS ASSESSMENT CHECKLIST

Task Performed	Possible Points	TASKS
❑	5	Washes hands and follows standard precautions.
❑	5	Has patient disrobe from waist down and put on gown.
❑	5	Assists patient to sit on the end of the examination table. Covers patient's lap and legs with drape.
❑	5	Assists patient to lie back on table while supporting patient's feet and back and extending foot of table.
❑	15	Positions stirrups level with the table and approximately one foot from edge of table. Locks stirrups into position.
❑	5	*Rationale:* Facilitates patient examination and ensures patient safety.
❑	5	Has patient move as close to edge of examination table as possible.
❑	10	Assists patient to bend knees and place feet in stirrups. Moves drape to diamond shape to ensure privacy.
❑	5	Places small pillow under patient's head.
❑	5	Upon completion of procedure, extends foot extension of table.
❑	5	Assists patient to slide toward head of table and place legs on foot extension.

SKILLS COMPETENCY ASSESSMENT — continued

Procedure 24–3: Positioning Patient in the Lithotomy Position

Task Performed	Possible Points	TASKS
❑	5	Assists patient to seated position while replacing foot extension.
❑	10	Has patient sit at end of table for a few minutes to prevent dizziness.
❑	15	Once patient is stable (checks color of patient's skin, checks pulse), gives further instructions as required.
❑	5	Completed the tasks within 5 minutes.
❑	15	Results obtained were accurate.

______		Earned	ADD POINTS OF TASKS CHECKED
	120	Points	TOTAL POINTS POSSIBLE
______		SCORE	DETERMINE SCORE (divide points earned by total points possible, multiply results by 100)

Actual Student Time Needed to Complete Procedure: ____________

Student's Initials: ____________ Instructor's Initials: ____________ Grade: ____________

Suggestions for Improvement: ____

____

____

____

Evaluator's Name (print) ____

Evaluator's Signature ____

Comments ____

SKILLS COMPETENCY ASSESSMENT

Procedure 24–4: Positioning Patient in the Fowler's Position

Student's Name: ______________________________ Date: __________

Objective: To safely and properly assist patient into the Fowler's position for examination of upper body and head; often used for patients with cardiovascular or respiratory problems.

Conditions: The student demonstrates the ability to position patient in the Fowler's position using the following equipment and supplies: examination table, drape, gown.

Time Requirements and Accuracy Standards: 2 minutes. Points assigned reflect importance of step to meeting objective: Important = (5) Essential = (10) Critical = (15). Automatic failure results if any of the **critical** tasks are omitted or performed incorrectly.

STANDARD PRECAUTIONS:

SKILLS ASSESSMENT CHECKLIST

Task Performed	Possible Points	TASKS
☐	5	Washes hands and follows standard precautions.
☐	5	Provides gown and assists to disrobe if necessary.
☐	5	Assists patient to sit on the end of the examination table. Covers lap and legs with drape.
☐	5	Assists patient to slide back on table leaning on back rest.
☐	5	Supports patient's feet while extending foot of table.
☐	10	Positions head of table at a 90° angle (45° for Semi-Fowler's).
☐	5	Covers patient with drape from shoulders to ankles.
☐	5	Upon completion of procedure, replaces foot extension.
☐	10	Has patient sit at end of table for a few minutes to prevent dizziness.
☐	15	Once patient is stable (checks color of patient's skin, checks pulse), gives further instructions as required.
☐	5	Completed the tasks within 2 minutes.
☐	15	Results obtained were accurate.

________	Earned	ADD POINTS OF TASKS CHECKED
90	Points	TOTAL POINTS POSSIBLE
________	SCORE	DETERMINE SCORE (divide points earned by total points possible, multiply results by 100)

Actual Student Time Needed to Complete Procedure: __________

Student's Initials: __________ Instructor's Initials: __________ Grade: __________

Suggestions for Improvement: ______________________________

Evaluator's Name (print) ______________________________

Evaluator's Signature ______________________________

Comments ______________________________

SKILLS COMPETENCY ASSESSMENT

Procedure 24–5: Positioning Patient in the Knee-Chest Position

Student's Name: ______________________________ Date: __________

Objective: To safely and properly assist patient in knee-chest position for examination of the rectum, sigmoid colon, and in some instances, the vagina.

Conditions: The student demonstrates the ability to position patient in the knee-chest position using the following equipment and supplies: examination table, drape, gown.

Time Requirements and Accuracy Standards: 5 minutes. Points assigned reflect importance of step to meeting objective: Important = (5) Essential = (10) Critical = (15). Automatic failure results if any of the **critical** tasks are omitted or performed incorrectly.

STANDARD PRECAUTIONS:

SKILLS ASSESSMENT CHECKLIST

Task Performed	Possible Points	TASKS
☐	5	Washes hands and follows standard precautions.
☐	5	Has patient completely undress. Provides gown.
☐	5	Instructs patient to sit on the end of the examination table with drape open over lap and legs.
☐	5	Instructs patient to lie back on table while supporting patient's feet and back and extending foot of table.
☐	5	Waits until physician is ready to begin examination to assist patient into knee-chest position.
☐	5	*Rationale:* Because this is an embarrassing and uncomfortable position for the patient, it is best to wait until the physician is ready to begin the examination.
☐	10	Assists patient to turn onto abdomen by turning the patient toward the medical assistant, being careful to stay in the center of the table to avoid a fall. Medical assistant places her/his left hand on the patient's back for support and guides the patient toward her/him. Adjusts drape.
☐	10	Assists patient to rise to knees by helping patient bend at the hips to place the chest on the table; keeps patient covered with drape.

Task Performed	Possible Points	TASKS
❑	10	Ensures that patient's arms are bent to each side of the head with hands placed under the head. If this position is uncomfortable, has patient rest on the elbows. Adjusts drape from shoulders to ankles.
❑	10	Upon completion of procedure, assists patient to lie flat on abdomen. Then, assists patient to turn onto the back (patient turns toward medical assistant) and return to seated position.
❑	10	Has patient sit at end of table for a few minutes to prevent dizziness.
❑	15	Once patient is stable (checks patient's skin color, checks pulse), gives further instructions as required.
❑	5	Completed the tasks within 5 minutes.
❑	15	Results obtained were accurate.

______	Earned	ADD POINTS OF TASKS CHECKED
115	Points	TOTAL POINTS POSSIBLE
______	SCORE	DETERMINE SCORE (divide points earned by total points possible, multiply results by 100)

Actual Student Time Needed to Complete Procedure: ____________

Student's Initials: ____________ Instructor's Initials: ____________ Grade: ____________

Suggestions for Improvement: ______________________________

____

____

____

Evaluator's Name (print) ______________________________

Evaluator's Signature ______________________________

Comments ______________________________

SKILLS COMPETENCY ASSESSMENT

Procedure 24–6: Positioning Patient in Prone Position

Student's Name: ______________________________ Date: ____________

Objective: To safely and properly position the patient into the prone position for examination of the posterior aspect of the body, including the back, spine, or legs.

Conditions: The student demonstrates the ability to position the patient in the prone position using the following equipment and supplies: examination table, drape, gown.

Time Requirements and Accuracy Standards: 2 minutes. Points assigned reflect importance of step to meeting objective: Important = (5) Essential = (10) Critical = (15). Automatic failure results if any of the **critical** tasks are omitted or performed incorrectly.

STANDARD PRECAUTIONS:

SKILLS ASSESSMENT CHECKLIST

Task Performed	Possible Points	TASKS
❑	5	Washes hands and follows standard precautions.
❑	5	Has patient undress. Provides gown.
❑	5	Assists patient to sit on the end of the examination table. Places drape over lap and legs.
❑	5	Assists patient to lie back on table while supporting patient's feet and back and extending foot of table.
❑	10	Assists patient to turn toward the medical assistant, then onto abdomen, being careful to stay in center of table to avoid a fall. Places pillow under patient's feet and head.
❑	5	Adjusts patient's drape from shoulders to ankles.
❑	10	Upon completion of procedure, assists patient to turn toward the medical assistant. Then, assists patient to seated position.
❑	10	Has patient sit at end of table for a few minutes to prevent dizziness.
❑	15	Once patient is stable (checks patient's skin color, checks pulse), gives further instructions as required.

Task Performed	Possible Points	TASKS
☐	5	Completed the tasks within 2 minutes.
☐	15	Results obtained were accurate.

________	Earned	ADD POINTS OF TASKS CHECKED
90	Points	TOTAL POINTS POSSIBLE
________	SCORE	DETERMINE SCORE (divide points earned by total points possible, multiply results by 100)

Actual Student Time Needed to Complete Procedure: ____________

Student's Initials: ____________ Instructor's Initials: ____________ Grade: ____________

Suggestions for Improvement: ____

____

____

____

Evaluator's Name (print) ____

Evaluator's Signature ____

Comments ____

SKILLS COMPETENCY ASSESSMENT

Procedure 24–7: Positioning Patient in the Sims' Position

Student's Name: ______________________________ Date: ____________

Objective: To safely and properly assist patient into Sims', or lateral, position for rectal examination, rectal temperature, proctoscopy, sigmoidoscopy, for an enema, and in some instances, for vaginal examination.

Condition: The student demonstrates the ability to position patient in the Sims' position using the following equipment and supplies: examination table, drape, gown.

Time Requirements and Accuracy Standards: 2 minutes. Points assigned reflect importance of step to meeting objective: Important = (5) Essential = (10) Critical = (15). Automatic failure results if any of the **critical** tasks are omitted or performed incorrectly.

STANDARD PRECAUTIONS:

SKILLS ASSESSMENT CHECKLIST

Task Performed	Possible Points	TASKS
☐	5	Washes hands and follows standard precautions.
☐	5	Has patient undress. Provides gown.
☐	5	Assists patient to sit on the end of the table. Places drape over lap and legs.
☐	10	Assists patient to lie back on table while supporting patient's feet and back and extending foot of table.
☐	10	Assists patient to turn toward the medical assistant onto the left side with the left arm behind the body, placing body weight on the chest. Adjusts drape.
☐	10	Assists patient to slightly flex left knee and flex right knee to a 90° angle for support.
☐	10	Ensures that patient's right arm is bent in front of body with hand toward head at an angle to provide support.
☐	5	Adjusts drape from shoulders to ankles creating triangle or diamond shape.
☐	10	Upon completion of procedure, instructs patient to turn toward the medical assistant, then onto back, then into seated position.
☐	10	Has patient sit at end of table for a few minutes to prevent dizziness.

Task Performed	Possible Points	TASKS
❑	15	Once patient is stable (checks patient's skin color, checks pulse), gives further instructions as required.
❑	5	Completed the tasks within 2 minutes.
❑	15	Results obtained were accurate.

________	Earned	ADD POINTS OF TASKS CHECKED
115	Points	TOTAL POINTS POSSIBLE
________	SCORE	DETERMINE SCORE (divide points earned by total points possible, multiply results by 100)

Actual Student Time Needed to Complete Procedure: ____________

Student's Initials: ____________ Instructor's Initials: ____________ Grade: ____________

Suggestions for Improvement: ____

____

____

____

Evaluator's Name (print) ____

Evaluator's Signature ____

Comments ____

SKILLS COMPETENCY ASSESSMENT

Procedure 24–8: Positioning Patient in the Trendelenburg Position

Student's Name: ______________________________ Date: __________

Objective: To safely and properly assist patient into Trendelenburg position for certain abdominal surgical procedures.

Condition: The student demonstrates the ability to position the patient in the Trendelenburg position using the following equipment and supplies: examination table, drape, gown.

Time Requirements and Accuracy Standards: 2 minutes. Points assigned reflect importance of step to meeting objective: Important = (5) Essential = (10) Critical = (15). Automatic failure results if any of the **critical** tasks are omitted or performed incorrectly.

STANDARD PRECAUTIONS:

SKILLS ASSESSMENT CHECKLIST

Task Performed	Possible Points	TASKS
❑	5	Washes hands and follows standard precautions.
❑	5	Assists patient to undress. Provides gown.
❑	5	Assists patient to sit on the end of the table. Places drape over lap and legs.
❑	5	Assists patient to lie back on table, with head at headboard. Adjusts drape.
❑	10	Ensures that patient's feet are flexed over the end of the table.
❑	5	May lower the head of table to a 45° angle, if necessary.
❑	5	Adjusts drape from shoulders to ankles to ensure privacy.
❑	10	Upon completion of procedure, assists patient to return to seated position.
❑	10	Allows patient to sit at end of table for a few minutes to prevent dizziness.
❑	15	Once patient is stable (checks patient's skin color, checks pulse), gives further instructions as required.
❑	5	Completed the tasks within 2 minutes.
❑	15	Results obtained were accurate.

______	Earned	ADD POINTS OF TASKS CHECKED
95	Points	TOTAL POINTS POSSIBLE
______	SCORE	DETERMINE SCORE (divide points earned by total points possible, multiply results by 100)

Actual Student Time Needed to Complete Procedure: __________

Student's Initials: __________ Instructor's Initials: __________ Grade: __________

Suggestions for Improvement: ______________________________

Evaluator's Name (print) ______________________________

Evaluator's Signature ______________________________

Comments ______________________________

SKILLS COMPETENCY ASSESSMENT

Procedure 24–9: Assisting with a Complete Physical Examination

Student's Name: ______________________________ Date: ____________

Objective: To assist the physician in a complete physical examination.

Conditions: The student demonstrates the ability to assist the physician in a complete physical examination using the following equipment and supplies: urine specimen bottle, laboratory request forms, balance beam scales, Snellen chart, patient gown and drape, thermometer, stethoscope, sphygmomanometer, examination lights, penlights, ophthalmoscope, tonometer, otoscope, tuning fork, nasal speculum, tongue depressors, laryngeal and pharyngeal mirrors, tape measure, percussion hammer, safety pins, cotton balls, kidney-shaped basin, gloves, lubricant, tissues, alcohol swabs, gauze sponges, biohazard and regular waste containers.

Time Requirements and Accuracy Standards: 15 minutes. Points assigned reflect importance of step to meeting objective: Important = (5) Essential = (10) Critical = (15). Automatic failure results if any of the **critical** tasks are omitted or performed incorrectly.

STANDARD PRECAUTIONS: 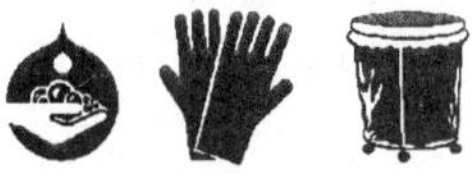

SKILLS ASSESSMENT CHECKLIST

Task Performed	Possible Points	TASKS
☐	5	Washes hands.
☐	5	Assembles equipment.
☐	10	Places instruments in easily accessible sequence for physician's use, making efficient use of time and space.
☐	5	Greets and identifies patient.
☐	5	Explains procedure to patient.
☐	5	*Rationale:* Explains procedure to obtain patient cooperation and allay apprehension.
☐	5	Reviews medical history with patient (see Procedure 22–1).
☐	5	*Rationale:* Reviewing medical history ensures that information is complete and current.
☐	15	Takes and records patient's vital signs, visual acuity, and hearing test results.
☐	10	Obtains a urine specimen (see chapter 18 for urine collection procedures).
☐	10	Obtains all required blood samples (see chapter 33, procedures 33–1 through 33–4, for blood specimen collection procedures and chapter 34, procedures 34–1 through 34–9, for blood analysis procedures).
☐	10	Obtains electrocardiogram if directed by physician (see Procedures 31–1 and 31–2).
☐	10	Provides patient with appropriate gown and drape.

SKILLS COMPETENCY ASSESSMENT — continued

Procedure 24–9: Assisting with a Complete Physical Examination

Task Performed	Possible Points	TASKS
❑	5	Assists patient to disrobe completely; explains where the opening for the gown is to be placed.
❑	5	*Rationale:* Assists patient in maintaining modesty, privacy, and warmth.
❑	5	Assists patient in sitting at the end of the table; drapes patient's lap and legs to maintain patient's modesty.
❑	5	Informs physician when patient is ready.
❑	5	When the physician arrives, remains by the patient ready to assist him or her and/or physician.
❑	5	Positions patient in a seated or supine position for the head, throat, eye, ear, and neck examination.
❑	5	Turns off lights to allow pupils to dilate for retinal examination, if necessary.
❑	5	Hands the physician instruments as required (some physicians will not require the medical assistant to hand the instruments).
❑	5	Has patient maintain the seated position for auscultation of the chest and heart and examination of the posterior aspect of the body.
❑	5	Maintains a quiet atmosphere to enhance the ability of the physician in hearing heart and lung sounds.
❑	5	*Rationale:* Understands that a quiet environment is necessary to accurately hear heart and lung sounds.
❑	5	Assists the patient into a supine position and drapes patient for examination of the chest. For female patients, see Procedure 30-7: Instructing Patient in Self-Breast Examination.
❑	5	Maintains patient in supine position and drapes patient for abdominal and extremities examinations.
❑	5	Gynecological examination may then be performed for female patients (see Procedure 30–6: Assisting with Gynecologic or Pelvic Examination and a Papanicolaou (Pap) Test). Assists patient into lithotomy position for gynecological and rectal examination.
❑	5	Testicular examination performed and rectal area examined for lesions and for size of prostate for male patients.
❑	5	Assists patient into Sims' position, if a more comprehensive rectal examination is necessary.
❑	5	Upon completion of the examination, assists patient to seated position and allows patient to sit at end of table for a few minutes to recover from any dizziness.
❑	5	Assures patient stability (checks color of skin, checks pulse) before allowing patient to stand up.

Task Performed	Possible Points	TASKS
❑	5	Assists patient in dressing; provides privacy.
❑	15	Charts any notes or patient instructions per physician's orders.
❑	5	Escorts patient to physician's office for discussion of examination results.
❑	5	Puts on disposable gloves.
❑	5	Disposes of gown and drape in a biohazard waste container.
❑	5	*Rationale:* Proper disposal prevents microorganism cross-contamination from patient body secretions.
❑	5	Disposes of contaminated materials in a biohazard container.
❑	5	*Rationale:* Prevents cross-contamination from bloodborne microorganisms and OPIM.
❑	5	Removes table paper and disposes in a biohazard waste container.
❑	5	*Rationale:* Prevents microorganism cross-contamination.
❑	5	Disinfects counters and examination table with a solution of 10 percent bleach.
❑	5	*Rationale:* Prevents microorganism cross-contamination by blood and OPIM.
❑	10	Cleans, sanitizes, disinfects, or sterilizes reusable instruments as instructed.
❑	5	Removes gloves, discards them in a biohazard waste container.
❑	5	*Rationale:* Prevents microorganism cross-contamination by blood and OPIM.
❑	5	Washes hands.
❑	10	Replaces table paper and equipment in preparation for the next patient.
❑	5	Completed the tasks within 15 minutes.
❑	15	Results obtained were accurate.

________	Earned	ADD POINTS OF TASKS CHECKED
300	Points	TOTAL POINTS POSSIBLE
________	SCORE	DETERMINE SCORE (divide points earned by total points possible, multiply results by 100)

Actual Student Time Needed to Complete Procedure: ____________

Student's Initials: ____________ Instructor's Initials: ____________ Grade: ____________

Suggestions for Improvement: ______________________________

Evaluator's Name (print) ______________________________

Evaluator's Signature ______________________________

Comments ______________________________

EVALUATION OF CHAPTER KNOWLEDGE

How has your instructor evaluated the knowledge you have achieved?

Knowledge	Instructor Evaluation *Good*	 *Average*	 *Poor*
Understands six methods used in physical examinations	_____	_____	_____
Demonstrates ability to place patients in eight positions used for physical examinations	_____	_____	_____
Understands draping techniques and the importance of patient privacy	_____	_____	_____
Identifies instruments and supplies necessary for examination of various body parts	_____	_____	_____
Identifies basic components of the physical examination	_____	_____	_____
Identifies sequence followed during a routine physical examination	_____	_____	_____
Recalls method of examination, instruments used, and positions for examination of at least eight body parts	_____	_____	_____
Understands quality control techniques and guidelines	_____	_____	_____
Observes all standard precautions and applies principles of aseptic technique	_____	_____	_____
Documents accurately, maintaining medical records and completing requisition forms	_____	_____	_____
Prepares patient for procedure	_____	_____	_____
Respects patient and attends to patient's emotional needs during physical examination	_____	_____	_____
Prepares and maintains examination and treatment areas	_____	_____	_____

Student's Initials: ______ Instructor's Initials: ______

Grade: _______

CHAPTER 25

Assisting With Minor Surgery

PERFORMANCE OBJECTIVES

Minor surgery is often performed in the ambulatory care setting by a physician with the help of a medical assistant. Medical assistants must be knowledgeable about surgical asepsis and sterile principles, surgical instruments, suture materials, surgical supplies and equipment, and basic surgery setup. Medical assistants should also know how to prepare patients for minor surgery, provide patient care, and assist the physician during common minor surgical procedures performed in the ambulatory care setting.

EXERCISES AND ACTIVITIES

Vocabulary Builder

A. Unscramble the following vocabulary words. Write the correct word in the space next to each scrambled word.

1. mmationinfla ______________________________
2. ineepinephr ______________________________
3. turealig ______________________________
4. diumso xidedrohy ______________________________
5. bechilens ______________________________
6. thesiaanes ______________________________
7. tabedine ______________________________
8. lversi ratenit ______________________________
9. propisoyl holcoal ______________________________
10. drohygen ideoxper ______________________________
11. turesstric ______________________________

12. nusatet ______________________________

13. calsurgi sispesa ______________________________

B. Match the vocabulary words below with their correct definitions.

_____ 1. Allergies

_____ 2. Antibacterial

_____ 3. Approximate

_____ 4. Bandage

_____ 5. Cautery

_____ 6. Contamination

_____ 7. Dressings

_____ 8. Infection

_____ 9. Informed Consent

_____ 10. Liquid Nitrogen

_____ 11. Mayo Stand/Instrument Tray

_____ 12. Ratchets

_____ 13. Surgery Cards

_____ 14. Suture

_____ 15. Swaged

A. To bring together the edges of a wound.

B. A written reference for surgeries and procedures.

C. Gauze or other material applied directly to a wound to absorb secretions and for protection.

D. When a surgical needle is attached to length of suture material.

E. Surgical material or thread; may describe the act of sewing with the surgical thread and needle.

F. Being sensitive to a normally harmless substance that causes an autoimmune reaction.

G. An invasion of pathogens into living tissue.

H. A voluntary agreement to have a procedure or surgery after a patient has been informed about the risks and benefits.

I. A portable metal tray table used for setting up sterile fields for minor surgery and procedures.

J. Capable of destroying bacteria.

K. Commonly and incorrectly referred to as "dry ice," it is a very volatile freezing agent used to destroy unwanted tissue such as warts.

L. The locking mechanisms on the handles of many surgical instruments.

M. The destruction of tissue by burning.

N. Gauze or other material applied over dressing to protect and immobilize.

O. To make something unclean, often used to describe a sterile area being made "unsterile" or exposing a clean area to a pathogenic substance.

LEARNING REVIEW/CASE STUDY

1. Identify each entry below as an example that follows strict sterile principles or an example in which the sterile area, field, or tray is contaminated by writing "sterile" or "contaminated" in the spaces provided.

_______________ A. Bruce Goldman, CMA, collects used instruments handed to him by Dr. Mark Woo during a minor surgical procedure to excise an infected sebaceous cyst by placing the instruments in a separate container or area out of view of the patient.

_______________ B. Ellen Armstrong, CMA, sets up a sterile field for a minor surgical procedure. After setting up the field, she remembers that a sterile solution is required and leaves the room to obtain the solution to be poured into a sterile cup.

_______________ C. Wanda Slawson, CMA, removes a dressing from a wound on a patient's arm and reaches over the sterile field to discard the used dressing in a biohazard waste container she has placed on the other side of the sterile field she set up for the procedure.

_______________ D. Patient Edith Leonard will not stop talking and asking questions as Liz Corbin, CMA, removes sutures from a small wound on Edith's arm sustained during a recent fall. The medical assistant is careful to time her responses to Edith so she is not talking when she is working directly over the sterile field.

_______________ E. Anna Preciado, CMA, applies sterile gloves in preparation to assist Dr. Lewis with a minor surgical procedure. During the procedure, she comforts the patient and assists the physician as required. When Anna's hands are not in use, she keeps them down at her sides, careful not to touch her gloved hands to her clothing or any other nonsterile item.

For each example above that represents a contamination of a sterile area, field, or tray, describe what went wrong and describe the correct sterile guidelines for each circumstance.

____

____

____

____

2. Identify each action that follows as an action appropriate to medical aseptic hand-washing technique (MAH), or surgical aseptic hand-washing technique (SAH).

_____ A. do not apply lotion

_____ B. glove for protection

_____ C. 2–3 minute duration

_____ D. scrub nails with brush and clean under each nail with cuticle stick

_____ E. apply lotion

_____ F. wash hands and wrists, and forearms to the elbows

_____ G. hands held down during rinsing

_____ H. 5–6 minute duration

3. Audrey Jones, CMA, will assist Dr. Lewis in suturing a long, deep, gaping laceration in Lenore McDonnell's leg, sustained when she fell while performing a wheelchair transfer from a car to the sidewalk on her campus. Audrey must prepare the examination room and assemble a sterile surgical tray for the physician's suturing procedure.

   A. From the selection that follows, identify each instrument by name. In the space below the instrument, give a brief description of what it is used for. Then, choose the correct instruments Audrey will need to prepare a sterile surgical tray for Dr. Lewis's suturing of the lacerated wound by placing an "X" in the appropriate boxes.

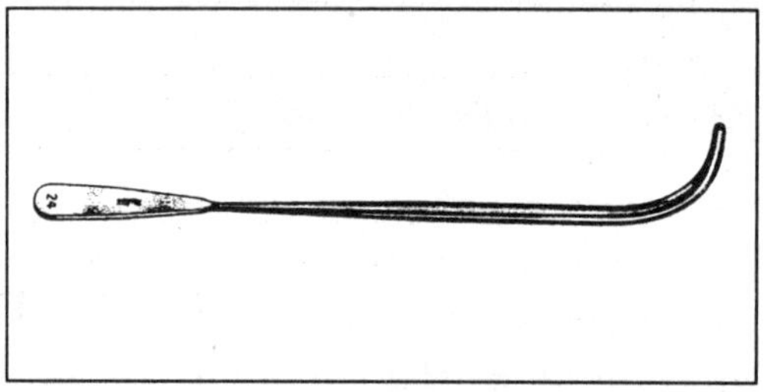

☐ A. ____________________

Purpose: ____________________

____

____

____

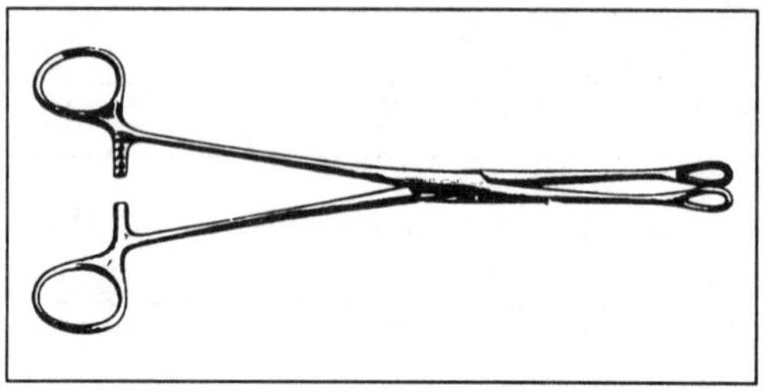

☐ B. ____________________

Purpose: ____________________

____

____

____

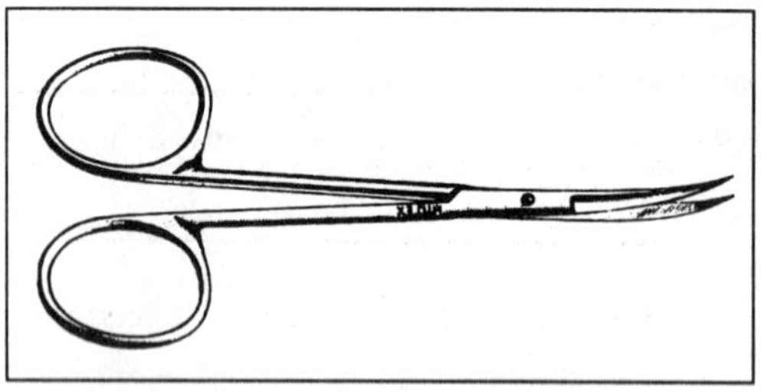

☐ C. ____________________

Purpose: ____________________

____

____

____

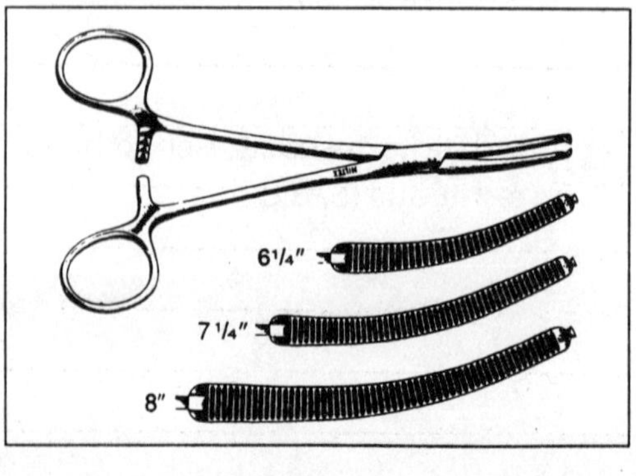

☐ D. ____________________

Purpose: ____________________

____

____

____

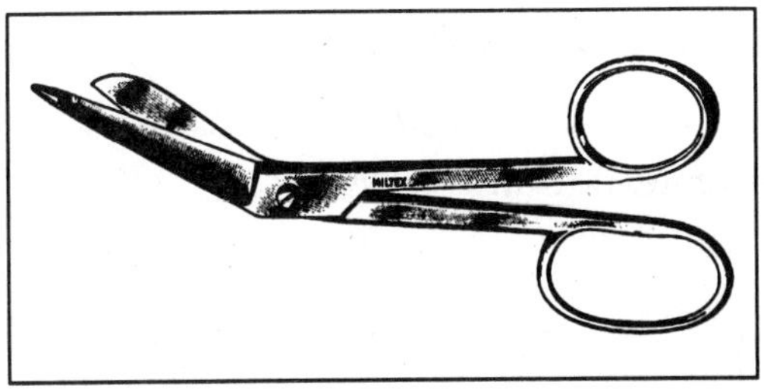

❑ E. ____________________

Purpose: ____________________

____

____

____

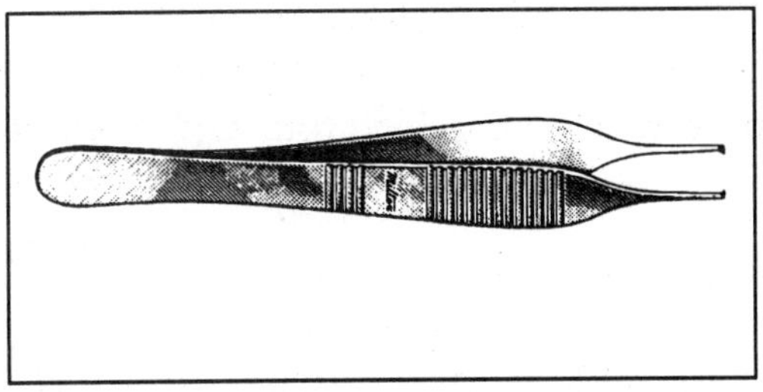

❑ F. ____________________

Purpose: ____________________

____

____

____

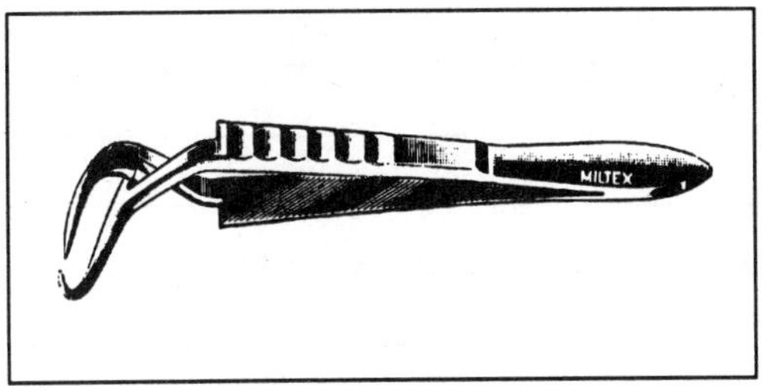

❑ G. ____________________

Purpose: ____________________

____

____

____

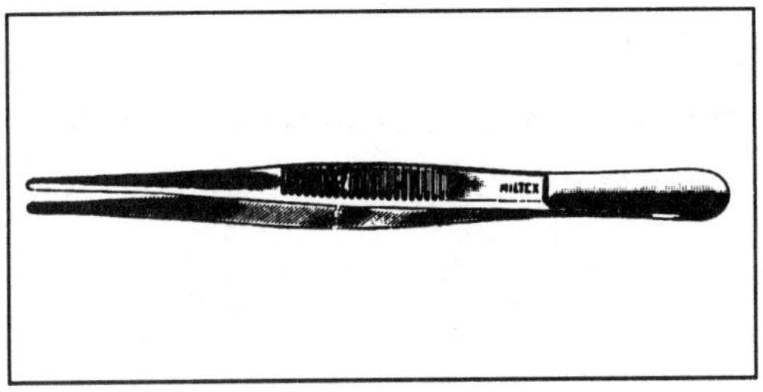

❑ H. ____________________

Purpose: ____________________

____

____

____

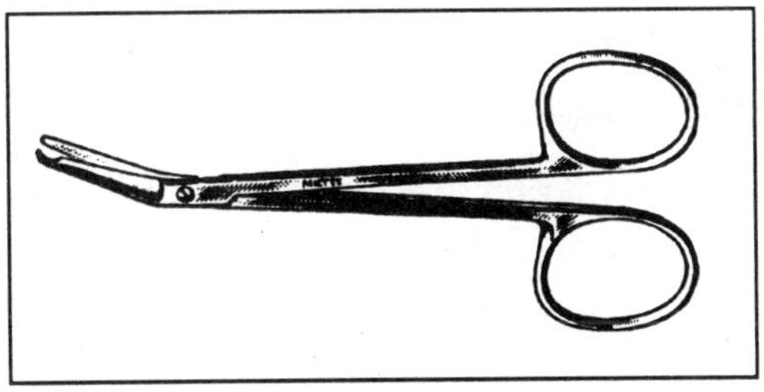

❑ I. ____________________

Purpose: ____________________

____

____

____

B. What other equipment will Audrey need to place on the sterile surgical tray for the physician's suturing of the lacerated wound? ____________________

____

What supplies will be needed for the side table? ____________________

____

C. When is suturing recommended? ____________________

____

____

What benefit does suturing provide the patient? ______________________________

____

Why must be done before a lacerated wound may be sutured? Why? ______________

____

4. When Lenore McDonnell returns to the physician's office to have sutures removed from her leg, Dr. Lewis checks the wound for the degree of healing and instructs Audrey Jones, CMA, to remove the sutures.

   A. From the selection of instruments shown in exercise #3A, which four will Audrey require for the suture removal procedure?

      (1) ______________________ (3) ______________________

      (2) ______________________ (4) ______________________

   B. What other equipment and supplies will Audrey assemble?

      ____

      ____

      ____

   C. What technique will Audrey use to perform the removal of the sutures?

      ____

      ____

      ____

   D. After removing the sutures, what additional patient care will Audrey give? Why?

      ____

      ____

      ____

SUPPLEMENTARY RESOURCES

Study Guide Disk: Additional practice exercises for this chapter are available on the study guide disk found in the textbook.

Medical Assisting Videos: Appropriate content is available on Delmar's Medical Assisting Videos, 2nd ed., for the following topics:

Tape 5: Set a Sterile Field
- Open a Sterile Pack
- Open a Peel Pack
- Use Disposable Trays of Instruments
- Perform Surgical Aseptic Procedures

Tape 6: Take Vital Signs

Tape 8: Assist Physician with Examination and Treatments
- Position and Drape the Patient
- Role of the Medical Assistant During the Examination

SKILLS COMPETENCY ASSESSMENT

Procedure 25–1: Chemical "Cold" Sterilization

Student's Name: ______________________________ Date: ____________

Objective: To sterilize heat-sensitive items such as fiber-optic endoscopes and delicate cutting instruments using an appropriate chemical solution.

Condition: The student demonstrates the ability to sterilize heat-sensitive items such as fiber-optic endoscopes and delicate cutting instruments using an appropriate chemical solution such as Cidex Steris System® (Percacetic acid) and the following equipment and supplies: airtight container, timer, sterile water, gloves (heavy-duty), sterile towel, plastic-lined sterile drapes.

Time Requirements and Accuracy Standards: 5 minutes. Points assigned reflect importance of step to meeting objective: Important = (5) Essential = (10) Critical = (15). Automatic failure results if any of the **critical** tasks are omitted or performed incorrectly.

STANDARD PRECAUTIONS:

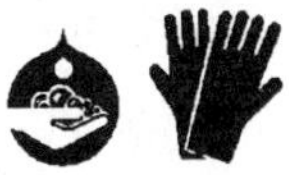

SKILLS ASSESSMENT CHECKLIST

Task Performed	Possible Points	TASKS
☐	10	Sanitizes items that require chemical sterilization (see Procedure 21–4). Rinses and dries items.
☐	5	*Rationale:* Recalls that debris and body proteins must be scrubbed from items prior to sterilization.
☐	5	Reads manufacturer's instructions on original container of chemical sterilization solution.
☐	5	*Rationale:* Understands that each brand of chemical sterilization solution has specific preparation instructions and germicidal properties. Keeps solution in original container to avoid accidental poisoning.
☐	5	Puts on gloves.
☐	5	*Rationale:* Understands that heavy-duty gloves help protect from sharp items puncturing the skin and from harsh chemicals.
☐	10	Prepares solution as indicated by manufacturer, places the date of opening or preparation on the container, and initials it.
☐	5	*Rationale:* Following the manufacturer's instructions ensures sterility.
☐	5	Pours solution into a container with an airtight lid; avoids splashing.
☐	5	*Rationale:* Understands that chemicals should not be left exposed to open air in order to prevent evaporation and loss of potency, exposure to environmental contaminants, accidental inhalation, or poisoning. Splashing may cause injury to skin or mucous membranes.

SKILLS COMPETENCY ASSESSMENT — continued

Procedure 25–1: Chemical "Cold" Sterilization

Task Performed	Possible Points	TASKS
❑	10	Places sanitized and dried items into the solution, completely submersing item(s). Avoids splashing when placing items into airtight container.
❑	5	*Rationale:* Understands that total immersion is necessary for sterilization to be achieved.
❑	5	Closes lid of containers, labels with name of solution, exposure time required per manufacturer, and initials.
❑	5	*Rationale:* Understands that exposure time is the required time indicated by the manufacturer to achieve sterility.
❑	10	Does not open lid or add additional items during the processing time.
❑	5	*Rationale:* Understands that adding to the container interrupts the sterilization process and limits effectiveness of the chemical.
❑	15	Follows the recommended processing time, lifts item(s) from the container using sterile gloved hands or sterile transfer forceps. Holds item carefully above sterile basin and pours copious amounts of sterile water over it and through it (endoscopes) until adequately rinsed of chemical solution.
❑	5	*Rationale:* Items, once they are processed, are sterile and must be handled appropriately. Chemicals are rinsed from both the outside and inside of equipment (endoscopes) because they can be caustic to tissues.
❑	10	Holds item(s) upright for a few seconds to allow excess sterile water to drip off.
❑	10	Places the sterile item on a sterile towel, which has been placed on a sterile field, and dries it with another sterile towel. Removes the towel used for drying from the sterile field. Plastic-lined sterile drapes are used for the sterile field.
❑	5	*Rationale:* Plastic-lined sterile drapes create a barrier to prevent moisture from drawing contaminants from the metal surgical instrument tray or countertop up into the sterile area. The wet towel used to dry the endoscope is removed to prevent contamination.
❑	5	Completed the tasks within 5 minutes.
❑	15	Results obtained were accurate.

______	Earned	ADD POINTS OF TASKS CHECKED
165	Points	TOTAL POINTS POSSIBLE
______	SCORE	DETERMINE SCORE (divide points earned by total points possible, multiply results by 100)

Actual Student Time Needed to Complete Procedure: ____________

Student's Initials: ____________ Instructor's Initials: ____________ Grade: ____________

Suggestions for Improvement: ______________________________

Evaluator's Name (print) ______________________________

Evaluator's Signature ______________________________

Comments ______________________________

SKILLS COMPETENCY ASSESSMENT

Procedure 25–2: Applying Sterile Gloves

Student's Name: ______________________________ Date: ____________

Objective: To provide direction on how to apply sterile gloves without compromising sterility.

Conditions: The student demonstrates the ability to apply sterile gloves without compromising sterility using a packaged pair of sterile gloves.

Time Requirements and Accuracy Standards: 5 minutes. Points assigned reflect importance of step to meeting objective: Important = (5) Essential = (10) Critical = (15). Automatic failure results if any of the **critical** tasks are omitted or performed incorrectly.

STANDARD PRECAUTIONS:

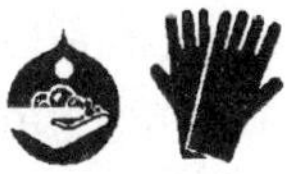

SKILLS ASSESSMENT CHECKLIST

Task Performed	Possible Points	TASKS
☐	5	Removes rings and watches. Washes hands using surgical asepsis.
☐	5	*Rationale:* Understands that jewelry can snag gloves, interfering with barrier protection.
☐	10	Inspects glove package for tears or stains.
☐	5	*Rationale:* Torn or stained gloves are not sterile and must be disposed of or used for nonsterile purpose.
☐	10	Places the glove package on a clean, dry, flat surface above waist level.
☐	5	*Rationale:* A contaminated surface would compromise sterility of the sterile package.
☐	10	Peels open the package taking care not to touch the sterile inner surface of the package. Does not allow the gloves to slide beyond the sterile inner border.
☐	15	Opens the gloves with the cuffs toward the body, the palms of the gloves face up, and the thumbs pointing outward. Turns the package around, being careful not to reach over the sterile area or touch the inner surface or the gloves, if the gloves are not positioned properly.
☐	15	Grasps the inner cuffed edge of the opposite glove with the index finger and thumb of the nondominant hand. Picks the glove straight up off the package surface without dragging or dangling the fingers over any nonsterile area.
☐	5	*Rationale:* This method prevents the outer glove from becoming contaminated.

SKILLS COMPETENCY ASSESSMENT — continued

Procedure 25–2: Applying Sterile Gloves

Task Performed	Possible Points	TASKS
☐	15	Slides the hand carefully into the glove with the palm up on the dominant hand. Does not allow the outside of the glove to come into contact with anything. Always holds the hands above the waist and away from the body.
☐	5	*Rationale:* Understands that palm-up orientation keeps glove sterile in the palm area if it rolls slightly on the back of the hand.
☐	15	Picks up the glove for the remaining hand with the gloved hand by slipping four fingers under the outside of the cuff. Lifts the second glove up, keeping it held above the waist and away from the body. Does not allow the glove to drag across the package or touch nonsterile surfaces.
☐	5	*Rationale:* Understands that outside of the other glove is sterile and may only be touched by another sterile surface.
☐	15	Slips the second hand into the glove with the palm up. Does not allow the outside of the gloves to touch nonsterile skin.
☐	15	Adjusts the gloves on the hands as needed, but avoids touching the wrist area. Keeps gloved hands above the waist and away from the body. Does not touch nonsterile surfaces with gloved hands.
☐	5	Completed the tasks within 5 minutes.
☐	15	Results obtained were accurate.

_______	Earned	ADD POINTS OF TASKS CHECKED
175	Points	TOTAL POINTS POSSIBLE
_______	SCORE	DETERMINE SCORE (divide points earned by total points possible, multiply results by 100)

Actual Student Time Needed to Complete Procedure: ____________

Student's Initials: ____________ Instructor's Initials: ____________ Grade: ____________

Suggestions for Improvement: ______________________________

____

____

____

Evaluator's Name (print) ______________________________

Evaluator's Signature ______________________________

Comments ______________________________

SKILLS COMPETENCY ASSESSMENT

Procedure 25–3: Setting Up and Covering a Sterile Field

Student's Name: ______________________________ Date: ____________

Objective: To set up and cover a sterile field.

Conditions: The student demonstrates the ability to use disposable sterile field drapes or sterile towels to isolate a sterile area or field as well as to cover the sterile field for use in minor office surgery and procedures using the following equipment and supplies: 2 disposable sterile field drapes or 2 sterile towels (muslin or linen with water-repellent finish), Mayo instrument tray/stand, sterile transfer forceps.

Time Requirements and Accuracy Standards: 10 minutes. Points assigned reflect importance of step to meeting objective: Important = (5) Essential = (10) Critical = (15). Automatic failure results if any of the **critical** tasks are omitted or performed incorrectly.

STANDARD PRECAUTIONS:

SKILLS ASSESSMENT CHECKLIST

Task Performed	Possible Points	TASKS
❑	5	Washes hands.
❑	10	Sanitizes and disinfects a Mayo instrument tray.
❑	5	Selects an appropriate disposable sterile field drape and places drape package on a clean, dry, flat surface, or removes a fan-folded sterile cloth towel from a canister using sterile forceps.
❑	5	*Rationale:* Sterile field drapes are fan-folded and positioned within the package to facilitate ease of use. Sterile towels are fan-folded and positioned within the canister for ease of use.
❑	10	If using disposable drape, peels open the package exposing the fan-folded drape. Turns package if necessary so cut corners of drape face toward the body. Or, removes sterile towel from canister using sterile transfer forceps.
❑	5	*Rationale:* The drape or towel will naturally unfold as it is lifted so care must be taken to ensure than it is lifted quickly and allowed to unfold without touching a nonsterile area.
❑	10	With thumb and forefinger of one hand, carefully grasps the top cut corner without touching the rest of the drape or towel and picks up the drape or towel high enough to assure that as it unfolds it does not drag across a nonsterile area.
❑	10	Holds the drape or towel above waist level and away from the body and grasps the opposing corner so both corners along the short edge of the drape are held.

SKILLS COMPETENCY ASSESSMENT — continued

Procedure 25–3: Setting Up and Covering a Sterile Field

Task Performed	Possible Points	TASKS
❑	15	Keeps the drape or towel above waist level and away from the body and reaches over the Mayo tray with the drape or towel. Takes care that the lower edge does not drag across the tray.
❑	5	*Rationale:* Sterile principle states that sterile items should be kept above the waist.
❑	15	Gently pulls the drape or towel toward the body as it is laid onto the tray. If adjusting to center on tray, does not touch the center of the drape or towel, or reach over the sterile field, but walks around or reaches underneath the tray to move it or make adjustments.
❑	5	*Rationale:* Understands that edges hanging over the tray are not sterile.
❑	15	Repeats procedure with a second drape or towel. Instead of pulling the drape toward the body, which would necessitate reaching over the sterile field, applies the covering drape or towel by holding it up in front of the field. Adjusts the lower edge so it is even with the lower edge of the field drape or towel. With a forward motion, carefully lays the cover over the sterile field.
❑	5	*Rationale:* Understands that reaching over sterile field will contaminate the tray.
❑	5	Completed the tasks within 10 minutes.
❑	15	Results obtained were accurate.

______	Earned	ADD POINTS OF TASKS CHECKED
140	Points	TOTAL POINTS POSSIBLE
______	SCORE	DETERMINE SCORE (divide points earned by total points possible, multiply results by 100)

Actual Student Time Needed to Complete Procedure: ____________

Student's Initials: ____________ Instructor's Initials: ____________ Grade: ____________

Suggestions for Improvement: ______________________________________

____

____

____

Evaluator's Name (print) ______________________________________

Evaluator's Signature ______________________________________

Comments ______________________________________

SKILLS COMPETENCY ASSESSMENT

Procedure 25–4: Opening Sterile Packages of Instruments and Applying Them to a Sterile Field

Student's Name: ______________________________ Date: ____________

Objective: To open sterile packages of surgical instruments and supplies and place them onto a sterile field using sterile technique.

Conditions: The student demonstrates the ability to open sterile packages of surgical instruments and supplies and place them onto a sterile field with sterile technique using the following equipment and supplies: Mayo instrument tray, sterile field drapes (2) or sterile towels (2), sterile gloves, wrapped-twice sterile surgical instruments, prepackaged sterile surgical supplies.

Time Requirements and Accuracy Standards: 10 minutes. Points assigned reflect importance of step to meeting objective: Important = (5) Essential = (10) Critical = (15). Automatic failure results if any of the **critical** tasks are omitted or performed incorrectly.

STANDARD PRECAUTIONS:

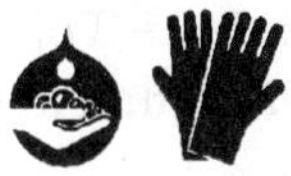

SKILLS ASSESSMENT CHECKLIST

Task Performed	Possible Points	TASKS
☐	5	Assembles supplies.
☐	5	Washes hands and sets up sterile field.
☐	10	Positions package of surgical instruments on palm of nondominant hand with outer envelope flap on top to facilitate opening the pack while protecting the sterile contents.
☐	5	*Rationale:* This will facilitate opening the pack while protecting the sterile contents.
☐	10	Grasps the taped end of the top flap and opens the first flap away from them. Does not touch the inside of the flap.
☐	10	Grasps just the folded back tips of the side flaps and pulls the right-sided flap to the right. Then pulls the left-sided flap to the left, taking care not to reach over the package.
☐	5	*Rationale:* Understands that pulling the tips of the flaps toward each side allows the inner portion of the package to be exposed without contamination.
☐	10	Pulls the last flap toward them by grasping the folded-back tip, taking care not to touch the inner contents of the package.
☐	5	*Rationale:* Understands that this method avoids reaching over the inner contents of the package.
☐	10	Gathers all of the loose edges together to obtain a snug covering over their nondominant hand. Closes their covered hand over the inner package and carefully applies the inner package to the sterile field.

SKILLS COMPETENCY ASSESSMENT — continued

Procedure 25–4: Opening Sterile Packages of Instruments and Applying Them to a Sterile Field

Task Performed	Possible Points	TASKS
❑	5	*Rationale:* Understands that gathering loose edges prevents dragging across the sterile field.
❑	15	Opens peel-apart packages using sterile techniques by grasping both edges of the flaps and pulling them apart in a rolling down motion, keeping both hands together. Gradually exposes the sterile item between the two peel-apart edges. Offers the sterile inner contents to the sterile-gloved physician or applies it to the sterile field using a flipping motion, taking care not to contaminate either the package contents or the field.
❑	15	Applies sterile gloves. Arranges instruments and supplies in an organized and logical manner according to the physician's preference. Points all handles toward the user. Separates instruments as much as possible within the space of the field so entanglement of instruments is not a problem.
❑	10	Applies the sterile field cover.
❑	5	*Rationale:* A sterile cover will need to be applied if the surgical tray will not be used immediately, needs to be moved, or if the medical assistant leaves the tray unattended.
❑	5	Completed the tasks within 10 minutes.
❑	15	Results obtained were accurate.

______	Earned	ADD POINTS OF TASKS CHECKED
145	Points	TOTAL POINTS POSSIBLE
______	SCORE	DETERMINE SCORE (divide points earned by total points possible, multiply results by 100)

Actual Student Time Needed to Complete Procedure: ____________

Student's Initials: ____________ Instructor's Initials: ____________ Grade: ____________

Suggestions for Improvement: ______________________________

____

____

____

Evaluator's Name (print) ______________________________

Evaluator's Signature ______________________________

Comments ______________________________

SKILLS COMPETENCY ASSESSMENT

Procedure 25–5: Pouring a Sterile Solution into a Cup on a Sterile Field

Student's Name: ______________________________ Date: ____________

Objective: To pour a sterile solution into a cup on a sterile tray in a sterile manner.

Conditions: The student demonstrates the ability to pour a sterile solution into a cup on a sterile tray in a sterile manner using the following equipment and supplies: covered sterile surgical tray with a sterile cup in upper-right corner, container of sterile solution.

Time Requirements and Accuracy Standards: 2 minutes. Points assigned reflect importance of step to meeting objective: Important = (5) Essential = (10) Critical = (15). Automatic failure results if any of the **critical** tasks are omitted or performed incorrectly.

SKILLS ASSESSMENT CHECKLIST

Task Performed	Possible Points	TASKS
☐	5	Transports the surgical tray into the surgical area before pouring the solution. Or: the surgical tray can be set up for immediate use in the surgical area.
☐	5	*Rationale:* Understands that solution may tip and spill during transport.
☐	5	Reads the label of the solution container and checks the expiration date.
☐	5	*Rationale:* To avoid pouring the wrong solution or using an outdated solution.
☐	10	Removes the cap from the solution container taking care not to touch the inner surface of the cap. Places the cap upside down on a nonsterile surface to avoid touching the inner surface of the cap with a nonsterile surface. Holds the cap right side up when it is held in the hand.
☐	5	*Rationale:* Understands that touching the inside of the cap with the hand or a nonsterile surface will contaminate the inside of an otherwise sterile container.
☐	15	Reads the label again to assure accuracy. Places palm over the label to protect the label from stains. Pours a small amount of the solution into a bowl or cup that is outside of the sterile field. If the sterile tray is set up in the surgical area, solution can be poured prior to covering the surgical tray with a sterile drape or towel.
☐	5	*Rationale:* This action cleanses container lip. NOTE: If the surgical tray is set up in the surgical area, the solution can be poured prior to voering the surgical ray with a sterile drape or towel.
☐	10	Pulls back carefully on the upper-right corner of the tray cover to expose the cup. Takes care to touch only the corner tip of the cover and to not reach over the exposed field.

SKILLS COMPETENCY ASSESSMENT — continued

Procedure 25–5: Pouring a Sterile Solution into a Cup on a Sterile Field

Task Performed	Possible Points	TASKS
❑	5	*Rationale:* Reaching over the sterile field or touching the underside of the cover will contaminate the sterile surgical tray.
❑	15	Approaches from the corner of the tray, and using the cleansed side of the lip of the container, pours the needed amount of solution into the sterile cup. Takes precautions to avoid splashing, spilling, reaching over the field, or touching any of the sterile surfaces.
❑	5	*Rationale:* Prevents contaminants from "wicking" from the metal tray into the sterile field. Polylined sterile field drapes will create a barrier.
❑	5	Replaces the cap of the solution container using sterile technique.
❑	10	Replaces the corner of the drape cover using sterile technique or covers with a sterile drape or towel.
❑	5	Completed the tasks within 2 minutes.
❑	15	Results obtained were accurate.

______		Earned	ADD POINTS OF TASKS CHECKED
	125	Points	TOTAL POINTS POSSIBLE
______		SCORE	DETERMINE SCORE (divide points earned by total points possible, multiply results by 100)

Actual Student Time Needed to Complete Procedure: ____________

Student's Initials: ____________ Instructor's Initials: ____________ Grade: ____________

Suggestions for Improvement: ______________________________

____

____

____

Evaluator's Name (print) ______________________________

Evaluator's Signature ______________________________

Comments ______________________________

SKILLS COMPETENCY ASSESSMENT

Procedure 25–6: Preparation of Patient Skin for Minor Surgery

Student's Name: ______________________________ Date: ____________

Objective: To remove as many microorganisms as possible from the patient's skin prior to surgery.

Conditions: The student demonstrates the ability to remove as many microorganisms as possible from the patient's skin prior to surgery using the following equipment and supplies: absorbent pad, drape, disposable prep kit (includes: antiseptic soap, several sponges, razor, and a container for water), sterile water, antiseptic solution, sterile bowl, sterile gloves for medical assistant and physician (2 pairs).

Time Requirements and Accuracy Standards: 10 minutes. Points assigned reflect importance of step to meeting objective: Important = (5) Essential = (10) Critical = (15). Automatic failure results if any of the **critical** tasks are omitted or performed incorrectly.

STANDARD PRECAUTIONS: 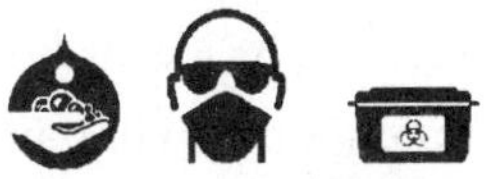

SKILLS ASSESSMENT CHECKLIST

Task Performed	Possible Points	TASKS
☐	5	Washes hands. Assembles equipment.
☐	5	Identifies patient. Explains the procedure, provides privacy, and drapes patient if appropriate.
☐	10	Provides good light source.
☐	5	Positions patient for comfort and preparation of site exposure.
☐	5	Washes hands.
☐	5	Protects area under preparation site with an absorbent pad.
☐	10	Puts on sterile gloves.
☐	10	Applies antiseptic soap (Betadine) with 4 × 4 sponges, beginning at operative site and moving outward in a circular motion from the center to away from the center of the prepared area.
☐	5	*Rationale:* Move from cleaner to least-clean areas to prevent contamination.
☐	5	Discards used sponges as necessary.

SKILLS COMPETENCY ASSESSMENT — continued

Procedure 25–6: Preparation of Patient Skin for Minor Surgery

Task Performed	Possible Points	TASKS
❑	15	Holds skin taut and uses razor to shave hair away from operative site, following hair growth pattern to prevent accidental nicks, which can cause infection.
❑	15	When hair has been removed, scrubs again in a circular fashion for about two to five minutes.
❑	10	Rinses shaved area with sterile water and dries with a sterile 4 × 4 gauze sponge.
❑	5	Covers with a sterile towel; instructs patient to not touch the area.
❑	5	Pours antiseptic solution (Betadine) into the sterile bowl. Physician will put on sterile gloves and using a sterile 4 × 4 gauze sponge will paint the operative site with the antiseptic solution. Lets dry, drapes patient with sterile drapes, and commences with the surgical procedure.
❑	5	Completed the tasks within 10 minutes.
❑	15	Results obtained were accurate.

______	Earned	ADD POINTS OF TASKS CHECKED
135	Points	TOTAL POINTS POSSIBLE
______	SCORE	DETERMINE SCORE (divide points earned by total points possible, multiply results by 100)

Actual Student Time Needed to Complete Procedure: ____________

Student's Initials: ____________ Instructor's Initials: ____________ Grade: ____________

Suggestions for Improvement: ____

____

____

____

Evaluator's Name (print) ____

Evaluator's Signature ____

Comments ____

SKILLS COMPETENCY ASSESSMENT

Procedure 25–7: Assisting with Minor Surgery

Student's Name: ______________________________ Date: ____________

Objective: To maintain sterility during minor surgical procedures that require surgical excision of a neoplasm.

Conditions: The student demonstrates the ability to maintain sterility during minor surgical procedures that require surgical excision of a neoplasm using the following equipment and supplies. Mayo stand: needles and syringe, Betadine solution, gauze sponges, scalpel and blades, dissecting scissors, operating scissors, forceps that hold the drapes or 4 sterile towels and 4 clamps, hemostats (2 curved and 2 straight), thumb forceps, suture material, tissue forceps, needle holder, skin retractor, transfer forceps. Side table: sterile gloves, labeled biopsy containers with formalin, appropriate laboratory requisition, anesthesia, alcohol wipes, dressing tape, bandages, biohazard container.

Time Requirements and Accuracy Standards: Time varies according to patient's condition and length of time required by the physician to complete the procedure. Points assigned reflect importance of step to meeting objective: Important = (5) Essential = (10) Critical = (15). Automatic failure results if any of the **critical** tasks are omitted or performed incorrectly.

STANDARD PRECAUTIONS:

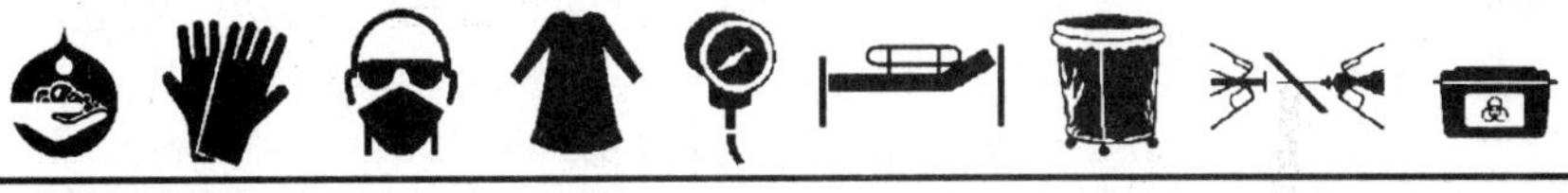

SKILLS ASSESSMENT CHECKLIST

Task Performed	Possible Points	TASKS
❑	5	Checks room for readiness and equipment for cleanliness.
❑	5	Washes hands.
❑	5	Sets up side table of nonsterile items.
❑	5	*Rationale:* Understands that nonsterile items will contaminate a sterile field.
❑	10	Performs surgical asepsis handwash.
❑	15	Sets up sterile field on a Mayo stand or on a clean, dry, flat surface. • Uses a commercially prepared sterile setup that is appropriate for the surgical procedure. Opens the setup creating a sterile field with the inside of the sterile wrap. Adds other articles such as instruments or supplies as needed by using sterile transfer forceps or peel-apart packages that can be opened in a sterile fashion. *or* • Removes a sterile fan-folded towel from a canister of sterile towels using sterile transfer forceps. Holds one edge of the sterile towel and allows it to become unfolded by gently shaking it. Grasps the other edge and gently places the towel on the Mayo stand from the farthest side to the side nearest the body. Adds sterile articles.
❑	10	Applies sterile gloves. Arranges instruments according to use.

SKILLS COMPETENCY ASSESSMENT — continued

Procedure 25–7: Assisting with Minor Surgery

Task Performed	Possible Points	TASKS
❑	10	Covers the sterile field with a sterile towel if not being used immediately. Gently places towel from the side nearest the body to the side farthest away from the body.
❑	5	Identifies patient, explains the procedure, and prepares the patient.
❑	5	Prepares patient's skin (see Procedure 25–6).
❑	15	Removes the sterile cover from the sterile setup as the physician applies sterile gloves. Lifts the towel by grasping the tip of the corner farthest away from the body and lifting toward the body. Does not allow arms to pass over sterile field.
❑	15	Assists the physician as necessary, being certain to follow the principles of surgical asepsis. The physician will inject local anesthetic, apply Betadine or another antiseptic to the surgical site, apply sterile drapes, and begin the surgery.
❑	15	The medical assistant will assist the physician during surgery in the following manner: • Holds the vial of anesthesia while the physician withdraws the appropriate dose. • Adjusts the instrument tray and equipment around the physician. • Assures a good light source. • Comforts and supports the patient emotionally. • Assists with the surgery as directed by the physician (sterile gloves must be worn). • Hands instruments to the physician and receives used instruments from the physician and places them in a basin or container out of the patient's sight. • Holds biopsy container to receive specimen being excised, if necessary. • Does not contaminate the inside of the container. • Holds the cover facing down. Tightly places cover on the container. • Assists with or applies sterile dressing to the operative site.
❑	5	Assists patient as necessary.
❑	15	Handles the specimen container with disposable gloves as recommended by standard precautions. Assures that the container is tightly covered, labeled with the patient's name, date, type, and source of specimen and sent to the laboratory recommended by the appropriate laboratory requisition.
❑	15	Cleans surgical or examination room while wearing appropriate personal protective equipment (PPE). • Disposes of used sponges in biohazard container and knife blades and other disposable sharps in puncture-proof sharps container. • Rinses used surgical instruments; soaks, sanitizes, and sterilizes for reuse. • Removes gloves and other PPE and disposes of per OSHA guidelines.

Task Performed	Possible Points	TASKS
☐	5	Washes hands.
☐	5	Documents in the patient's record that the specimen was sent to the laboratory.
☐	5	Completed the tasks within the time constraint identified by the instructor.
☐	15	Results obtained were accurate.
______	Earned	ADD POINTS OF TASKS CHECKED
	185 Points	TOTAL POINTS POSSIBLE
______	SCORE	DETERMINE SCORE (divide points earned by total points possible, multiply results by 100)

Actual Student Time Needed to Complete Procedure: ____________

Student's Initials: ____________ Instructor's Initials: ____________ Grade: ____________

Suggestions for Improvement: ____

____

____

____

Evaluator's Name (print) ____

Evaluator's Signature ____

Comments ____

DOCUMENTATION

Chart the procedure in the patient's medical record.

Date: ____________________

Charting: ____

____

____

Student's Initials: ____________

SKILLS COMPETENCY ASSESSMENT

Procedure 25–8: Suturing of Laceration or Incision Repair

Student's Name: ______________________________ Date: ____________

Objective: To assist the physician in wound cleaning and suture repair of a laceration or incision-type wound.

Conditions: The student demonstrates the ability to assist the physician in wound cleaning and suture repair of a laceration or an incision-type wound, using the following equipment and supplies. Surgical tray: syringe and needle for anesthetic, hemostats (curved), Adson or tissue forceps, Iris scissors (curved), suture material and needle, needle holder, gauze sponges. Side table: anesthetic, as ordered by the physician, dressings, bandages, tape, splint/brace/sling (optional), sterile gloves.

Time Requirements and Accuracy Standards: 10 minutes. Points assigned reflect importance of step to meeting objective: Important = (5) Essential = (10) Critical = (15). Automatic failure results if any of the **critical** tasks are omitted or performed incorrectly.

STANDARD PRECAUTIONS:

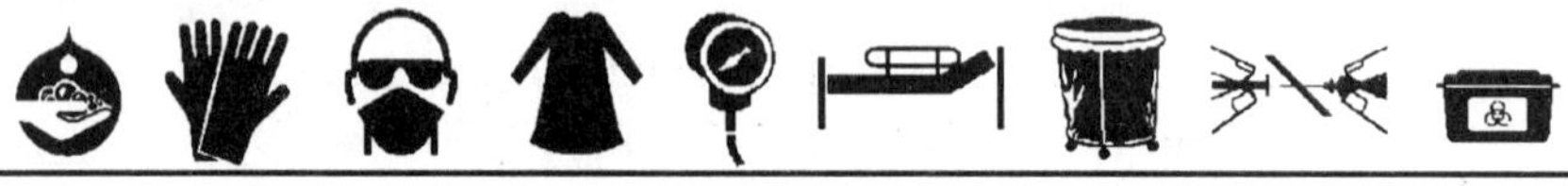

SKILLS ASSESSMENT CHECKLIST

Task Performed	Possible Points	TASKS
❑	5	Washes hands.
❑	10	Identifies the patient and explains the procedure. Checks for signed consent forms.
❑	5	Reassures and comforts the patient as needed.
❑	15	Assesses cause of wound and its severity. • Determines any known allergies and last tetanus booster • Identifies any health concerns to avoid possible complications • Soaks wound in an antiseptic solution as ordered by the physician • Cleans and dries wound • Positions patient comfortably, lying down
❑	5	Assists the physician as needed.
❑	5	Supports the patient as needed.
		Postoperative Care
❑	5	Applies sterile gloves.
❑	5	Cleans area around the wound.
❑	5	Dresses/bandages/splints wound following the physician's preference.
❑	5	Removes gloves, washes hands.

Task Performed	Possible Points	TASKS
❑	15	Checks patient's vital signs.
❑	15	Explains wound care to the patient (and caregiver) and provides written instructions, including symptoms of infection.
❑	5	Assists the patient with any concerns or questions.
❑	5	Arranges for follow-up appointment and medication, as ordered.
❑	10	Disposes of supplies per OSHA guidelines. Cleans room, sanitizes instruments, sterilizes for reuse.
❑	5	Washes hands; documents the procedure.
❑	5	Completed the tasks within 10 minutes.
❑	15	Results obtained were accurate.

______	Earned	ADD POINTS OF TASKS CHECKED
140	Points	TOTAL POINTS POSSIBLE
______	SCORE	DETERMINE SCORE (divide points earned by total points possible, multiply results by 100)

Actual Student Time Needed to Complete Procedure: ____________

Student's Initials: ____________ Instructor's Initials: ____________ Grade: ____________

Suggestions for Improvement: ______________________________

Evaluator's Name (print) ______________________________

Evaluator's Signature ______________________________

Comments ______________________________

DOCUMENTATION

Chart the procedure in the patient's medical record.

Date: ____________________

Charting: ______________________________

____

____

Student's Initials: ______________

SKILLS COMPETENCY ASSESSMENT

Procedure 25–9: Dressing Change

Student's Name: ______________________________ Date: ____________

Objective: To remove a wound dressing and apply a dry sterile dressing.

Conditions: The student demonstrates the ability to remove a wound dressing and apply a dry sterile dressing using the following equipment and supplies. Sterile field: several sterile gauze sponges and other dressing material as needed, sterile bowl with Betadine solution, sterile dressing forceps. Side area: nonsterile gloves, sterile gloves, container of hydrogen peroxide or sterile water, cotton-tipped applicators, sterile adhesive strips (optional), antibacterial ointment/cream as ordered, tape, bandage scissors (2), waterproof waste bag, biohazard waste container.

Time Requirements and Accuracy Standards: 10 minutes. Points assigned reflect importance of step to meeting objective: Important = (5) Essential = (10) Critical = (15). Automatic failure results if any of the **critical** tasks are omitted or performed incorrectly.

STANDARD PRECAUTIONS:

SKILLS ASSESSMENT CHECKLIST

Task Performed	Possible Points	TASKS
☐	5	Washes hands.
☐	10	Prepares sterile field. Adds gauze sponges, bowl with solution, and forceps.
☐	5	Positions a waterproof bag away from sterile area.
☐	5	Pours Betadine solution into sterile bowl.
☐	5	Identifies the patient and explains the procedure.
☐	5	Reassures and comforts the patient as needed.
☐	5	Loosens tape on dressing or cuts off bandage if necessary.
☐	5	Puts on nonsterile gloves or uses forceps.
☐	10	Removes bandage carefully, places in biohazard waste container. Does not pass over sterile field.
☐	15	Removes dressing, taking care not to cause stress on the wound. If stuck to the wound, pours small amounts of sterile water or hydrogen peroxide over dressing; allows to soak for a short time. Removes dressing when loose enough to remove without resistance.
☐	10	Places used dressing in waterproof bag without touching inside or outside of bag.
☐	10	Assesses wound and notes any drainage or signs of infection. Removes and discards gloves in waterproof bag.

Task Performed	Possible Points	TASKS
☐	10	Washes hands, applies sterile gloves.
☐	5	Cleans the wound with Betadine solution.
☐	5	Disposes of used gauze in waterproof bag.
☐	10	Using forceps, applies sterile gauze sponge (s) to wound.
☐	5	Removes gloves and disposes of in waterproof bag.
☐	5	Secures dressing with adhesive tape, roller bandage, or elastic bandage.
☐	5	Disposes of waterproof bag in biohazard container.
☐	5	Washes hands.
☐	15	Documents procedure and describes wound appearance (i.e., discharge, signs of infection, healing, etc.)
☐	5	Completed the tasks within 10 minutes.
☐	15	Results obtained were accurate.

_______	Earned	ADD POINTS OF TASKS CHECKED
175	Points	TOTAL POINTS POSSIBLE
_______	SCORE	DETERMINE SCORE (divide points earned by total points possible, multiply results by 100)

Actual Student Time Needed to Complete Procedure: ____________

Student's Initials: ____________ Instructor's Initials: ____________ Grade: ____________

Suggestions for Improvement: ________________________________

Evaluator's Name (print) ________________________________

Evaluator's Signature ________________________________

Comments________________________________

DOCUMENTATION

Chart the procedure in the patient's medical record.

Date:____________________

Charting: ________________________________

____

____

Student's Initials:____________

SKILLS COMPETENCY ASSESSMENT

Procedure 25–10: Suture Removal

Student's Name: ______________________________ Date: ____________

Objective: To remove sutures from a healed minor surgical wound (as per physician).

Conditions: The student demonstrates the ability to remove sutures from a healed minor surgical wound (as per physician) using the following equipment and supplies: gauze sponges, biohazard waste container, tape, suture removal kit (suture scissors or staple remover and thumb forceps), sterile latex gloves, Betadine solution or wash.

Time Requirements and Accuracy Standards: 10 minutes. Points assigned reflect importance of step to meeting objective: Important = (5) Essential = (10) Critical = (15). Automatic failure results if any of the **critical** tasks are omitted or performed incorrectly.

STANDARD PRECAUTIONS:

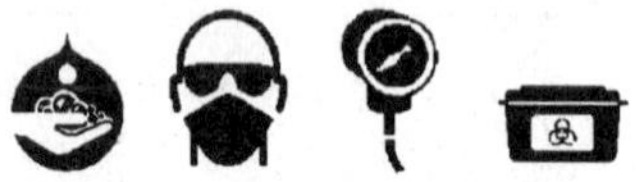

SKILLS ASSESSMENT CHECKLIST

Task Performed	Possible Points	TASKS
☐	5	Identifies patient. Washes hands.
☐	5	Opens suture removal kit.
☐	10	Applies sterile gloves.
☐	10	Uses thumb forceps to gently pick up one knot of a suture. Pulls gently upward.
☐	15	Uses suture removal scissors to cut one side of the suture as close to skin as possible.
☐	5	*Rationale:* This technique ensures that the suture will be pulled out from under the skin, avoiding contamination of the wound.
☐	15	Removes all sutures in the same manner, noting number of sutures removed. Disposes of the sutures on a sterile gauze sponge.
☐	5	Examines the wound to be sure all sutures have been removed.
☐	5	Applies Betadine solution to area.
☐	5	Applies dry sterile dressing if ordered by physician.
☐	5	Removes gloves. Disposes of used items per OSHA guidelines.
☐	5	Washes hands.
☐	15	Checks patient's vital signs.

Task Performed	Possible Points	TASKS
☐	10	Explains wound care; provides written instructions.
☐	5	Arranges follow-up appointment if necessary.
☐	5	Documents the procedure.
☐	5	Completed the tasks within 10 minutes.
☐	15	Results obtained were accurate.

_______	Earned	ADD POINTS OF TASKS CHECKED
145	Points	TOTAL POINTS POSSIBLE
_______	SCORE	DETERMINE SCORE (divide points earned by total points possible, multiply results by 100)

Actual Student Time Needed to Complete Procedure: ____________

Student's Initials: ____________ Instructor's Initials: ____________ Grade: ____________

Suggestions for Improvement: ______________________________

____

____

____

Evaluator's Name (print) ______________________________

Evaluator's Signature ______________________________

Comments ______________________________

DOCUMENTATION

Chart the procedure in the patient's medical record.

Date: ____________________

Charting: ______________________________

____

____

Student's Initials: ____________

SKILLS COMPETENCY ASSESSMENT

Procedure 25–11: Application of Sterile Adhesive Skin Closure Strips

Student's Name: ______________________________ Date: __________

Objective: To approximate the edges of a wound after the removal of sutures. Sometimes used in lieu of sutures or to give additional support along with sutures.

Conditions: The student demonstrates the ability to approximate the edges of a wound after the removal of sutures using the following equipment and supplies. Surgical tray: suture removal instruments, sterile adhesive skin closure strips, Iris scissors (straight), tincture of benzoin (optional) in sterile cup, sterile cotton-tipped applicators (for tincture of benzoin). Side area: sterile gloves, dressings, bandages, tape.

Time Requirements and Accuracy Standards: 5 minutes. Points assigned reflect importance of step to meeting objective: Important = (5) Essential = (10) Critical = (15). Automatic failure results if any of the **critical** tasks are omitted or performed incorrectly.

STANDARD PRECAUTIONS:

SKILLS ASSESSMENT CHECKLIST

Task Performed	Possible Points	TASKS
☐	5	Identifies the patient and explains the procedure. Positions patient comfortably.
☐	5	Washes hands and applies gloves.
☐	5	Removes bandages and dressings.
☐	5	Cleans and dries wound.
☐	10	Removes sutures (as per physician's orders).
☐	5	Assesses the need for skin closure strips and alerts the physician as indicated.
☐	10	Removes gloves, washes hands, opens container of tincture of benzoin, applies sterile gloves.
☐	10	Applies tincture of benzoin to edges of wound if directed. Uses sterile cotton-tipped applicator, taking care not to let it come into contact with the actual wound.
☐	15	Removes strips from packaging one at a time. Applies one end of a skin closure strip to one side of the wound. Places the first strip over the center of the wound.
☐	10	Secures the end to the skin by carefully pressing.
☐	10	Stretches the strip across the edge of the wound and secures it on the other side in the same manner. The motion should bring the edges together without puckering the skin.
☐	10	Applies the next two closure strips at halfway points between the first strip and each end of the wound.

Task Performed	Possible Points	TASKS
❑	15	Continues in this manner until the edges are approximated.
		Postoperative care
❑	5	Dresses and bandages if necessary.
❑	5	Disposes of used items per OSHA guidelines.
❑	5	Removes gloves and washes hands.
❑	15	Checks the patient's vital signs.
❑	15	Explains wound care to the patient (and caregiver) and provides written instructions, including symptoms of infection.
❑	5	Assists the patient with any concerns or questions.
❑	5	Arranges for follow-up appointment and medication, as ordered.
❑	5	Documents the procedure.
❑	5	Completed the tasks within 5 minutes.
❑	15	Results obtained were accurate.

______	Earned	ADD POINTS OF TASKS CHECKED
195	Points	TOTAL POINTS POSSIBLE
______	SCORE	DETERMINE SCORE (divide points earned by total points possible, multiply results by 100)

Actual Student Time Needed to Complete Procedure: ____________

Student's Initials: ____________ Instructor's Initials: ____________ Grade: ____________

Suggestions for Improvement: ______________________________

Evaluator's Name (print) ______________________________

Evaluator's Signature ______________________________

Comments ______________________________

DOCUMENTATION

Chart the procedure in the patient's medical record.

Date: ____________________

Charting: ______________________________

____

____

Student's Initials: ____________

SKILLS COMPETENCY ASSESSMENT

Procedure 25–12: Sebaceous Cyst Excision

Student's Name: ______________________________ Date: __________

Objective: To remove an inflamed or infected sebaceous cyst. To remove a sebaceous cyst that is not inflamed or infected but is located on an area of the body where the cyst is unsightly or where it may become irritated from rubbing.

Conditions: The student demonstrates the ability to assist in the removal of an inflamed or infected sebaceous cyst or to remove a sebaceous cyst that is not inflamed or infected using the following equipment and supplies. Surgical tray: syringe/needle for anesthesia, Iris scissors (curved), mosquito hemostat (curved), scalpel blades and handle, suture material with needle, Mayo scissors (curved). Side area: skin prep supplies, tissue forceps (2), gauze sponges (many), needle holder, fenestrated drape, antiseptic solution (Betadine), gloves (sterile and nonsterile), personal protective equipment, anesthesia as directed, dressing, bandages, tape, specimen container/requisition (optional), biohazard waste container, extra gauze squares, safety razor (optional), alcohol pledgets, culturette (optional).

Time Requirements and Accuracy Standards: Time varies according to patient's condition and the time required by the physician to complete the procedure. Points assigned reflect importance of step to meeting objective: Important = (5) Essential = (10) Critical = (15). Automatic failure results if any of the **critical** tasks are omitted or performed incorrectly.

STANDARD PRECAUTIONS:

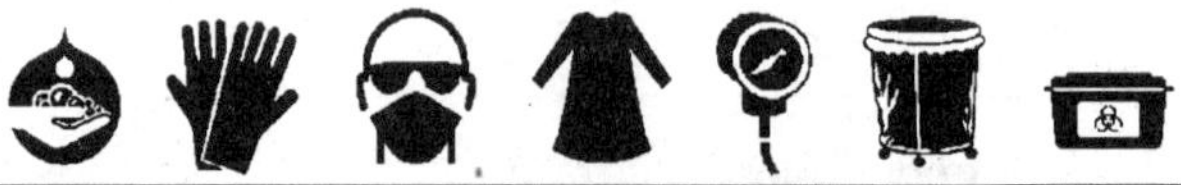

SKILLS ASSESSMENT CHECKLIST

Task Performed	Possible Points	TASKS
☐	10	Washes hands. Identifies the patient and explains the procedure.
☐	5	Reassures and comforts the patient as needed.
☐	15	Determines any known allergies and last tetanus booster. Checks for signed consent form.
☐	5	Identifies any health concerns to avoid possible complications.
☐	5	Positions the patient comfortably, lying down.
☐	5	Performs the skin preparation, as directed.
☐	5	Wears appropriate PPE if cyst is infected.
☐	5	*Rationale:* Purulent material may drain out of the wound.
☐	15	Assists physician to inject the anesthesia by holding the vial while the physician withdraws the appropriate amount of anesthesia. Continues to assist while the physician incises the cyst, removes it, and sutures the surgical incision. The physician will place the specimen in a container with a preservative to be sent to the pathology lab for analysis.
☐	5	Supports patient during surgery.

Task Performed	Possible Points	TASKS
		Postoperative Care
❑	5	Applies sterile gloves.
❑	5	Cleans area around the wound.
❑	5	Dresses and bandages, as directed.
❑	5	Disposes of items per OSHA guidelines. Removes gloves.
❑	5	Washes hands.
❑	15	Checks the patient's vital signs.
❑	15	Explains wound care to the patient (and caregiver) and provides written instructions, including symptoms of infection.
❑	5	Assists the patient with any concerns or questions.
❑	5	Arranges for follow-up appointment and medication, as ordered.
❑	5	Documents the procedure.
❑	5	Completed the tasks within the time constraint identified by the instructor.
❑	15	Results obtained were accurate.

______	Earned	ADD POINTS OF TASKS CHECKED
165	Points	TOTAL POINTS POSSIBLE
______	SCORE	DETERMINE SCORE (divide points earned by total points possible, multiply results by 100)

Actual Student Time Needed to Complete Procedure: ____________

Student's Initials: ____________ Instructor's Initials: ____________ Grade: ____________

Suggestions for Improvement: ______________________________

Evaluator's Name (print) ______________________________

Evaluator's Signature ______________________________

Comments ______________________________

DOCUMENTATION

Chart the procedure in the patient's medical record.

Date: ____________________

Charting: ______________________________

____

____

Student's Initials: ____________

SKILLS COMPETENCY ASSESSMENT

Procedure 25–13: Incision and Drainage of Localized Infections

Student's Name: ______________________________ Date: __________

Objective: To incise and drain an abscess or other localized infection.

Conditions: The student demonstrates the ability to assist in the incision and drainage of localized infections using the following equipment and supplies. Surgical tray: syringe/needle for anesthesia, scalpel blades and handle, thumb forceps, mosquito hemostat (optional), gauze sponges (many), fenestrated drape, tissue forceps (2), Mayo scissors, Iris scissors, antiseptic solution, such as Betadine in a sterile cup. Side area: skin prep supplies, gloves (sterile and nonsterile), personal protective equipment, anesthesia as directed, dressing, bandages, tape, specimen container with preservative/requisition (optional), biohazard waste container, extra gauze sponges, Iodoform gauze wick or penrose drain, alcohol pledget, antiseptic solution, culturette (optional).

Time Requirements and Accuracy Standards: Time varies according to patient condition and the time required by the physician to complete the procedure. Points assigned reflect importance of step to meeting objective: Important = (5) Essential = (10) Critical = (15). Automatic failure results if any of the **critical** tasks are omitted or performed incorrectly.

STANDARD PRECAUTIONS:

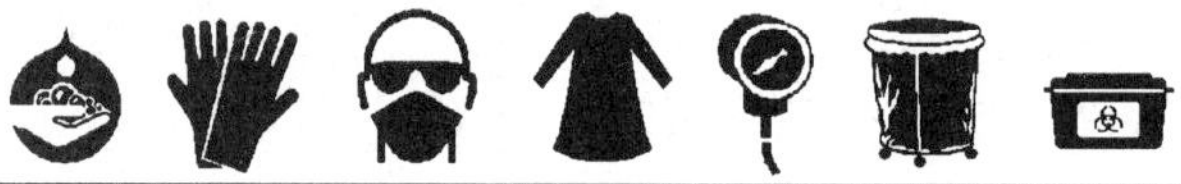

SKILLS ASSESSMENT CHECKLIST

Task Performed	Possible Points	TASKS
❑	5	Washes hands.
❑	5	Identifies the patient and explains the procedure.
❑	5	Reassures and comforts the patient as needed.
❑	15	Determines any known allergies and last tetanus booster.
❑	15	Checks for signed consent form.
❑	5	Identifies any health concerns to avoid possible complications.
❑	5	Positions the patient comfortably, lying down.
❑	5	Puts on PPE.
❑	15	Performs the skin preparation as directed.
❑	15	Assists the physician as needed to inject the anesthesia by holding the vial while the appropriate amount is aspirated for injection. The physician will incise the abscess and either Iodoform gauze or a penrose drain will be inserted into the wound to encourage drainage.
❑	5	Supports the patient as needed.

Task Performed	Possible Points	TASKS
		Postoperative Care
❑	5	Applies sterile gloves.
❑	5	Cleans area around the wound.
❑	10	Dresses and bandages as directed. Several thicknesses of dressing material may be needed to absorb exudate.
❑	5	Disposes of items per OSHA guidelines. Removes gloves, washes hands.
❑	15	Checks the patient's vital signs.
❑	15	Explains wound care to the patient (and caregiver) and provides written instructions such as apply warm moist compresses to wound. Explains to watch for symptoms of infection.
❑	5	Assists the patient with any concerns or questions.
❑	5	Arranges for follow-up appointment and medication, as ordered.
❑	10	Documents the procedure.
❑	5	Completed the tasks within the time constraint identified by the instructor.
❑	15	Results obtained were accurate.

________	Earned	ADD POINTS OF TASKS CHECKED
180	Points	TOTAL POINTS POSSIBLE
________	SCORE	DETERMINE SCORE (divide points earned by total points possible, multiply results by 100)

Actual Student Time Needed to Complete Procedure: ____________

Student's Initials: ____________ Instructor's Initials: ____________ Grade: ____________

Suggestions for Improvement: ________________________________

Evaluator's Name (print) ________________________________

Evaluator's Signature ________________________________

Comments ________________________________

DOCUMENTATION

Chart the procedure in the patient's medical record.

Date: ____________________

Charting: ________________________________

____

____

Student's Initials: ____________

SKILLS COMPETENCY ASSESSMENT

Procedure 25–14: Aspiration of Joint Fluid

Student's Name: ______________________________ Date: __________

Objective: To remove excess synovial fluid from a joint following injury.

Conditions: The student demonstrates the ability to assist the physician in removing excess synovial fluid from a joint following injury using the following equipment and supplies. Surgical tray: syringe/needle for anesthesia, gauze sponges, sterile basin for aspirated fluid, fenestrated drape (optional), syringe/needle for drainage. Side area: skin prep supplies, gloves (sterile and nonsterile), personal protective equipment, anesthesia as directed, cortisone medication as directed, culturette (optional), pathology requisition, specimen container, biohazard waste container, extra gauze sponges (sterile, unopened), alcohol pledgets, dressing and bandages.

Time Requirements and Accuracy Standards: Time varies according to patient condition and the time required by the physician to complete the procedure. Points assigned reflect importance of step to meeting objective: Important = (5) Essential = (10) Critical = (15). Automatic failure results if any of the **critical** tasks are omitted or performed incorrectly.

STANDARD PRECAUTIONS:

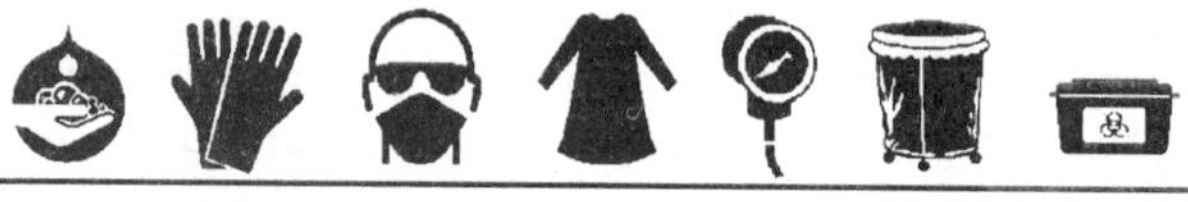

SKILLS ASSESSMENT CHECKLIST

Task Performed	Possible Points	TASKS
☐	5	Washes hands.
☐	5	Identifies the patient and explains the procedure. Reassures and comforts the patient as needed.
☐	15	Determines any known allergies and last tetanus booster.
☐	15	Checks for signed consent form. Identifies any health concerns to avoid possible complications.
☐	5	Positions the patient comfortably, lying down.
☐	5	Puts on PPE if needed.
☐	5	Performs the skin preparation as directed.
☐	15	Assists the physician by holding the vial as anesthesia is aspirated. The physician will insert the needle into the synovial sac and aspirate fluid with the syringe. The aspirated fluid will be put into a sterile bowl as the syringe fills with fluid. The process continues until excess fluid is removed.
☐	5	Supports the patient as needed.
		Postoperative care
☐	5	Applies sterile gloves.
☐	5	Cleans area around the wound.

Task Performed	Possible Points	TASKS
❑	10	Dresses and bandages as directed.
❑	5	Disposes of items per OSHA guidelines. Removes gloves.
❑	5	Washes hands.
❑	15	Checks the patient's vital signs.
❑	15	Explains wound care to the patient (and caregiver) and provides written instructions, including symptoms of infection.
❑	5	Assists the patient with any concerns or questions.
❑	5	Arranges for follow-up appointment and medication, as ordered.
❑	10	Sends labeled specimen to the pathology lab, if directed.
❑	5	Documents the procedure.
❑	5	Completed the tasks within the time constraint identified by the instructor.
❑	15	Results obtained were accurate.
______	Earned	ADD POINTS OF TASKS CHECKED
180	Points	TOTAL POINTS POSSIBLE
______	SCORE	DETERMINE SCORE (divide points earned by total points possible, multiply results by 100)

Actual Student Time Needed to Complete Procedure: ____________

Student's Initials: ____________ Instructor's Initials: ____________ Grade: ____________

Suggestions for Improvement: ________________________________

Evaluator's Name (print) ________________________________

Evaluator's Signature ________________________________

Comments ________________________________

DOCUMENTATION

Chart the procedure in the patient's medical record.

Date: ____________________

Charting: ________________________________

____

____

Student's Initials: ____________

SKILLS COMPETENCY ASSESSMENT

Procedure 25–15: Hemorrhoid Thrombectomy

Student's Name: ______________________________ Date: ____________

Objective: To excise inflamed hemorrhoids.

Conditions: The student demonstrates the ability to assist the physician in excising inflamed hemorrhoids using the following equipment and supplies. Surgical tray: syringe/needle for anesthesia, mosquito hemostat (curved), sterile basin, gauze sponges, fenestrated drape. Side area: skin prep supplies, gloves (sterile and nonsterile), personal protective equipment, anesthesia as directed, biohazard waste container, extra gauze sponges, soft absorbent pad (similar to sanitary napkin), T-bandage (to hold pad in place).

Time Requirements and Accuracy Standards: Time varies according to patient's condition and the time required by the physician to complete the procedure. Points assigned reflect importance of step to meeting objective: Important = (5) Essential = (10) Critical = (15). Automatic failure results if any of the **critical** tasks are omitted or performed incorrectly.

STANDARD PRECAUTIONS:

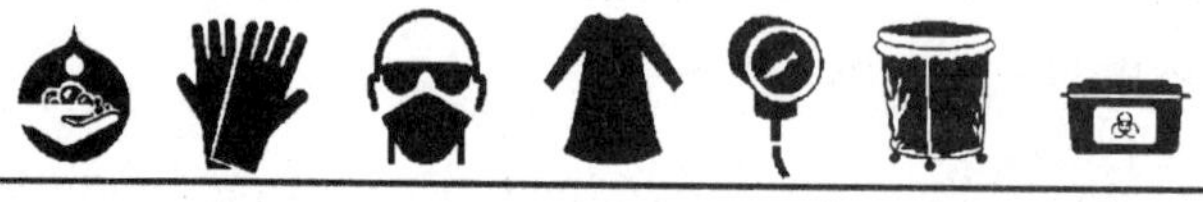

SKILLS ASSESSMENT CHECKLIST

Task Performed	Possible Points	TASKS
☐	5	Washes hands.
☐	5	Identifies the patient and explains the procedure. Reassures and comforts the patient as needed.
☐	15	Determines any known allergies and last tetanus booster.
☐	15	Checks for signed consent form.
☐	10	Identifies any health concerns to avoid possible complications.
☐	10	Positions the patient comfortably, according to physician preference; usually lithotomy position is used.
☐	5	Assists with adequate draping for patient comfort.
☐	5	Applies PPE if necessary.
☐	5	Performs the skin preparation as directed.
☐	10	Assists the physician to aspirate the appropriate amount of local anesthesia. The physician will excise the hemorrhoids with a scalpel and remove the clot within with a hemostat forceps.
☐	5	Supports the patient as needed.
		Postoperative Care
☐	10	Applies sterile gloves.

Task Performed	Possible Points	TASKS
❑	10	Assists the physician in placing the soft absorbent pad against the wound. It may be held in place with a T-shaped bandage.
❑	5	Disposes of used items per OSHA guidelines. Removes gloves and washes hands.
❑	5	Assists the patient as needed.
❑	15	Checks the patient's vital signs.
❑	15	Explains wound care to the patient (and caregiver) per physician. Sitting in a tub of warm water is soothing and aids healing. Provides written instructions, including signs of complications such as excessive bleeding or pain.
❑	5	Assists the patient with any concerns or questions.
❑	5	Arranges for follow-up appointment and medication, as ordered.
❑	5	Documents the procedure.
❑	5	Completed the tasks within the time constraint identified by the instructor.
❑	15	Results obtained were accurate.

_______	Earned	ADD POINTS OF TASKS CHECKED
185	Points	TOTAL POINTS POSSIBLE
_______	SCORE	DETERMINE SCORE (divide points earned by total points possible, multiply results by 100)

Actual Student Time Needed to Complete Procedure: __________

Student's Initials: __________ Instructor's Initials: __________ Grade: __________

Suggestions for Improvement: ______________________________

Evaluator's Name (print) ______________________________

Evaluator's Signature ______________________________

Comments ______________________________

DOCUMENTATION

Chart the procedure in the patient's medical record.

Date: __________________

Charting: ______________________________

____

____

Student's Initials: __________

EVALUATION OF CHAPTER KNOWLEDGE

How has your instructor evaluated the knowledge you have achieved?

Knowledge	**Instructor Evaluation** *Good*	*Average*	*Poor*
Defines surgical asepsis and differentiates between surgical asepsis and medical asepsis	_____	_____	_____
Lists basic rules to follow to protect sterile areas	_____	_____	_____
Explains the sizing standards of suture material and the criteria used to select the most appropriate type and size	_____	_____	_____
Is able to identify and describe the intended use of a wide variety of surgical instruments	_____	_____	_____
Demonstrates the ability to select the most appropriate type of dressings for a given situation	_____	_____	_____
States advantages and disadvantages of Betadine, Hibeclens, isopropyl alcohol, and hydrogen peroxide when each is used as a skin antiseptic	_____	_____	_____
Defines anesthesia and explains the advantages and disadvantages of epinephrine as an additive to injectable anesthetics	_____	_____	_____
Recalls preoperative issues to be addressed in patient preparation and education	_____	_____	_____
Identifies postoperative concerns to be addressed with the patient and the caregiver	_____	_____	_____
Demonstrates procedure for applying sterile gloves	_____	_____	_____
Demonstrates ability to set up a surgical tray, including laying the field, supplies and instruments, pouring a sterile solution, using transfer forceps, and covering the sterile tray	_____	_____	_____
Explains what is meant by alternative surgical methods	_____	_____	_____
Documents accurately	_____	_____	_____
Attends to patient's emotional needs	_____	_____	_____

Student's Initials: ______ Instructor's Initials: ______

Grade: _______

CHAPTER 26

Rehabilitation Medicine

PERFORMANCE OBJECTIVES

Rehabilitation medicine is a field of medicine that specializes in both preventing disease or injury and restoring patients' physical function, using a combination of physical and mechanical agents to aid in the diagnosis and treatment. The goal of rehabilitation medicine is to help restore the functions that have been affected by a patient's condition. The role of the medical assistant is to assist the physician or rehabilitation therapist in enabling a patient to regain normal or near-normal function after an illness or injury. A medical assistant might assist a patient in learning to safely ambulate following a period of sedentary recuperation; in learning the correct use of assistive devices, such as crutches, a cane, or a walker; or in performing therapeutic exercises. Range of motion exercises, designed to maintain a patient's joint mobility, are often performed by the medical assistant. In addition to therapeutic exercise, a variety of therapeutic modalities such as heat, cold, light, electricity, and water can be used as part of the patient's rehabilitation program, and the medical assistant should be familiar with how these modalities act on the body and understand the safety precautions associated with each. It is very important for the medical assistant to understand the goals and objectives of the rehabilitation program designed by the physician or therapist. A medical assistant's duties in the field of rehabilitation medicine often involve physical strength and coordination, such as when performing wheelchair transfers. It is important to follow proper procedures at all times to protect both the patient and the medical assistant from injury. Therapeutic communication between medical assistants and rehabilitation patients is essential to providing encouragement and support for patients who face difficult, uncomfortable, or frustrating physical challenges.

EXERCISES AND ACTIVITIES

Vocabulary Builder

A. Rehabilitation Medicine Terminology

Match each of the following key vocabulary terms to the example that best describes it.

A. Vasoconstriction
B. Thermotherapy
C. Muscle testing
D. Contractures
E. Goniometer
F. Body mechanics
G. Atrophy
H. Rehabilitation medicine
I. Goniometry
J. Ambulation
K. Gait
L. Ultrasound
M. Activities of daily living (ADL)
N. Hemiplegia
O. Range of motion (ROM)
P. Modality
Q. Cryotherapy
R. Gait belt
S. Vasodilation
T. Assistive devices

_____ 1. Patient Lenore McDonell, confined to a wheelchair since early childhood, receives continuing physical therapy to minimize the effects of any decrease of ability or size in her legs caused by inactivity.

_____ 2. Clinical medical assistant Anna Preciado enjoys working with patients to help them restore their bodies to normal or near-normal function following an illness or injury. Her interest has led her to pursue advanced training in this field of medical discipline.

_____ 3. When examining a new patient, a physical therapist must determine which of the physical agents, such as heat, cold, light, water, and electricity, will be most beneficial in treating the patient's condition.

_____ 4. As Margaret Thomas, diagnosed with Parkinson's disease, began to develop balance problems and difficulties in walking, her physical therapist prescribed the use of high-frequency sound waves to generate heat in the deep tissue of her right leg, producing a therapeutic effect.

_____ 5. Cold applications are used to constrict blood vessels and slow or stop the flow of blood to an area.

_____ 6. Lenny Taylor, suffering the early stages of dementia from Alzheimer's, works with an occupational therapist to practice methods of making everyday tasks easier to perform.

_____ 7. Heat is a modality that creates a therapeutic effect by causing blood vessels to dilate, thereby increasing circulation to an area and speeding up the healing process.

_____ 8. When construction worker Jaime Carrera suffers a shoulder injury on the job, Dr. James Whitney performs this process for assessing the motion, strength, and task potential of the muscle group, tendons, and associated tissues.

_____ 9. Joe Guerrero, CMA, instructs patient Martin Gordon on the correct method of ambulating while using a three-point gait and axillary crutches.

_____ 10. Dr. Winston Lewis recommends this heat modality to help relieve Herb Fowler's chronic lower back pain, caused by strain on the back muscles created by the patient's overweight condition.

_____ 11. When patient Dottie Tate comes to Inner City Health Care complaining of a sore back and several recent falls, clinical medical assistant Bruce Goldman secures a gait belt around Dottie's waist and asks her to walk across the room. Staying a step behind her and slightly to the side, Bruce carefully observes Dottie's progress when performing this task.

_____ 12. As a muscle atrophies, shrinking and losing its strength, joints become stiff and develop these deformities. Without constant exercise, the musculoskeletal system deteriorates.

_____ **13.** Dr. Susan Rice recommends that patient Dottie Tate begin to use a walker at home to prevent further falls. Bruce Goldman, CMA, secures this safety device around Dottie's waist and positions her inside the walker as he gives her verbal instructions to begin the procedure of learning to ambulate with a walker.

_____ **14.** Elderly patient Abigail Johnson is afraid that because she has diabetes mellitus she is at increased risk for stroke. "I don't want to end up a vegetable and a burden to my family," she tells Dr. Elizabeth King, "all paralyzed on one side like that."

_____ **15.** Clinical medical assistant Joe Guerrero employs this practice of using certain key muscle groups together with correct body alignment to avoid injury when assisting patient Lenore McDonell in performing a transfer from her wheelchair to the examination table.

_____ **16.** Margaret Thomas's neurologist uses this instrument to measure the angle of her shoulder joint's range of motion during a follow-up examination for Parkinson's disease.

_____ **17.** Dr. Mark Woo chooses this cold modality to treat the sprained wrist of an emergency patient, reducing inflammation.

_____ **18.** Canes, walkers, and crutches are examples of walking aids.

_____ **19.** When lying flat with arms at the sides, the average person should be able to move from a 20° hyperextension of the elbow joint to a 150° flexion.

_____ **20.** A physical therapist uses the measurement of joint motion to help evaluate a patient's range of motion.

B. Joint Movement Terminology

Unscramble each term of joint movement to reveal the correct spelling. Then match the term to its correct definition.

A. CIUDBANOT _______________

B. SIONTXEEN _______________

C. VSOIREEN _______________

D. RSIONHTXEEENYP _______________

E. TIONNOARP _______________

F. VRSEINNOI _______________

G. TATORION _______________

H. XELIONF _______________

I. PINUSITAON _______________

J. SRDOXELFIINO _______________

K. ARPNTLA XELIONF _______________

L. UCTIONADD _______________

M. UMDIONTCUCRIC _______________

_____ **1.** Moving the arm so the palm is up.

_____ **2.** Moving a body part outward.

_____ 3. Straightening of a body part.
_____ 4. Motion toward the midline of the body.
_____ 5. Moving a body part inward.
_____ 6. Turning a body part around its axis.
_____ 7. A position of maximum extension, or extending a body part beyond its normal limits.
_____ 8. Motion away from the midline of the body.
_____ 9. Circular motion of a body part.
_____ 10. Moving the arm so the palm is down.
_____ 11. Moving the foot downward at the ankle.
_____ 12. Moving the foot upward at the ankle joint.
_____ 13. Bending of a body part.

Learning Review

1. Some patients require assistive devices in order to ambulate. Three broad types of assistive devices are listed below. For each assistive device, name the various styles available and one identifying feature of each style. Also, name the physical conditions each style is best suited to be used with as part of a physician's treatment plan.

CANES

(1) ______________________________

____

(2) ______________________________

____

(3) ______________________________

____

WALKERS

(1) ______________________________

____

(2) ______________________________

____

CRUTCHES

(1) ______________________________

____

(2) ______________________________

____

(3) ______________________________

____

2. Therapeutic exercise helps patients restore their bodies, protect their bodies from further damage, and prevent against the development of respiratory and circulatory complications caused by inactivity. Medical assistants need to understand the goals and objectives of therapeutic exercise programs. Patients will need support and encouragement to stick to their programs.

   Name four types of exercise programs that are employed for therapeutic or preventative purposes. Then match each one to the example that best describes it.

   ____ 1. ____

   ____ 2. ____

   ____ 3. ____

   ____ 4. ____

   A. Patient Jim Marshall, suffering a sports injury to the muscles surrounding the knee, performs exercises in a therapy pool.

   B. Lourdes Austen performs self-directed exercises at home to improve the range of motion and increase strength in her left arm, following lumpectomy and axillary lymph node dissection.

   C. Lenore McDonell, confined to a wheelchair and unable to move her legs voluntarily, works regularly with a physical therapist to avoid atrophy and contractures in the legs and to improve overall circulation.

   D. Jaime Carrera, recovering from a shoulder injury, rebuilds upper body strength with a daily regimen of push-ups: first against the wall and then on the floor.

3. A. List six precautionary measures that should be observed when performing range of motion exercises on a patient.

   (1) ____

   ____

   (2) ____

   ____

   (3) ____

   ____

   (4) ____

   ____

   (5) ____

   ____

   (6) ____

   ____

B. For each illustration below, identify the range of motion exercise being performed.

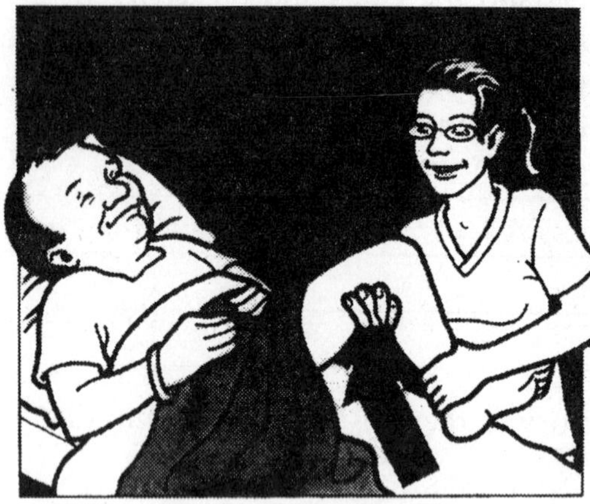

1. ______________________

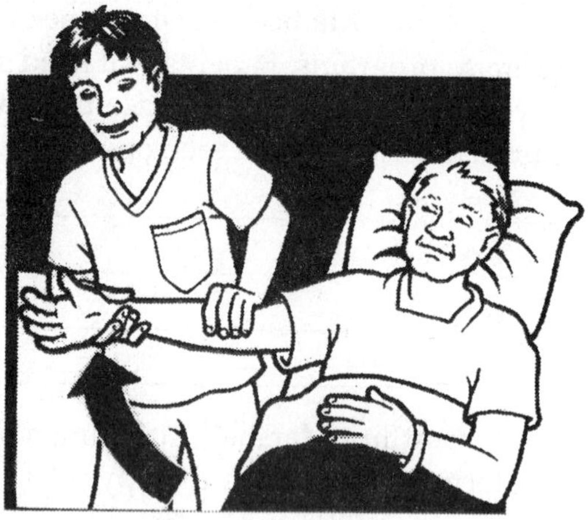

2. ______________________

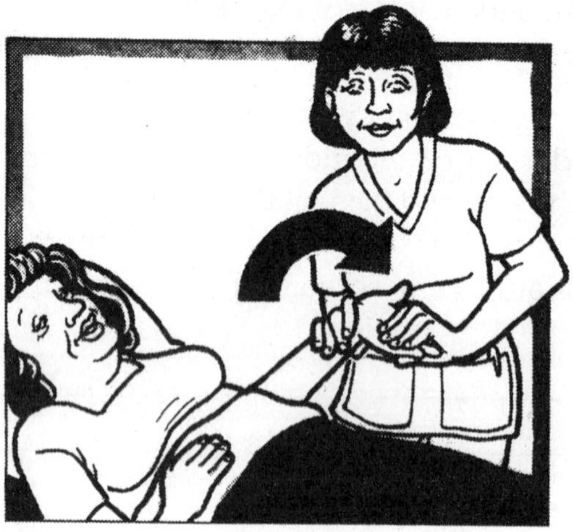

3. ______________________

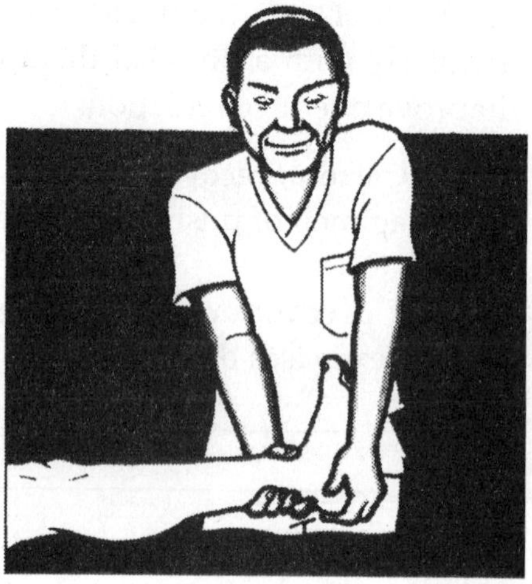

4. ______________________

4. Therapeutic exercise is not the only way to treat painful joints or tissues. Many patients respond well to the therapeutic modalities of heat and cold, thermotherapy and cryotherapy. List six precautions that medical assistants must take when applying heat or cold modalities.

(1) ______________________

____

(2) ______________________

____

(3) ______________________

____

(4) ______________________

____

(5) ______________________

____

(6) ______________________________

____

5. Identify each modality listed below as either a dry heat therapy (DHT), a moist heat therapy (MHT), a moist cold therapy (MCT) or a dry cold therapy (DCT) by placing the proper letters in the space provided. Then identify whether the modality can be performed at home by the patient, with or without caregiver assistance, or whether the modality must be performed in a clinical setting under the supervision of a health care professional. List any special precautions or concerns.

_______ A. Ice pack ______________________________

____

_______ B. Paraffin wax bath ______________________________

____

_______ C. Cold compress ______________________________

____

_______ D. Hot water bottle ______________________________

____

_______ E. Hot compress ______________________________

____

_______ F. Whirlpool bath ______________________________

____

_______ G. Heating pad ______________________________

____

_______ H. Hot soak of one extremity ______________________________

____

_______ I. Hot pack ______________________________

____

_______ J. Total body immersion in a Hubbard tank ______________________________

____

6. For each of the following, identify the proper temperature and correct amount of time the modality should be administered to the patient.

A. Aquamatic K-Pad for an elderly patient ______________________________

B. Paraffin wax bath for a patient with rheumatoid arthritis ______________________________

C. An ice pack for a patient with an ankle sprain ______________________________

D. Hot water bottle for an adult patient ______________________________

E. A hot compress to drain pus from a patient's skin infection ______________________________

F. Hot soak of the arm and hand for a patient with osteoarthritis ______________________________

7. How do ultrasound waves travel best? What are the special concerns of ultrasound treatment, how long can ultrasound be administered, and who is authorized to perform ultrasound procedures on patients?

____

____

____

____

Investigation Activity

It is important to remember that patients undergoing rehabilitative medicine may be coping with the consequences of a serious accident or illness. Patients may no longer be able to perform activities of daily living, and they may feel frustrated, angry, or depressed at this loss of ability. Other patients, however, may have a strong sense of willpower and determination. Individuals will react differently. Similarly, friends and family members who serve as caregivers may be more or less willing, physically able, or temperamentally inclined to assist the patient in maintaining a program of rehabilitative care and treatment. The medical assistant can serve as an educator for the patient and caregiver, instructing both in methods that can make treatment easier and increase the chances of success. The medical assistant is also a strong source of support and encouragement.

Using a family member or friend in the role of caregiver, the student should play the role of a patient who has recently suffered a serious accident and is unable to walk or use his or her right arm and hand. Substitute a kitchen chair for a wheelchair placed in a stationary position with the breaks locked. Remain in the chair while the caregiver helps you put on a change of clothing, eat a full meal, and make a telephone call. Be alternately feisty or polite, determined or depressed, mentally focused or unable to concentrate; gauge the reaction of your caregiver to each emotional standpoint.

Consider the following.

1. How can an understanding of proper body mechanics and methods for assisting patients help caregivers and their loved ones who are suffering some kind of physical restriction? How easily did you and your caregiver perform each task?
2. What emotions did both you and your caregiver display? How did the encouragement or lack of encouragement displayed on either side affect the success of each task?
3. Ask your caregiver to write a brief paragraph or two describing the experience and how he or she felt about assisting you.

CASE STUDIES

Medical assistants must practice good body mechanics to protect themselves and their patients from injury. Often called on to lift heavy objects, perform patient transfers, and assist patients in ambulation, medical assistants need to know how to execute their duties safely and efficiently.

For each situation below, discuss the following.

1. What is the best action of the medical assistant?
2. What is the best therapeutic response of the medical assistant?
3. Could the situation have been avoided? If so, how? If not, why not?

Case 1

Ellen Armstrong, CMA, performs the annual task of assembling and moving inactive patient files into a storage filing area for safekeeping. It is the end of the day and Ellen is tired and eager to finish the job; this task has never been one of Ellen's favorites. When she gets to filling the last of three cartons of files, Ellen moves the carton to a shelf, about shoulder-high, in the storage room. She returns and decides to take both of the remaining cartons in one trip. Fatigued, she bends at the waist to pick them up.

Case 2

After explaining the procedure to the patient and her son, Wanda Slawson, CMA, performs the transfer of Mary Craig, an elderly blind patient with diabetes mellitus who is suffering from atrophy of the legs, from a car to a wheelchair in the parking lot of Inner City Health Care. Unfortunately, because of Mary's position in the car, the patient must be transferred with her weaker side closest to the wheelchair. The patient panics during the transfer and throws her arms around Wanda's neck as she is lifting and pivoting Mary to the right to position her in the wheelchair. The patient's son John rushes forward to grab onto his mother.

Case 3

Dr. Susan Rice asks Bruce Goldman, CMA, to instruct patient Dottie Tate in the use of a walker to prevent further falls at home. Dottie is silent as Dr. Rice leaves the examination room and Bruce proceeds to set the walker correctly. However, when Dottie sees that Bruce must once again put Dottie in a gait belt for her protection—the belt was used earlier in the examination to assess Dottie's ability to ambulate—the patient gets feisty. She is visibly tired and ready to go home. "I'll learn to use the walker if I have to, but I won't wear that infernal contraption. It makes me feel like a baby. And it's such a bother. Who wants to go through all that? We just don't need it."

SUPPLEMENTARY RESOURCES

Study Guide Disk: Additional practice exercises for this chapter are available on the study guide disk found in the back of the textbook.

Medical Assisting Videos: Appropriate content is available on Delmar's Medical Assisting Videos, 2nd ed., Tape 9, for the following topics:

- Introduction to Body Mechanics
- Body Mechanics
- Transfer Wheelchair to Examination Table and Back
- Ultrasound Procedures
- Rehabilitative Care
- Passive Range of Motion Exercises
- Instructing Patients with Special Needs

SKILLS COMPETENCY ASSESSMENT

Procedure 26–1: Transferring Patient from Wheelchair to Examination Table

Student's Name: ______________________________ Date: ____________

Objective: To safely transfer a patient from a wheelchair to an examination table

Conditions: The student demonstrates the ability to transfer a patient from a wheelchair to an examination table using the following equipment and supplies: wheelchair, examination table, gait belt, stool with rubber tips and a handle for gripping.

Time Requirements and Accuracy Standards: 5 minutes. Points assigned reflect importance of step to meeting objective: Important = (5) Essential = (10) Critical = (15). Automatic failure results if any of the **critical** tasks are omitted or performed incorrectly.

STANDARD PRECAUTIONS:

SKILLS ASSESSMENT CHECKLIST

Task Performed	Possible Points	TASKS
☐	5	Washes hands.
☐	5	Identifies patient, introduces self, explains procedure.
☐	10	Places the wheelchair next to the examination table and locks the brakes.
☐	5	*Rationale:* Understands that patient must be placed on his or her strongest side nearest the examination table to allow him or her to balance on that leg during transfer.
☐	5	Places the gait belt securely around the patient's waist. Tucks excess under belt.
☐	5	Moves the wheelchair footrests up and out of the way. Has patient place feet firmly on floor.
☐	5	Positions the stool in front of the examination table as close to the wheelchair as possible and instructs the patient to move to the edge of the wheelchair.
☐	15	Stands directly in front of the patient with feet slightly apart. Bends at the hips and knees, grasps the gait belt, and instructs the patient to place both hands on the armrests of the wheelchair.
☐	5	*Rationale:* If patient does not have strength in the arms to push upward, instructs the patient to rest hands at sides.
☐	10	Gives a signal and lifts the gait belt upward, pushing with the knees. If patient has strength in the good leg, ask patient to push up with that leg and both arms.
☐	15	Grasps gait belt and instructs the patient to step onto the stool with the foot closest to the examination table, pivoting so the patient's back is to the examination table. Makes sure the buttocks are slightly higher than the bed. Supports patient's outer leg with the leg furthest from the examination table.

Task Performed	Possible Points	TASKS
❑	5	Instructs patient to grasp stool handle and place other hand on examination table.
❑	5	Eases the patient to a seated position on examination table.
❑	5	Places the patient in proper examination position on the table.
❑	5	Moves the wheelchair and stool out of the way.
		Modification: Two-Person Transfer
❑	5	Places gait belt snugly around the patient's waist and tucks excess end under the belt.
❑	5	One person stands in front of the patient and the other to the side, next to the examination table.
❑	10	Both persons grasp the gait belt from underneath. Has patient place both hands on the wheelchair armrests.
❑	10	On one person's signal, both persons pull the patient upward. Has patient push up with both hands, if upper body strength is sufficient; if not, asks patient to rest arms at sides.
❑	15	Person nearest the examination table moves wheelchair out of the way, while the other pivots the patient and has the patient place the stronger leg on the stool. Asks patient to grasp the stool handle, if upper body strength is sufficient.
❑	5	On one person's signal, both persons lift the patient onto the examination table.
❑	5	Places the patient in the proper examination position on the table.
❑	5	Completed the tasks within 5 minutes.
❑	15	Results obtained were accurate.

_______	Earned	ADD POINTS OF TASKS CHECKED
	Points	TOTAL POINTS POSSIBLE SINGLE 105 DOUBLE 75
_______	SCORE	DETERMINE SCORE (divide points earned by total points possible, multiply results by 100)

Actual Student Time Needed to Complete Procedure: ____________

Student's Initials: ____________ Instructor's Initials: ____________ Grade: ____________

Suggestions for Improvement: ______________________________

Evaluator's Name (print) ______________________________

Evaluator's Signature ______________________________

Comments ______________________________

SKILLS COMPETENCY ASSESSMENT

Procedure 26–2: Transferring Patient from Examination Table to Wheelchair

Student's Name: ______________________________ Date: __________

Objective: To safely transfer a patient from the examination table to a wheelchair

Conditions: The student demonstrates the ability to transfer a patient safely from the examination table to a wheelchair using the following equipment and supplies: wheelchair, stool with rubber tips and gripping handle, gait belt, examination table.

Time Requirements and Accuracy Standards: 5 minutes. Points assigned reflect importance of step to meeting objective: Important = (5) Essential = (10) Critical = (15). Automatic failure results if any of the **critical** tasks are omitted or performed incorrectly.

STANDARD PRECAUTIONS:

SKILLS ASSESSMENT CHECKLIST

Task Performed	Possible Points	TASKS
☐	5	Washes hands.
☐	5	Identifies the patient and explains procedure.
☐	15	Positions the wheelchair next to the examination table and locks the brakes.
☐	5	*Rationale:* Places wheelchair close to the patient's strongest side, so the patient can transfer weight to strong leg and foot when stepping down.
☐	5	Positions the stool next to the wheelchair.
☐	10	Assists the patient to rise to a seated position; places the gait belt snugly around the patient's waist and tucks excess end under the belt.
☐	15	Places one arm under the patient's arm and around the patient's shoulders, and the other arm under the patient's knees. Pivots the patient so the legs are dangling over the side of the examination table.
☐	15	Keeps a hand on the patient, moves directly in front of patient and grasps the patient by placing hands under gait belt. Plants feet shoulder's width apart and bends knees to have a greater base of support.
☐	10	Gives signal and pulls the patient slightly forward so the patient's feet come down onto the stool. Instructs the patient to push off examination table and grasp the stool handle for support.
☐	10	Still grasping gait belt, instructs the patient to step to the floor with the strong leg, pivoting at the same time so the patient's back is to the wheelchair.

Task Performed	Possible Points	TASKS
☐	5	Has the patient grasp the armrests of the wheelchair.
☐	5	Bends from knees and hips and lowers the patient into the wheelchair, making sure the patient is seated comfortably.
☐	5	Lowers footrests and places the patient's feet on them.
☐	5	Completed the tasks within 5 minutes.
☐	15	Results obtained were accurate.

______	Earned	ADD POINTS OF TASKS CHECKED
130	Points	TOTAL POINTS POSSIBLE
______	SCORE	DETERMINE SCORE (divide points earned by total points possible, multiply results by 100)

Actual Student Time Needed to Complete Procedure: ______________

Student's Initials: ______________ Instructor's Initials: ______________ Grade: ______________

Suggestions for Improvement: ______________________________

Evaluator's Name (print) ______________________________

Evaluator's Signature ______________________________

Comments ______________________________

SKILLS COMPETENCY ASSESSMENT

Procedure 26–3: Assisting the Patient to Stand and Walk

Student's Name: ______________________________________ Date: ____________

Objective: To help a patient ambulate safely.

Conditions: The student demonstrates the ability to help a patient stand and walk safely using the following equipment and supplies: gait belt and chair or wheelchair.

Time Requirements and Accuracy Standards: 5 minutes. Points assigned reflect importance of step to meeting objective: Important = (5) Essential = (10) Critical = (15). Automatic failure results if any of the **critical** tasks are omitted or performed incorrectly.

STANDARD PRECAUTIONS:

SKILLS ASSESSMENT CHECKLIST

Task Performed	Possible Points	TASKS
		One Person Assist with Ambulation
☐	5	Washes hands.
☐	10	Identifies the patient and explains procedure.
☐	15	Locks the brakes on the wheelchair if the patient is using one; places the patient's feet on the floor and moves the foot plates out of the way.
☐	15	Instructs the patient to slide forward in the chair; places the gait belt around the patient's waist and tucks excess under the belt.
☐	5	Stands directly in front of the patient, grasps the gait belt from underneath and assists the patient to stand on signal; instructs the patient to push up on the armrests of the wheelchair.
☐	15	Steadies the patient and watches for balance, strength, and skin color. Takes pulse, if necessary.
☐	5	*Rationale:* Can triage, or assess, the patient's physical state, looking for signs of potential unsteadiness or syncope, for example.
☐	5	If the patient is steady, proceeds by standing slightly behind and to the side of the patient's weaker side.
☐	10	Grasps the gait belt with one hand and places the other on the patient's bent arm for support. Gait belt is grasped with the fingers under the belt, palm up and elbow bent.
☐	5	Starts with the same foot as the patient and keeps in step with the patient.
☐	15	Documents the procedure; includes, date, time, duration of ambulation, response of patient, and instructions given. Initials report.
☐	5	Completed the tasks within 5 minutes.
☐	15	Results obtained were accurate.

________	Earned	ADD POINTS OF TASKS CHECKED
125	Points	TOTAL POINTS POSSIBLE
________	SCORE	DETERMINE SCORE (divide points earned by total points possible, multiply results by 100)

Task Performed	Possible Points	TASKS
		Modification: Two-Person Assist with Ambulation
❑	45	Performs the first four steps of the One-Person Assist Procedure.
❑	5	Has a person stand on either side of the patient. Grasps the gait belt from underneath with one hand, and places the other hand on the patient's back for support.
❑	5	During ambulation, both persons remain on either side of the patient and slightly behind. Both persons grasp the gait belt throughout the ambulation.
❑	15	Documents procedure including date, time, duration of ambulation, response of the patient, and instructions given. Initials report.
❑	5	Completed the tasks within 5 minutes.
❑	15	Results obtained were accurate.

_______	Earned	ADD POINTS OF TASKS CHECKED
90	Points	TOTAL POINTS POSSIBLE
_______	SCORE	DETERMINE SCORE (divide points earned by total points possible, multiply results by 100)

Actual Student Time Needed to Complete Procedure: ____________

Student's Initials: ____________ Instructor's Initials: ____________ Grade: ____________

Suggestions for Improvement: ______________________________

Evaluator's Name (print) ______________________________

Evaluator's Signature ______________________________

Comments ______________________________

DOCUMENTATION

Chart the procedure in the patient's medical record.

Date: __________

Charting for One-Person Assist: ______________________________

____

____

____

Charting for Two-Person Assist: ______________________________

____

____

Student's Initials: _______

SKILLS COMPETENCY ASSESSMENT

Procedure 26–4: Care of the Falling Patient

Student's Name: ______________________________ Date: ____________

Objective: To help the patient fall safely in order to avoid injury.

Conditions: The student demonstrates the ability to help the patient fall safely to avoid injury using the following equipment and supplies: gait belt already secured to patient.

Time Requirements and Accuracy Standards: 5 minutes. Points assigned reflect importance of step to meeting objective: Important = (5) Essential = (10) Critical = (15). Automatic failure results if any of the **critical** tasks are omitted or performed incorrectly.

SKILLS ASSESSMENT CHECKLIST

Task Performed	Possible Points	TASKS
❑	15	Keeps a firm hand on the gait belt.
❑	5	*Rationale:* Clothing can shift, providing an unstable handhold.
		Falling backward
❑	15	If the patient falls backward, widens stance to become a better base of support. Student allows the patient to fall against his or her body and guides the patient to the floor.
❑	5	Calls for assistance and takes the patient's pulse.
________		Points 40
		Falling to either side
❑	15	If the patient falls to either side, student steadies the patient back onto the feet by moving his or her foot in the direction in which the patient is falling.
❑	10	Asks whether the patient would like to stop the ambulation session; checks the patient for signs of fatigue. If necessary, calls for assistance and takes the patient's pulse.
________		Points 25
		Falling forward
❑	15	Supports the patient around the middle if the patient falls forward. Steps forward with outer leg and gently lowers the patient to the floor while protecting the patient from injury.
❑	10	Calls for assistance and takes the patient's pulse.
❑	15	Has the patient examined by a nurse or doctor before moving the patient again.
❑	15	Documents the fall in an incident report.
________		Points 55

Task Performed	Possible Points	TASKS
❑	5	Completed the tasks within 5 minutes.
❑	15	Results obtained were accurate.
______		Points 20

______		Earned	ADD POINTS OF TASKS CHECKED
	140	Points	TOTAL POINTS POSSIBLE
______		SCORE	DETERMINE SCORE (divide points earned by total points possible, multiply results by 100)

Actual Student Time Needed to Complete Procedure: __________

Student's Initials: __________ Instructor's Initials: __________ Grade: __________

Suggestions for Improvement: __________

Evaluator's Name (print) __________

Evaluator's Signature __________

Comments __________

DOCUMENTATION

Chart the procedure in the patient's medical record.

Date: __________

Charting: __________

____

____

____

____

____

Student's Initials: __________

SKILLS COMPETENCY ASSESSMENT

Procedure 26–5: Assisting a Patient to Ambulate with a Walker

Student's Name: ______________________________ Date: ____________

Objective: To help a patient ambulate safely and independently with a walker.

Conditions: The student demonstrates the ability to help a patient ambulate independently and safely with a walker using the following equipment and supplies: walker, gait belt.

Time Requirements and Accuracy Standards: 10 minutes. Points assigned reflect importance of step to meeting objective: Important = (5) Essential = (10) Critical = (15). Automatic failure results if any of the **critical** tasks are omitted or performed incorrectly.

STANDARD PRECAUTIONS:

SKILLS ASSESSMENT CHECKLIST

Task Performed	Possible Points	TASKS
☐	5	Washes hands.
☐	5	Identifies the patient and explains procedure.
☐	5	Applies the gait belt snugly around the patient's waist and tucks excess under belt.
☐	10	Checks the walker to be sure the rubber suction tips are secure on all the legs; checks the handrests for rough or damaged edges. Tightens all adjustments.
☐	10	Checks to make sure the patient is wearing good walking shoes with a rubber sole.
☐	5	Checks the height of the walker.
☐	5	*Rationale:* Walker must be adjusted to the correct position for the patient's height.
☐	5	Positions the patient inside the walker and instructs the patient to hold onto the handles while keeping the walker in front of the body.
☐	5	Stands behind and slightly to the side of the patient.
☐	15	Instructs the patient to lift the walker and place all four legs of the walker out in front so the back legs are even with the patient's toes.
☐	15	Instructs the patient to lean forward and transfer weight so that the patient steps into the walker, first with the stronger leg, then with the weaker leg. Makes sure the patient brings the stronger leg past the weaker leg.
☐	10	Monitors the patient carefully, alert to signs of fatigue in the patient. Stands ready to catch the patient in the event of a fall.

Task Performed	Possible Points	TASKS
❑	10	If the walker has rollers, watches the patient roll the walker ahead a comfortable distance from the body, then walk into it. The patient can also walk normally with a rolling walker by simply rolling it in front and leaning into the gait, using the walker for support.
❑	15	Documents the date, time, duration of ambulation, response of the patient, and instructions given. Initials the report.
❑	5	Completed the tasks within 10 minutes.
❑	15	Results obtained were accurate.
______	Earned	ADD POINTS OF TASKS CHECKED
140	Points	TOTAL POINTS POSSIBLE
______	SCORE	DETERMINE SCORE (divide points earned by total points possible, multiply results by 100)

Actual Student Time Needed to Complete Procedure: ____________

Student's Initials: ____________ Instructor's Initials: ____________ Grade: ____________

Suggestions for Improvement: ____________

Evaluator's Name (print) ____________

Evaluator's Signature ____________

Comments ____________

DOCUMENTATION

Chart the procedure in the patient's medical record.

Date: ________

Charting: ____________

____

____

____

____

____

Student's Initials: _______

SKILLS COMPETENCY ASSESSMENT

Procedure 26–6: Teaching the Patient to Ambulate with Axillary Crutches

Student's Name: ______________________________ Date: __________

Objective: To teach the patient how to ambulate safely using axillary crutches.

Conditions: The student demonstrates the ability to teach the patient how to ambulate safely using axillary crutches with the following equipment and supplies: axillary crutches and gait belt.

Time Requirements and Accuracy Standards: 10 minutes. Points assigned reflect importance of step to meeting objective: Important = (5) Essential = (10) Critical = (15). Automatic failure results if any of the **critical** tasks are omitted or performed incorrectly.

STANDARD PRECAUTIONS:

SKILLS ASSESSMENT CHECKLIST

Task Performed	Possible Points	TASKS
❑	5	Washes hands.
❑	5	Identifies the patient and explains procedure.
❑	10	Assembles the axillary crutches and makes sure they are in good condition and good working order.
❑	15	Checks the measurement of the crutches.
❑	10	Applies the gait belt; assists the patient to stand and places the crutches under the patient's armpits.
❑	15	Instructs the patient to carry weight completely on the hands and not on the armpits.
❑	10	Instructs the patient to put all weight on the good leg and bend the weak leg slightly so it will not drag on the floor while walking.
❑	5	Assists the patient with the required gait.
❑	15	Teaches the patient how to inspect the crutches daily for safety. • Check wing nuts. • Check crutch tips for wear and tear. • Check foam pads of hand grips and armpit rests for tears. • Wear comfortable shoes, preferably with rubber soles. • Never use crutches on waxed floors or loose rugs.
❑	5	Washes hands.

Task Performed	Possible Points	TASKS
☐	15	Documents the date, time, duration of ambulation, and instructions given. Initials the report.
☐	5	Completed the tasks within 10 minutes.
☐	15	Results obtained were accurate.
________	Earned	ADD POINTS OF TASKS CHECKED
130	Points	TOTAL POINTS POSSIBLE
________	SCORE	DETERMINE SCORE (divide points earned by total points possible, multiply results by 100)

Actual Student Time Needed to Complete Procedure: ____________

Student's Initials: ____________ Instructor's Initials: ____________ Grade: ____________

Suggestions for Improvement: ____

Evaluator's Name (print) ____

Evaluator's Signature ____

Comments ____

DOCUMENTATION

Chart the procedure in the patient's medical record.

Date: _________

Charting: ____

____

____

____

____

____

Student's Initials: _______

SKILLS COMPETENCY ASSESSMENT

Procedure 26–7: Assisting a Patient to Ambulate with a Cane

Student's Name: ______________________________ Date: __________

Objective: To teach patients how to walk safely with a cane.

Conditions: The student demonstrates the ability to teach patients how to walk safely with a cane using the following equipment and supplies: appropriate cane for patient, gait belt.

Time Requirements and Accuracy Standards: 5 minutes. Points assigned reflect importance of step to meeting objective: Important = (5) Essential = (10) Critical = (15). Automatic failure results if any of the **critical tasks are** omitted or performed incorrectly.

STANDARD PRECAUTIONS:

SKILLS ASSESSMENT CHECKLIST

Task Performed	Possible Points	TASKS
☐	5	Washes hands.
☐	5	Ascertains what type of cane the patient will be using and assembles the equipment.
☐	10	Identifies the patient and explains procedure.
☐	10	Checks the cane to be sure the bottom has a rubber suction tip(s).
☐	10	Applies the gait belt snugly around the patient's waist and assists the patient to a standing position.
☐	10	Places the cane 6 inches in front and slightly to the side of the foot of the strong leg. Adjusts the cane so the handle is at the level of the patient's hip joint.
☐	5	*Rationale:* Knows the proper angle to which the patient's elbow should be flexed during weightbearing.
☐	15	Instructs the patient to move the cane forward 10 to 18 inches, depending on the patient's ability.
☐	15	Instructs the patient to move the weak leg forward while transferring body weight to the cane.
☐	15	Instructs the patient to move the strong leg forward past the cane.
☐	5	Follows along behind and to the side of the patient's weak side.
☐	5	Washes hands.

Task Performed	Possible Points	TASKS
☐	15	Documents the date, time, duration of ambulation, response of the patient, and instructions given. Initials report.
☐	5	Completed the tasks within 5 minutes.
☐	15	Results obtained were accurate.
________	Earned	ADD POINTS OF TASKS CHECKED
145	Points	TOTAL POINTS POSSIBLE
________	SCORE	DETERMINE SCORE (divide points earned by total points possible, multiply results by 100)

Actual Student Time Needed to Complete Procedure: ____________

Student's Initials: ____________ Instructor's Initials: ____________ Grade: ____________

Suggestions for Improvement: ____________

Evaluator's Name (print) ____________

Evaluator's Signature ____________

Comments ____________

DOCUMENTATION

Chart the procedure in the patient's medical record.

Date: ________

Charting: ____________

____

____

____

____

____

Student's Initials: _______

SKILLS COMPETENCY ASSESSMENT

Procedure 26–8: Range of Motion Exercises, Upper Body

Student's Name: ______________________________ Date: ____________

Objective: To maintain or increase joint mobility in a patient's upper extremities and to prevent contractures.

Conditions: The student demonstrates the ability to perform range of motion exercises to maintain or increase joint mobility in a patient's upper body. This procedure is best done with the patient in the supine position. Repeat each motion several times.

Time Requirements and Accuracy Standards: 15 minutes. Points assigned reflect importance of step to meeting objective: Important = (5) Essential = (10) Critical = (15). Automatic failure results if any of the **critical** tasks are omitted or performed incorrectly.

STANDARD PRECAUTIONS:

SKILLS ASSESSMENT CHECKLIST

Task Performed	Possible Points	TASKS
		PREPROCEDURE TASKS
❑	5	Washes hands.
❑	10	Identifies the patient and explains procedure.
		PROCEDURE TASKS *Shoulder Flexion*
❑	5	Keeps the patient's arm straight and holds the arm at the wrist and elbow.
❑	10	Lifts the patient's arm straight over the patient's head until it rests flat on the bed or table above the patient's head.
❑	5	Bends the patient's elbow if there is not enough room on the bed.
❑	5	Brings the arm back to the patient's side.
		Shoulder Abduction and Adduction
❑	10	Keeps the patient's arm straight by the patient's side with the palm of the hand facing up; supports the arm at the wrist and elbow.
❑	5	Keeps the patient's arm straight; brings it out at a right angle to the patient's body.
❑	10	Brings the arm back to the patient's side. Keeping the arm straight, brings it across the patient's body.
❑	5	Returns the patient's arm to a position parallel to the body.

Task Performed	Possible Points	TASKS
		Internal and External Shoulder Rotation
❑	5	Brings the patient's arm out at a right angle from the body.
❑	5	Bends the elbow at a right angle and keeps the patient's upper arm on the bed.
❑	10	Keeping the patient's arm at a right angle, presses down on the shoulder with one hand while holding the patient's wrist with the other.
❑	5	Moves the hand gently back until it touches the bed next to the patient's head.
❑	5	Brings the patient's hand back down until the palm of the patient's hand touches the bed.
		Elbow Flexion and Extension
❑	10	Holding the patient's arm by the patient's side, palm up, flexes and extends the elbow.
		Wrist Extension and Flexion
❑	5	Supports the patient's arm above the wrist.
❑	5	Holding the palm of the patient's hand, extends the patient's wrist, then straightens it.
❑	10	Places hand over the patient's hand while supporting the patient's wrist; bends or flexes the hand.
		Wrist Inversion and Eversion
❑	5	Grasps the patient's wrist with one hand and grasps the patient's hand with the other.
❑	5	Slowly bends the patient's hand toward the patient's body, then away from the body.
		Wrist Supination and Pronation
❑	5	Grasps the patient's wrist with one hand and grasps the patient's hand with the other.
❑	5	Slowly turns the patient's hand toward the patient's feet, then toward the face.
		Finger Flexion and Extension
❑	10	Supports the patient's wrist with one hand. Covers the patient's fingers with the other hand and curls them over to make a fist.
❑	5	Uncurls the patient's fingers and straightens them.
		Finger and Thumb Abduction and Adduction
❑	10	Holds the patient's hand flat; pulls each finger away from the thumb, then pulls the finger back straight.
❑	5	Pulls the thumb away from the rest of the fingers, then pulls it back straight.

SKILLS COMPETENCY ASSESSMENT — continued

Procedure 26-8: Range of Motion Exercises, Upper Body

Task Performed	Possible Points	TASKS
		Thumb Opposition
❑	5	Supports the patient's hand.
❑	5	Touches each finger with the patient's thumb.
		POSTPROCEDURE TASKS
❑	15	Documents the date, time, limbs given ROM, and response of the patient. Initials report.
❑	5	Completed the tasks within 15 minutes.
❑	15	Results obtained were accurate.
______	Earned	ADD POINTS OF TASKS CHECKED
225	Points	TOTAL POINTS POSSIBLE
______	SCORE	DETERMINE SCORE (divide points earned by total points possible, multiply results by 100)

Actual Student Time Needed to Complete Procedure: ____________

Student's Initials: ____________ Instructor's Initials: ____________ Grade: ____________

Suggestions for Improvement: ____________

Evaluator's Name (print) ____________

Evaluator's Signature ____________

Comments ____________

DOCUMENTATION

Chart the ROM procedure indicated by the instructor in the patient's medical record.

Date: ____________

Charting: ____________

____

____

____

____

Student's Initials: ________

SKILLS COMPETENCY ASSESSMENT

Procedure 26–9: Range of Motion Exercises, Lower Body

Student's Name: ______________________________ Date: ____________

Objective: To maintain or increase joint mobility in the patient's lower extremities and to prevent contractures.

Conditions: The student demonstrates the ability to maintain or increase joint mobility in the lower extremities and to prevent contractures. This procedure is best done with the patient in the supine position. Repeat each movement several times.

Time Requirements and Accuracy Standards: 15 minutes. Points assigned reflect importance of step to meeting objective: Important = (5) Essential = (10) Critical = (15). Automatic failure results if any of the **critical** tasks are omitted or performed incorrectly.

STANDARD PRECAUTIONS:

SKILLS ASSESSMENT CHECKLIST

Task Performed	Possible Points	TASKS
		PREPROCEDURE TASKS
☐	5	Washes hands.
☐	10	Identifies the patient and explains procedure.
		PROCEDURE TASKS
		Hip Abduction and Adduction
☐	5	Supports the patient's knee and ankle.
☐	10	Keeping the patient's leg straight, moves the entire leg away from the body.
☐	15	Moves the patient's leg back, toward the midline of the body.
		Hip and Knee Flexion and Extension
☐	5	Supports the patient's knee and ankle.
☐	15	Bends the patient's knee and raises it as far toward the patient's chest as the patient's tolerance and comfort will allow.
☐	10	Lowers and straightens the patient's leg.
		Hip Rotation
☐	5	Supports the patient's leg at the knee and ankle.
☐	10	Rolls the patient's leg in a circular motion, away from the body.
☐	10	Rolls the patient's leg in a circular motion, toward the body.

SKILLS COMPETENCY ASSESSMENT — continued

Procedure 26–9: Range of Motion Exercises, Lower Body

Task Performed	Possible Points	TASKS
		Ankle Dorsiflexion and Plantar Flexion
❑	10	Keeps the patient's leg flat on the bed, with the knee slightly bent if more comfortable for the patient. Grasps the patient's ankle with one hand and the heel of the patient's foot with the other.
❑	10	With the hand holding the patient's heel, flexes the patient's foot and rests the bottom of the patient's foot against the student's forearm, keeping the elbow straight.
❑	10	Dorsiflexes the ankle by pushing the patient's foot toward the patient's knee with student's arm.
❑	5	Returns the foot to its flexed position against the student's forearm.
❑	10	Keeping one hand on the patient's ankle, plantar flexes the ankle by drawing the foot down toward the foot of the bed.
		Foot Inversion and Eversion
❑	5	Grasps the patient's ankle with one hand and the arch of the foot with the other.
❑	5	Turns the patient's foot inward.
❑	10	Returns the patient's foot to the midline, then gently turns it outward.
		Toe Flexion and Extension
❑	10	Holds the patient's ankle in one hand and places fingers over the patient's toes with the other hand.
❑	5	Bends the toes, then straightens them.
		Toe Abduction and Adduction
❑	5	Moves each toe one at a time away from the second toe.
❑	5	Moves each toe one at a time toward the second toe.
		POSTPROCEDURE TASKS
❑	15	Documents the date, time, limbs given ROM, and response of the patient. Initials the report.
❑	5	Completed the tasks within 15 minutes.

Task Performed	Possible Points	TASKS
❑	15	Results obtained were accurate.

________	Earned	ADD POINTS OF TASKS CHECKED
225	Points	TOTAL POINTS POSSIBLE
________	SCORE	DETERMINE SCORE (divide points earned by total points possible, multiply results by 100)

Actual Student Time Needed to Complete Procedure: ____________

Student's Initials: ____________ Instructor's Initials: ____________ Grade: ____________

Suggestions for Improvement: ________________________________

Evaluator's Name (print) ________________________________

Evaluator's Signature ________________________________

Comments ________________________________

DOCUMENTATION

Chart the procedure indicated by the instructor in the patient's medical record.

Date: __________

Charting: ________________________________

____

____

____

____

____

Student's Initials: _______

EVALUATION OF CHAPTER KNOWLEDGE

How has your instructor evaluated the knowledge you have gained?

Knowledge	**Instructor Evaluation** *Good*	*Average*	*Poor*
Knows the definition of rehabilitation medicine and its importance in patient care	_____	_____	_____
Understands the importance of correct posture and body mechanics and how to safely transfer patients and lift or move large objects using correct body mechanics	_____	_____	_____
Knows how to care for the falling patient	_____	_____	_____
Knows how to help a patient safely stand and walk	_____	_____	_____
Knows the three types of assistive devices and how to teach patients to ambulate using each	_____	_____	_____
Understands how to measure patients for axillary crutches	_____	_____	_____
Describes the ambulation gaits used with crutches	_____	_____	_____
Understands the function of joint range of motion and how to measure joint movement	_____	_____	_____
Understands how therapeutic exercise is used in rehabilitation medicine and knows the types of therapeutic exercises	_____	_____	_____
Knows the definitions of the body movements used in range of motion exercises	_____	_____	_____
Knows the types of therapeutic modalities, can explain how the body reacts to each, and can describe the situation in which each modality would be used	_____	_____	_____
Understands how ultrasound works			

Student's Initials: _______ Instructor's Initials: _______

Grade: ________

CHAPTER 27

Nutrition in Health and Disease

PERFORMANCE OBJECTIVES

Nutrition is the study of the intake of nutrients into the body and how the body uses these nutrients. A proper balance of nutrients is required for optimum health. As individuals progress through each stage of the life span, their diets must be modified to adapt to the body's changing needs. Particular disease states may also require a change from a normal diet to control the progress of the disease and help return the patient to good health. Medical assistants who recognize the type and quantity of nutrients required to maintain good health and who understand how the diet should be changed in response to various disease states or to changes in physical development can use their knowledge of nutritional principles to encourage patients to adopt healthy, nutritional habits. Addressing the patient's eating habits and concerns also helps ensure that the patient will comply with the physician's treatment plan regarding diet and nutrition. Medical assisting students can use this chapter to learn about the vital importance of good nutrition in promoting and maintaining health.

EXERCISES AND ACTIVITIES

Vocabulary Builder

A. Vitamins are a class of nutrients in which each specific vitamin has a function entirely of its own. These complex molecules are required by the body in minute quantities. What are the two functions of vitamins in the body?

(1) ______________________________

(2) ______________________________

B. *Identify the correct chemical name for each vitamin listed. Then describe what each vitamin does in the body to promote good health.*

______________________ A. One of the B-complex vitamins, also called nicotinic acid

____

________________ B. Vitamin B_1

____

________________ C. Vitamin E

____

________________ D. Vitamin D

____

________________ E. One of the B-complex vitamins, also called folacin

____

________________ F. Vitamin A

____

________________ G. Vitamin B_{12}

____

________________ H. Vitamin C

____

________________ I. Vitamin B_2

____

________________ J. Vitamin B_6

____

C. *Fill in the blank with the correct key vocabulary term from the list below.*

Absorption	Diuretics	Metabolism
Amino acids	Electrolytes	Nutrients
Antioxidant	Elimination	Nutrition
Basal metabolic rate (BMR)	Extracellular	Oxidation
Calories	Fat-soluble	Preservatives
Catalyst	Glycogen	Processed foods
Cellulose	Homeostasis	Saturated fats
Coenzyme	Ingestion	Trace minerals
Digestion	Major minerals	Water soluble

1. Artificial flavors, colors, and ________________, chemicals that keep food fresh longer, are nonnutritive substances commonly added to processed foods.
2. ________________ is the study of the intake of nutrients into the body and how the body processes and uses these nutrients.
3. Toxicity is most likely to occur with ________________ vitamins because they are stored in tissues composed of lipids and in the liver and are not carried easily into the bloodstream.

4. The best source of complete proteins are meats and animal products such as milk and eggs; complete proteins contain all eight of the essential ______________________.
5. Beverages that contain caffeine and alcohol, which are ______________________, will cause the body to increase urinary output and lose water. These substances should be avoided when performing activities, such as a good physical workout, and entering environments, such as an airplane passenger cabin, that promote dehydration.
6. A ______________________ is a nonprotein substance that acts with a catalyst to facilitate chemical reactions in the body.
7. ______________________ is the process of the digestive system involving the transfer of nutrients from the gastrointestinal tract into the bloodstream.
8. Chlorine (Cl) is a mineral with an important ______________________ function, one that takes place outside the cells of body tissues in the spaces between layers or groups of cells.
9. The total of all changes, or energy, chemical and physical, that takes place in the body is called ______________________.
10. Some minerals are considered ______________________ in that they become ionized and carry a positive or negative charge; these minerals must be carefully balanced in the body.
11. ______________________ begins at the mouth with chewing and progresses through the gastrointestinal tract to the small intestine.
12. ______________________ are ingested substances that help the body maintain a state of homeostasis.
13. The process of ______________________ maintains a constant internal environment of the human body, including such functions as heartbeat, blood pressure, respiration, and body temperature.
14. A ______________________ facilitates chemical reactions by speeding up the reaction time without the need for a high energy output.
15. It is always important to analyze the nutritional labels on ______________________ purchased in the supermarket.
16. Lard is one example of ______________________, which have been found to raise the level of fats and cholesterol in the blood and are hydrogenated, or contain hydrogen.
17. The ability to reduce ______________________ is a characteristic of vitamin E that has led some researchers to suggest that vitamin E may slow the aging process, although its true effectiveness has not yet been demonstrated.
18. The excretion of waste through the anus is called ______________________, the final step of the digestive process.
19. The amount of energy a substance is able to supply is measured in large ______________________.
20. Potassium is one of the seven ______________________ found in the body.

21. Vitamins that are __________________________ must be constantly ingested to maintain proper blood levels, as these vitamins are not easily stored in the body.
22. Vitamin E is a fat-soluble vitamin that belongs to a group of compounds called __________________________, which counteract the damaging effects of oxidation. Beta-carotene is another substance in this group.
23. Despite their name, __________________________ are vital to body functioning, and include molybdenum and fluorine.
24. ____________________ begins the digestive process when we put food in our mouths to eat.
25. Children, pregnant women, and people with a lean body mass will have a higher __________________________ because it takes more energy to fuel the muscles than it does to store fat.
26. A type of carbohydrate, __________________________, is derived from a plant source and supplies fiber in the human diet.
27. Ingested only in small quantities, __________________________ is an important carbohydrate form for storage of glucose in the body.

Learning Review

1. Identify each organ of the digestive system in the diagram below. Describe the healthy functioning of each organ in the space provided. Then, using a medical dictionary or encyclopedia, look up each organ and list one common disorder that would adversely affect the digestive process.

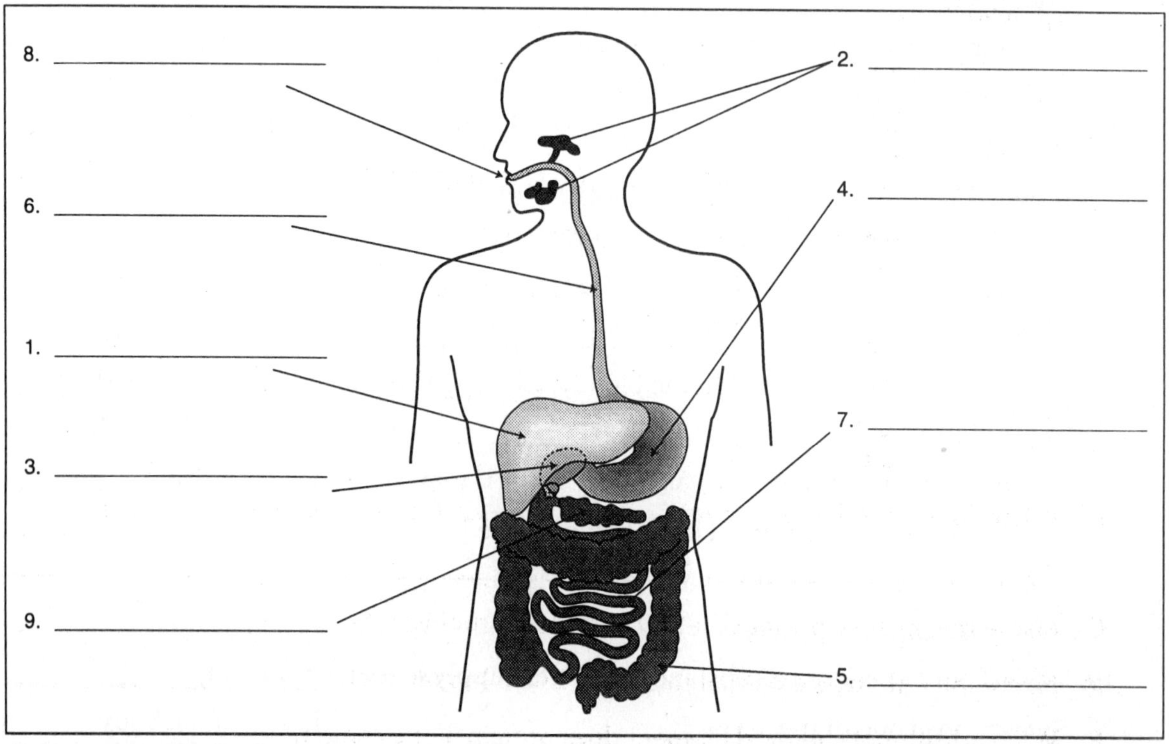

(1) Healthy function: ____________________
____________________ Common disorder: ____________________

(2) Healthy function: ____________________
____________________ Common disorder: ____________________

(3) Healthy function: ____________________
____________________ Common disorder: ____________________

(4) Healthy function: ____________________
____________________ Common disorder: ____________________

(5) Healthy function: ____________________
____________________ Common disorder: ____________________

(6) Healthy function: ____________________
____________________ Common disorder: ____________________

(7) Healthy function: ____________________
____________________ Common disorder: ____________________

(8) Healthy function: ____________________
____________________ Common disorder: ____________________

(9) Healthy function: ____________________
____________________ Common disorder: ____________________

2. A. Nutrients are divided into two groups: those that provide energy and those that do not.

Identify the nutrients listed below as providing energy or not providing energy by checking the appropriate box.

Energy	**No Energy**	
❑	❑	(1) Vitamins
❑	❑	(2) Carbohydrates
❑	❑	(3) Fiber
❑	❑	(4) Minerals
❑	❑	(5) Lipids (Fats)
❑	❑	(6) Proteins
❑	❑	(7) Water

B. What three chemical elements do carbohydrates, fats, and proteins all contain?

(1) ____________________ (2) ____________________ (3) ____________________

C. Name the most important dietary complex carbohydrate. ____________________

D. Name the only true essential fatty acid in the human diet. ____________________

E. What additional chemical element does protein alone contain? ____________________

F. When the body does not have enough carbohydrates or fats in supply as an energy source, what happens and what effect does this have on the body? ______________________

____

G. What does the acronym PEM stand for, and what usually occurs with this deficiency?

____

____

H. Name two diseases associated with deficiencies in protein.

(1) ______________________ (2) ______________________

3. A. List two distinct ways in which minerals differ from vitamins.

(1) ____

(2) ____

B. For each food source, list the mineral or minerals that each provides.

(1) Eggs ____

(2) Milk ____

(3) Cheese ____

(4) Salmon ____

(5) Bananas ____

(6) Green vegetables ____

4. For each of the following, identify the substance as a water-soluble vitamin (WSV), fat-soluble vitamin (FSV), a major mineral (MM), or a trace mineral (TM). Then match the substance to the response that best fits its character or properties.

____ 1. Sulfur	____ 6. Pyridoxine
____ 2. Vitamin B_{12}	____ 7. Iodine
____ 3. Iron	____ 8. Biotin
____ 4. Vitamin K	____ 9. Retinol
____ 5. Sodium	____ 10. Vitamin D

____ A. This substance works with potassium to maintain proper water balance and proper pH balance; the two also are involved in nervous muscular conduction and excitability.

____ B. This substance is part of the pigment rhodopsin found in the eye and is responsible in part for vision, especially night vision.

____ C. This substance is vital to life because of its role in the heme molecule, which carries oxygen to every cell in the body.

____ D. Rickets and osteomalacia are diseases caused by deficiencies in this substance; when deficiencies occur, usually in childhood, malformation of the skeleton is seen.

____ E. This member of the B-complex, along with pantothenic acid, is generally responsible for energy metabolism.

____ F. Because this substance is only found in foods from animal sources, such as liver, kidney, and dairy products, pernicious anemia, the result of deficiencies, may be a problem for some vegetarians.

____ G. This substance, found in rice, beans, and yeast, is important to protein metabolism.

____ H. This substance is a component of one of the amino acids and is found in protein; it is also involved in energy metabolism.

____ I. About half of the body's requirement for this substance is fulfilled through synthesis by intestinal bacteria; bile is required for its absorption into the bloodstream.

____ J. This substance is only found in the thyroid hormones; without it, the thyroid gland would be unable to regulate the overall metabolism of the body.

5. A. List six types of fiber that are carbohydrates.

(1) ____________________ (3) ____________________

(2) ____________________ (4) ____________________

(3) ____________________ (6) ____________________

B. What important fiber is not a carbohydrate? ____________________

Americans generally do not consume enough fiber. How much fiber should be consumed each day? ____________________ Why does brown rice contain more fiber than white rice? ____________________

6. A. What happens when the body takes in more calories than will be expended by the body as energy? ____________________

What happens when the body uses more energy than the calories it takes in will produce?

____

What is the ideal percentage of total calories that should be consumed as carbohydrates, fats, and proteins? Carbohydrates: __________ Fats: __________ Proteins: __________

B. An 8-fluid-ounce serving of 1% fat soy milk contains 110 calories with 2 grams of total fat, 20 grams of total carbohydrates, and 4 grams of total protein. Calculate the total number of calories from each energy nutrient; show your calculations in the spaces provided below.

Number of calories from fat: ________ Number of calories from carbohydrates: ________
Number of calories from protein: ________

Now calculate the percentage of total calories due to each energy nutrient.

Percent of calories from fat: ________ Percent of calories from carbohydrates: ________
Percent of calories from protein: ________

C. Compare the percentages of total Calories due to fat, carbohydrates, and protein found in soy milk to the percentages you calculated for one serving of peanut butter in your textbook's critical thinking question # 9.

Percent of Total Calories	Peanut Butter	Soy Milk
Fat		
Carbohydrates		
Protein		

How do the percentages relate to the ideal percentages for optimum energy balance in the body? ____________________

____

____

7. Dr. Elizabeth King has confirmed that patient Mary O'Keefe is pregnant with her third child.

   A. Name two minerals that Mary must increase amounts of in her diet.

   (1) ____________ (2) ____________

   B. Name three reasons why a woman needs to increase her intake of nutrients and calories when she is pregnant.

   (1) __________ (2) __________ (3) __________

   C. What dietary supplement usually needs to be added to a baby's diet? __________

8. When helping patients modify their diets, medical assistants need to be knowledgeable about the nutrients in the food we eat. The nutritional analysis label on the back or side of a food package is helpful when figuring out the levels of fat, cholesterol, sodium, carbohydrates, protein, and vitamins contained in a particular food.

   A. The percent of daily values listed on a label report the amount of a nutrient obtained by eating how many servings of a product? __________ The percentages are based on a __________ calorie diet. The listing for total carbohydrates is broken down into what two additional listings? (1) __________ (2) __________

   Which type of carbohydrate is more beneficial and why? __________

   ____

   A patient should look for a food product in which the sodium content is relatively low. What is the greatest number of milligrams of sodium a person should eat each day? __________

   What is the total amount of cholesterol a person should eat each day? __________

   Why is a high-fiber diet important? __________

   ____

   ____

B. Compare Figure 27–2, the nutrition food label from a box of muesli with fruit, nuts, and seeds, to Figure 27–3, the label from a package of pretzel snacks. Which is more nutritious and why? Note that one serving of the muesli, ½ cup or 55 grams, is roughly equivalent to two servings of pretzels, 14 pretzels or 60 grams.

Muesli

Nutrition Facts

Serving Size: 1/2 cup (55g)
Servings Per Container: about 8

Amount Per Serving	Cereal	Cereal + 125 mL Vitamin A & D fortified skim milk
Calories	210	250
Calories from Fat	30	35
	% Daily Value**	
Total Fat 3g*	5%	5%
Saturated Fat 0.5g	3%	3%
Cholesterol 0mg	0%	0%
Sodium 30mg	1%	4%
Total Carbohydrate 40g	13%	15%
Dietary Fiber 5g	21%	21%
Sugars 13g		
Protein 6g		
Vitamin A	0%	8%
Vitamin C	8%	8%
Calcium	4%	20%
Iron	35%	35%
Vitamin D	0%	10%
Thiamine	35%	40%
Riboflavin	25%	35%
Niacin	2%	2%
Vitamin B_6	15%	20%
Folate	10%	10%
Pantothenic Acid	4%	10%

*Amount in Cereal. One half cup skim milk contributes an additional 40 calories. 65 mg sodium. 6g total carbohydrate (6g sugars). and 4g protein.

**Percent Daily Values are based on a 2.000 calorie diet. Your daily values may be higher or lower depending on your calorie needs.

	Calories	2.000	2.500
Total Fat	Less than	65g	80g
Sat Fat	Less than	20g	25g
Cholesterol	Less than	300mg	300mg
Sodium	Less than	2.400mg	2.400mg
Total Carbohydrate		300g	375g
Dietary Fiber		25g	30g

Calories per gram:
Fat 9 • Carbohydrate 4 • Protein 4

Pretzels

Nutrition Facts

Serving Size: 7 Pretzels (30g)
Servings Per Container: 9.4

Amount Per Serving	
Calories 120	
Calories from Fat 10	
	% Daily Value*
Total Fat 1g	2%
Saturated Fat 0g	0%
Cholesterol 0g	0%
Sodium 360mg	15%
Total Carbohydrate 24g	8%
Dietary Fiber 1g	4%
Sugars 1g	
Protein 3g	

Vitamin A 0% Σ Vitamin C 0%
Calcium 0% Σ Iron 2%

*Percent Daily Values are based on a 2,000 calorie diet. Your daily values may be higher or lower depending on your calorie needs:

	Calories	2,000	2,500
Total Fat	Less than	65g	80g
Sat Fat	Less than	20g	25g
Cholesterol	Less than	300mg	300mg
Sodium	Less than	2,400mg	2,400mg
Total Carbohydrate		300g	375g
Dietary Fiber		25g	30g

Calories per gram:
Fat 9 Σ Carbohydrate 4 Σ Protein 4

Ingredients: Unbleached Wheat Flour, Water, Corn Syrup, Partially Hydrogenated Vegetable Oil (Soybean), Yeast Salt, Bicarbonates and Carbonates of Sodium.

9. Compare the advantages and disadvantages of the following diets: U. S. southern, Jewish, and Japanese.

Investigation Activity

Many of the foods we eat today are processed foods. We rely on the labels on the cans, bottles, and boxes lining grocery store shelves to tell us what nutrients are inside. However, many of us do not actually read the labels, but instead use the shape or color of a package or advertisements to make our decisions about purchasing food products.

Go into your family kitchen and choose your three favorite food or beverage products—anything from milk to salsa to fruit juice, frozen macaroni and cheese, or ice cream. Base your choices on the foods that are the best tasting and most satisfying, ones you purchase frequently at the grocery store. Remove the nutrition facts labels from each product and tape or glue them in the spaces below.

Product Name: ____________ Product Name: ____________ Product Name: ____________

Now look for one food or beverage item in your kitchen that attracted you solely on the basis of the product's packaging. Remove the nutrition facts label from the product and tape or glue it in the space provided.

Product Name: ______________________________

What is it about this packaging that attracts you to the product? Describe the package.

____

____

____

What kind of mood does the packaging put you in?

____

____

____

What does the packaging suggest about the product? For example, is the packaging trying to look healthy, fun, wholesome, convenient, traditional? Does the product inside the package live up to its packaging promise?

____

____

____

Does the packaging make any claims or promises? If so, what are they?

____

____

____

Is this product nutritious? Give your analysis of the information on the nutrition facts label.

____

____

____

CASE STUDY

Lourdes Austen, a breast cancer survivor, regularly attends a support group for breast cancer patients and survivors held once a month. Lourdes finds the group a great source of encouragement, information, and support—a safe place to discuss her feelings and concerns about breast cancer. The group is planning a session to talk about nutrition issues, and Lourdes asks clinical medical assistant Audrey Jones if she would like to attend the meeting with her to contribute to the group's discussion. With permission from office manager Marilyn Johnson and Lourdes's physician Dr. Elizabeth King, Audrey attends the meeting. The group members are enthusiastic and ask Audrey many questions, including the following. "Why is good nutrition important for cancer patients?" "I don't have much of an appetite any more and get nauseous all the time. What can I do?" "I keep hearing about those macrobiotic diets? Are they any good? Should I try them?"

Discuss the following:

1. What information can Audrey give in answer to the question regarding the importance of good nutrition for cancer patients?
2. What suggestion can Audrey offer to patients who have no appetite, nausea, or vomiting?
3. What can Audrey tell the group about macrobiotic diets?
4. What is the role of the medical assistant in attending the breast cancer support group meeting?

SUPPLEMENTARY RESOURCES

Study Guide Disk: Additional practice exercises for this chapter are available on the study guide disk found in the back of the textbook.

Medical Assisting Videos: Appropriate content is available on Delmar's Medical Assisting Videos, 2nd ed., Tape 8, for the following topics:

Take an In-Depth Patient History

Introduction to Health Promotion, Disease Prevention, and Self-Responsibility

Name of Product:	
Indications:	
Form of Drug and Dosage:	
Directions for Adults:	
Side effects:	
Contraindications:	

Name of Product:	
Indications:	
Form of Drug and Dosage:	
Directions for Adults:	
Side effects:	
Contraindications:	

Name of Product:	
Indications:	
Form of Drug and Dosage:	
Directions for Adults:	
Side effects:	
Contraindications:	

1. Where are medications stored in your home? Are they stored in more than one location? Is your medicine cabinet orderly or disorganized?

up / down stairs bathrooms - yes - down/yes up/no

2. Are there children in your household? Are drugs properly stored so children cannot reach them? What methods can be used to keep drugs away from children?

not small children - yes - locks, keeping out of reach....

3. How often do you clean out your medicine cabinet at home? How does your family dispose of medications? Why is maintaining an orderly medicine cabinet in the home important?

hardly ever - throw away - so you don't use wrong med.

CASE STUDY

While Anna Preciado, a clinical medical assistant newly hired at the offices of Drs. Lewis and King, is performing her shift duties, she notices a fellow employee exhibiting strange behavior. Audrey

CHAPTER 29

Dosage Calculation and Administration

PERFORMANCE OBJECTIVES

To safely administer medications to patients, medical assistants must possess a fundamental knowledge of pharmacology, have the ability to calculate doses of medication, and be competent in various methods of medication administration, including oral and parenteral. Medical assistants must also be aware of the legal and ethical aspects of medication administration. It is the responsibility of all health care professionals to provide care only within the scope of practice of their training and knowledge, and within legal and ethical boundaries. Only a physician has the legal authority to prescribe medications for patients. Medical assistants prepare and administer medications as directed by the physician, accurately documenting and reporting according to the facility's established policies and procedures. All standard precautions and OSHA guidelines are observed to protect health care professionals, patients, and visitors from the transmission of pathogens.

EXERCISES AND ACTIVITIES

Vocabulary Builder

Supply a brief definition for each key vocabulary term.

1. Apnea ~~apnea~~ appsence of breath
2. BSA
3. Hypoxemia lack of oxygen the blood
4. Meniscus
5. Nomogram
6. Parenteral a injection
7. Precipitate form of particals that separates the sol.
8. Taut to pull or draw tight
9. Unit Dose premeasured amount of med
10. Wheal slight elevation of skin produced by an [illegible]

Learning Review

1. The prescription is a written legal document that gives directions for compounding, dispensing, and administering a medication to a patient. In the spaces below, "decode" the physicians' written prescriptions for medication in lay person's terms and answer the questions that follow.

A. Dr. King prescribes an adult dosage for a fever.

LEWIS & KING, MD
2501 CENTER STREET
NORTHBOROUGH, OH 12345

Name Lourdes Austin

Address 821 Spring Lane, Apt. 12 Date 3/1/--

℞

Dilantin 100 mg tab
#90
Sig 100 mg p.o. tid

Generic Substitution Allowed Elizabeth King M.D.

Dispense As Written ______ M.D.

REPETATUR 0 1 2 3 p.r.n.

☑ LABEL

How many grains are in each dose? ______

______

How days of medication are dispensed? ______

______

B. Dr. Lewis prescribes a child's dosage for an ear infection.

LEWIS & KING, MD
2501 CENTER STREET
NORTHBOROUGH, OH 12345

Name Felicia Lawrence

Address 362 Owen's View Way Date 3/1/--

℞

Amoxicillin 250 mg/5cc
150cc
Sig 5cc p.o. tid

Generic Substitution Allowed Winston Lewis M.D.

Dispense As Written ______ M.D.

REPETATUR 0 1 2 3 p.r.n.

☑ LABEL

Perform the conversion:

______ 5 cc = ______ teaspoons

How many doses are included in the amount dispensed? ______

2. A. Identify the following measures as weight (W) or volume (V). Then name the measure each abbreviation stands for and what system of measurement it belongs to.

Weight	Volume	Abbreviation	Measure	System
❑	❑	Gm		
❑	❑	gr		
❑	❑	qt		
❑	❑	tbsp		
❑	❑	mL		
❑	❑	fldr		
❑	❑	gt		
❑	❑	μg		

B. Perform the following conversions:

(1) 4 tsp = ________ mL

(2) 3.5 in = ________ cm

(3) 1,200 mg = ________ Gm

(4) 30 mg = ________ gr

(5) 8 mL = ________ gtt

C. What are proportions? How are proportions useful in calculating dosages of medication?

3. A. Identify the type of syringe typically used for each of the following; list the size and calibration as well.

(1) Venipunture: ________________________________

(2) Insulin administration: ________________________________

(3) Allergy testing: ________________________________

B. For each syringe-needle combination below, identify the most likely parenteral route: Subcutaneous injection (SC), Intramuscular injection (IM), or Intradermal injection (ID). Also identify the proper angle of injection.

	Angle of injection
_____ 1. 3-cc syringe/22G, 1 1/2 inch needle	____________
_____ 2. 1-cc syringe/25G, 5/8 inch needle	____________
_____ 3. U-100 (1cc)/26G, 1/2 inch needle	____________
_____ 4. 3-cc syringe/25G, 5/8 inch needle	____________

Investigation Activity

Under the law, health care professionals who administer medications are expected to be knowledgeable about the drugs they administer and the effects the drug(s) may and/or will have on the patient.

A. List three medications that are commonly prescribed to patients in the ambulatory care setting.

Three commonly prescribed medications:

(1) ________________ (2) ________________ (3) ________________

B. Choose one of the medications listed above and research it, consulting the *PDR*, a medical encyclopedia, and a nurse's drug reference. Complete the chart on the next page.

Drug name (generic and brand)	
Action	Uses
Contraindications	Warnings when indicated
Adverse reactions	Common dosages and routes
Implications for patient care	
Patient teaching	Special considerations

CASE STUDY

Louise Kipperley comes to the urgent care center at Inner City Health Care when she experiences the third severe migraine headache in only one month. The headache has lasted two days and Louise has experienced symptoms of nausea and vomiting. Dr. Rice gives written orders to administer Imitrex 25 mg IM stat, along with a prescription for the patient to fill and use at home. Liz Corbin, CMA, makes a medicine card from the physician's order sheet of Louise's medical record and prepares the stat dosage for Louise according to the correct procedure for administering oral medications. Liz is about to transport the medication to Louise in examination room #3 when she reads the physician's written order for Louise, which calls for 25 mg IM stat. The written prescription is for Imitrex every 4 hours as needed. Liz discards the dosage she has prepared for the patient and instead gives Louise Dr. Rice's prescription and tells her to have it filled immediately.

Discuss the following:

1. What medication error has Liz made? What effect will the error likely have on the patient?
2. What should Liz do? What standard procedures should be followed when a medication error occurs?

SUPPLEMENTARY RESOURCES

Study Guide Disk: Additional practice exercises for this chapter are available on the study guide disk found in the back of the textbook.

Medical Assisting Videos: Appropriate content is available on Delmar's Medical Assisting Videos, 2nd ed., for the following topics:

Tape 2: Practice Risk Management Measure to Prevent Professional Liability
- Dispose of Controlled Substances in Compliance With Government Regulations
- Perform Within Ethical Boundaries

Tape 5: Infections in the Office

Tape 11: Prepare and Administer Medication As Directed By Physician
- Administer Oral Medications

Tape 12: Prepare and Administer Parenteral Medications
- Cartridge Injection Systems
- Safety Syringe
- Withdraw Parenteral Medication from Vial
- Initial Procedures Common To All Injections
- Administer Intramuscular Injections
- Administer Subcutaneous Injections
- Administer Intradermal Injections
- Completion Procedures Following Injections
- OSHA Regulations for Needles and "Sharps"
- Accidental Needlesticks

SKILLS COMPETENCY ASSESSMENT

Procedure 29–1: Administration of Oral Medications

Student's Name: ______________________________ Date: ____________

Objective: To correctly administer an oral medication after receiving a physician's order.

Conditions: The student demonstrates the ability to correctly administer an oral medication after receiving a physician's order, and using the following equipment and supplies: proper medication, medicine card, water, milk, or juice for patient.

Time Requirements and Accuracy Standards: 10 minutes. Points assigned reflect importance of step to meeting objective: Important = (5) Essential = (10) Critical = (15). Automatic failure results if any of the **critical** tasks are omitted or performed incorrectly.

STANDARD PRECAUTIONS:

SKILLS ASSESSMENT CHECKLIST

Task Performed	Possible Points	TASKS
☐	5	Verifies the physician's order.
☐	15	Follows the "Six Rights" (see textbook Figure 12–10A).
☐	5	Performs medical asepsis hand wash.
☐	5	Works in a well-lighted, quiet, clean area.
☐	5	Assembles equipment and supplies.
☐	15	Obtains the correct medication using the medicine card.
☐	15	Compares the medication label with the medicine card (first time).
☐	10	Checks the expiration date.
☐	15	Calculates dosage, if necessary.
☐	15	Correctly prepares: • Multiple dose solid medication • Unit dose medication • Liquid medication
☐	15	Compares medicine label with medicine card (second time).
☐	15	Returns medication to shelf and checks label (third time).
☐	5	Properly transports the medicine.
☐	5	Identifies the patient and explains the procedure.

Task Performed	Possible Points	TASKS
❑	10	Assesses patient. Takes vital signs if indicated.
❑	5	Assists patient to a comfortable position.
❑	10	Provides water, milk, or juice (unless contraindicated).
❑	15	Administers the medication. Makes sure the patient takes the medicine.
❑	10	Provides for the patient's safety by observing the patient for any adverse reactions.
❑	5	Documents the procedure in the patient's chart using the medicine card.
❑	5	Cares for equipment and supplies according to OSHA guidelines.
❑	5	Washes hands.
❑	5	Completed the tasks within 10 minutes.
❑	15	Results obtained were accurate.

_______	Earned	ADD POINTS OF TASKS CHECKED
230	Points	TOTAL POINTS POSSIBLE
_______	SCORE	DETERMINE SCORE (divide points earned by total points possible, multiply results by 100)

Actual Student Time Needed to Complete Procedure: __________

Student's Initials: __________ Instructor's Initials: __________ Grade: __________

Suggestions for Improvement: ______________________________

Evaluator's Name (print) ______________________________

Evaluator's Signature ______________________________

Comments ______________________________

DOCUMENTATION

Chart the procedure in the patient's medical record.

Date: ________

Charting: ______________________________

____

____

____

____

Student's Initials: ________

SKILLS COMPETENCY ASSESSMENT

Procedure 29–2: Administration of Subcutaneous, Intramuscular, and/or Intradermal Injections

Student's Name: ______________________________ Date: ____________

Objective: To properly administer subcutaneous, intramuscular, and/or intradermal injections.

Conditions: The student demonstrates the ability to properly administer subcutaneous, intramuscular, and/or intradermal injections using the following equipment and supplies: medication, as ordered by the physician, and medicine card, appropriately sized needle-syringe unit, antiseptic wipes, disposable gloves, sharps container.

Time Requirements and Accuracy Standards: 10 minutes. Points assigned reflect importance of step to meeting objective: Important = (5) Essential = (10) Critical = (15). Automatic failure results if any of the **critical** tasks are omitted or performed incorrectly.

STANDARD PRECAUTIONS:

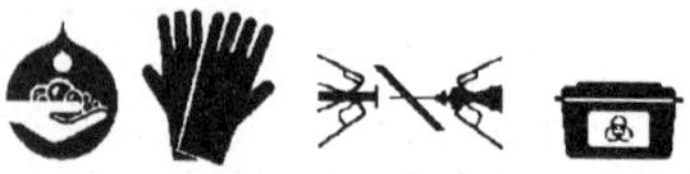

SKILLS ASSESSMENT CHECKLIST

Task Performed	Possible Points	TASKS
☐	10	Verifies the physician's order. Makes out medicine card taking information from physician's order sheet in the patient record.
☐	15	Follows the "Six Rights."
☐	5	Performs medical asepsis hand wash. Adheres to OSHA guidelines.
☐	5	Works in a well-lighted, quiet, clean area.
☐	10	Obtains the appropriate syringe-needle unit and alcohol swab.
☐	15	Obtains the correct medication.
☐	15	Compares the medication label with the medicine card (first time).
☐	10	Checks expiration date on medicine.
☐	15	Calculates dosage, if necessary.
☐	5	Prepares syringe-needle unit for use.
☐	5	Withdraws medication from container.
☐	15	Compares medicine label with the medicine card (second time).
☐	15	Places filled syringe-needle unit on the medicine tray with medicine card. Checks the medication label with the medicine card (third time).

Task Performed	Possible Points	TASKS
❑	5	Correctly transports the medicine to the patient.
❑	5	Identifies the patient. Explains the procedure.
❑	5	Assesses the patient. Puts on gloves.
❑	5	Prepares the patient for the injection (drapes, positions, allays apprehension).
❑	10	Selects an appropriate injection site. Follows a rotating schedule, if appropriate.
❑	10	Cleanses the injection site with a sterile antiseptic swab. Uses a circular motion, working from the center out to about two inches beyond the planned injection site.
❑	5	Allows the skin to dry.
❑	5	Administers the injection (aspirates to be certain needle is not in a blood vessel). Immediately disposes of syringe-needle unit in a puncture-proof sharps container.
❑	10	Massages injection site unless contraindicated (insulin, Imferon, heparin).
❑	5	Observes the patient for signs of difficulty.
❑	5	Inspects the injection site for bleeding, applies Band-Aid if necessary.
❑	5	Properly disposes of used equipment and supplies. Removes gloves.
❑	5	Performs medical asepsis hand wash.
❑	10	Correctly documents the procedure.
❑	5	Completed the tasks within 10 minutes.
❑	15	Results obtained were accurate.

________	Earned	ADD POINTS OF TASKS CHECKED
150	Points	TOTAL POINTS POSSIBLE
________	SCORE	DETERMINE SCORE (divide points earned by total points possible, multiply results by 100)

Procedure to follow should the medical assistant sustain an accidental needlestick after the injection:

❑	10	Thoroughly washes the site where the stick occurred.
❑	5	Cleanses the skin with an antiseptic.
❑	15	Reports the incident.
❑	10	Documents the incident and retains a copy of the incident report.
❑	15	Obtains medical attention and is tested for HBV and HIV.

SKILLS COMPETENCY ASSESSMENT — continued

Procedure 29–2: Administration of Subcutaneous, Intramuscular, and/or Intradermal Injections

Task Performed	Possible Points	TASKS
☐	10	Fills out appropriate OSHA paperwork (200 form).

______	Earned	ADD POINTS OF TASKS CHECKED
65	Points	TOTAL POINTS POSSIBLE
______	SCORE	DETERMINE SCORE (divide points earned by total points possible, multiply results by 100)

Actual Student Time Needed to Complete Procedure: ____________

Student's Initials: ____________ Instructor's Initials: ____________ Grade: ____________

Suggestions for Improvement: ______________________________

Evaluator's Name (print) ______________________________

Evaluator's Signature ______________________________

Comments ______________________________

DOCUMENTATION

Chart the procedure in the patient's medical record.

Date: __________

Charting: ______________________________

____

____

____

____

____

Student's Initials: _______

SKILLS COMPETENCY ASSESSMENT

Procedure 29–3: Withdrawing (Aspirating) Medication from a Vial

Student's Name: ______________________________ Date: ____________

Objective: To withdraw (aspirate) medication from a vial.

Conditions: The student demonstrates the ability to withdraw (aspirate) medication from a vial into a syringe for parenteral injection using the following equipment and supplies: medication order, medicine card, appropriate syringe and needle with cover, vial of medication, antiseptic wipes or sponges, disposable gloves, puncture-proof sharps container.

Time Requirements and Accuracy Standards: 10 minutes. Points assigned reflect importance of step to meeting objective: Important = (5) Essential = (10) Critical = (15). Automatic failure results if any of the **critical** tasks are omitted or performed incorrectly.

STANDARD PRECAUTIONS:

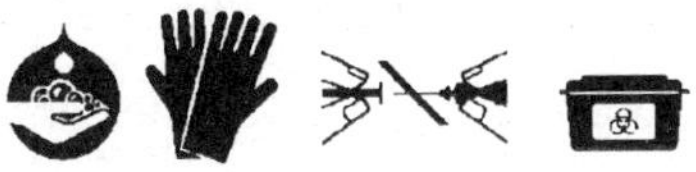

SKILLS ASSESSMENT CHECKLIST

Task Performed	Possible Points	TASKS
☐	15	Reads the medication order and assembles equipment. Checks for the "Six Rights." Reads the vial label by holding it next to the medicine card (first time).
☐	5	Washes hands, applies gloves.
☐	10	Selects the proper size needle and syringe for the medication and the route. If necessary, attaches the needle to the syringe.
☐	15	Checks the vial label against the medicine card (second time).
☐	5	Removes the metal or plastic cap from the vial. If the vial has been opened previously, cleans the rubber stopper by applying a disinfectant wipe in a circular motion.
☐	5	Removes the needle cover, pulling it straight off.
☐	15	Injects air into the vial as follows: • Holds the syringe pointed upward at eye level. Pulls back the plunger to take in a quantity of air equal to the ordered dose of medication. • Holds the vial upright (inverted) according to personal preference. Takes care not to touch the rubber stopper. • Inserts the needle through the rubber stopper of the vial. Injects air by pushing in the plunger.
☐	15	Withdraws the medication: Holds the vial and syringe steady. Pulls back on the plunger to withdraw the measured dose of medication. Measures accurately. Keeps the tip of the needle below the surface of the liquid to prevent air from entering the syringe. Keeps syringe at eye level.
☐	10	Checks the syringe for air bubbles. Removes air bubbles by tapping sharply on the syringe.
☐	5	Removes the needle from the vial. Replaces the sterile needle cover.

SKILLS COMPETENCY ASSESSMENT — continued

Procedure 29–3: Withdrawing (Aspirating) Medication from a Vial

Task Performed	Possible Points	TASKS
❑	15	Checks the vial label against the medicine card (third time).
❑	5	Places the filled needle and syringe on a medicine tray or cart with an antiseptic wipe and the medicine card. The dose is now ready for injection.
❑	5	Returns multiple-dose vials to the proper storage area (cabinet or refrigerator). Disposes of unused medication in a single-dose vial according to facility procedure. (Disposal of a controlled substance must be witnessed and the proper forms signed.)
❑	5	Discards used syringe-needle unit immediately after use in a sharps container.
❑	5	Removes gloves and disposes in biohazard waste container.
❑	5	Washes hands.
❑	5	Documents the procedure.
❑	5	Completed the tasks within 10 minutes.
❑	15	Results obtained were accurate.

______	Earned	ADD POINTS OF TASKS CHECKED
165	Points	TOTAL POINTS POSSIBLE
______	SCORE	DETERMINE SCORE (divide points earned by total points possible, multiply results by 100)

Actual Student Time Needed to Complete Procedure: ______________

Student's Initials: ______________ Instructor's Initials: ______________ Grade: ______________

Suggestions for Improvement: ______________________________

Evaluator's Name (print) ______________________________

Evaluator's Signature ______________________________

Comments ______________________________

DOCUMENTATION

Chart the procedure in the patient's medical record.

Date: __________

Charting: ______________________________

____

____

____

Student's Initials: ________

SKILLS COMPETENCY ASSESSMENT

Procedure 29–4: Withdrawing (Aspirating) Medication from an Ampule

Student's Name: ______________________________ Date: ____________

Objective: To withdraw (aspirate) medication from an ampule.

Conditions: The student demonstrates the ability to withdraw (aspirate) medication from an ampule into a syringe for parenteral injection using the following equipment and supplies: medicine tray, medicine card, ampule of medication, alcohol wipes, sterile gauze sponges, sharps container, sterile needle-syringe unit, gloves.

Time Requirements and Accuracy Standards: 5 minutes. Points assigned reflect importance of step to meeting objective: Important = (5) Essential = (10) Critical = (15). Automatic failure results if any of the **critical** tasks are omitted or performed incorrectly.

STANDARD PRECAUTIONS:

SKILLS ASSESSMENT CHECKLIST

Task Performed	Possible Points	TASKS
☐	10	Checks the physician's order. Writes out medicine card.
☐	5	Washes hands and gathers equipment. Puts on gloves.
☐	15	Obtains ampule of medication. Reads label and checks medicine card for correct medication, dose, route, and time (first time). Checks medication expiration date.
☐	5	Flicks ampule of medication, using a sharp flick of the wrist to force all of the medication down below the neck of the ampule into the body of the ampule.
☐	5	*Rationale:* Understands that if some medication remains trapped in ampule, an incorrect dosage may be administered to the patient.
☐	15	Thoroughly disinfects the neck with an alcohol swab. Checks label (second time).
☐	5	*Rationale:* Understands that ampule neck must be disinfected, as it may come into contact with the needle when the needle is inserted into the ampule.
☐	10	Wipes dry the neck of the ampule with a sterile gauze. Completely surrounds the ampule with the gauze and forcefully snaps off the top of the ampule by pushing the top away from the body.
☐	15	Sets opened ampule on medicine tray. Checks label (third time).
☐	15	With prepared sterile syringe-needle unit, aspirates the required dose into syringe. Covers needle with sheath and transports on the medicine tray to the patient.
☐	5	Identifies patient and administers medication.

SKILLS COMPETENCY ASSESSMENT — continued

Procedure 29–4: Withdrawing (Aspirating) Medication from an Ampule

Task Performed	Possible Points	TASKS
❑	5	Discards syringe-needle unit into sharps container. Discards alcohol swabs and gauze in biohazard waste container.
❑	5	Washes hands.
❑	5	Documents procedure.
❑	5	Completed the tasks within 5 minutes.
❑	15	Results obtained were accurate.
______	Earned	ADD POINTS OF TASKS CHECKED
140	Points	TOTAL POINTS POSSIBLE
______	SCORE	DETERMINE SCORE (divide points earned by total points possible, multiply results by 100)

Actual Student Time Needed to Complete Procedure: ____________

Student's Initials: ____________ Instructor's Initials: ____________ Grade: ____________

Suggestions for Improvement: ________________________________

Evaluator's Name (print) ________________________________

Evaluator's Signature ________________________________

Comments ________________________________

DOCUMENTATION

Chart the procedure in the patient's medical record.

Date: ________

Charting: ________________________________

____

____

____

____

____

Student's Initials: ______

SKILLS COMPETENCY ASSESSMENT

Procedure 29–5: Administering a Subcutaneous Injection

Student's Name: ______________________________ Date: ____________

Objective: To correctly administer a subcutaneous injection.

Conditions: The student demonstrates the ability to correctly administer a subcutaneous injection after receiving a physician's order, using the following equipment and supplies: medication ordered by physician, medicine card, appropriately sized needle-syringe unit, antiseptic wipe, disposable gloves, sharps container.

Time Requirements and Accuracy Standards: 5 minutes. Points assigned reflect importance of step to meeting objective: Important = (5) Essential = (10) Critical = (15). Automatic failure results if any of the **critical** tasks are omitted or performed incorrectly.

STANDARD PRECAUTIONS:

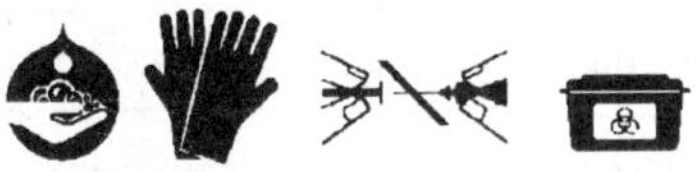

SKILLS ASSESSMENT CHECKLIST

Task Performed	Possible Points	TASKS
☐	10	Verifies the physician's order. Makes out a medicine card.
☐	15	Follows the "Six Rights."
☐	5	Performs medical asepsis hand wash. Adheres to OSHA guidelines.
☐	5	Works in a well-lighted, quiet, clean area.
☐	5	Obtains the appropriate equipment and supplies.
☐	15	Obtains the correct medication.
☐	15	Compares the medication label with the medicine card (first time).
☐	15	Checks expiration date on medicine.
☐	15	Calculates dosage, if necessary.
☐	15	Correctly prepares the parenteral medication.
☐	15	Compares medication label with the medicine card (second time).
☐	5	Replaces medication in an appropriate area (shelf, refrigerator). Compares the medication label (third time).
☐	5	Correctly transports the medicine to the patient.
☐	5	Identifies the patient. Explains the procedure.
☐	5	Assesses the patient. Puts on gloves.
☐	5	Prepares the patient for the injection (drapes, positions, allays apprehension).
☐	15	Checks label for third time.
☐	15	Selects an appropriate injection site.
☐	15	Correctly cleanses the site using a circular motion starting with the injection site and moving outward to a two-inch diameter. Allows skin to dry.

SKILLS COMPETENCY ASSESSMENT — continued

Procedure 29–5: Administering a Subcutaneous Injection

Task Performed	Possible Points	TASKS
❑	5	Removes needle guard.
❑	10	Grasps skin to form a one-inch fold.
❑	15	Inserts needle quickly at a 45-degree angle.
❑	15	Aspirates to be certain needle is not in a blood vessel.
❑	10	Slowly injects the medicine.
❑	5	Correctly removes the needle and syringe.
❑	5	Immediately disposes of needle and syringe in a sharps container.
❑	15	Covers site. Massages (unless contraindicated), as with insulin, Imferon, and heparin.
❑	5	Removes gloves and washes hands.
❑	5	Provides for patient's safety.
❑	5	Documents the procedure.
❑	5	Completed the tasks within 5 minutes.
❑	15	Results obtained were accurate.

______	Earned	ADD POINTS OF TASKS CHECKED
315	Points	TOTAL POINTS POSSIBLE
______	SCORE	DETERMINE SCORE (divide points earned by total points possible, multiply results by 100)

Actual Student Time Needed to Complete Procedure: ____________

Student's Initials: ____________ Instructor's Initials: ____________ Grade: ____________

Suggestions for Improvement: ____

Evaluator's Name (print) ____

Evaluator's Signature ____

Comments ____

DOCUMENTATION

Chart the procedure in the patient's medical record.

Date: __________

Charting: ____

____

____

____

Student's Initials: _______

SKILLS COMPETENCY ASSESSMENT

Procedure 29–6: Administering an Intramuscular Injection

Student's Name: ______________________________ Date: ____________

Objective: To correctly administer an intradermal injection.

Conditions: The student demonstrates the ability to correctly administer an intradermal injection after receiving a physician's order, using the following equipment and supplies: medication as ordered by physician, with medication card, appropriately sized needle-syringe unit, antiseptic wipe, disposable gloves, sharps container.

Time Requirements and Accuracy Standards: 5 minutes. Points assigned reflect importance of step to meeting objective: Important = (5) Essential = (10) Critical = (15). Automatic failure results if any of the **critical** tasks are omitted or performed incorrectly.

STANDARD PRECAUTIONS: 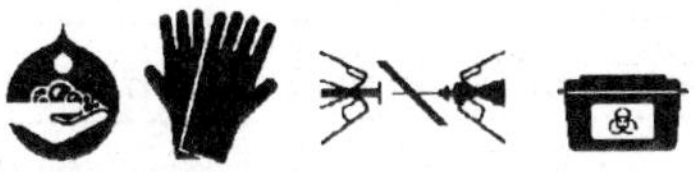

SKILLS ASSESSMENT CHECKLIST

Task Performed	Possible Points	TASKS
❑	10	Verifies the physician's order. Makes out a medicine card.
❑	15	Follows the "Six Rights."
❑	5	Performs medical asepsis hand wash. Adheres to OSHA guidelines.
❑	5	Works in a well-lighted, quiet, clean area.
❑	5	Obtains the appropriate equipment and supplies.
❑	15	Obtains the correct medication.
❑	15	Compares the medication label with the medicine card (first time). Checks expiration date.
❑	15	Calculates dosage, if necessary.
❑	15	Correctly prepares the parenteral medication.
❑	15	Compares medicine label with the medicine card (second time).
❑	15	Replaces medication on an appropriate shelf and compares medication label with medicine card (third time).
❑	5	Correctly transports the medicine to the patient.
❑	5	Identifies the patient. Explains the procedure.
❑	5	Assesses the patient. Puts on gloves.
❑	5	Prepares the patient for the injection (drapes, positions, allays apprehension).
❑	10	Selects an appropriate injection site.
❑	10	Correctly cleanses the site using a circular motion and covering a two-inch diameter. Allows the skin to dry.
❑	5	Removes needle guard.

SKILLS COMPETENCY ASSESSMENT — continued

Procedure 29–6: Administering an Intramuscular Injection

Task Performed	Possible Points	TASKS
❑	5	Stretches the skin taut, pulling it tight.
❑	10	Using a dart-like motion, inserts needle to the hub at a 90-degree angle.
❑	5	Releases the skin.
❑	15	Aspirates to check for blood.
❑	5	Injects the medicine slowly.
❑	5	Correctly removes the needle and syringe.
❑	10	Immediately disposes of needle and syringe in a sharps container.
❑	15	Covers site. Massages (unless contraindicated), as with insulin, Imferon, and heparin.
❑	5	Disposes of equipment. Removes gloves.
❑	5	Washes hands.
❑	5	Observes the patient for signs of difficulty.
❑	5	Provides for patient's safety.
❑	5	Documents the procedure.
❑	5	Completed the tasks within 5 minutes.
❑	15	Results obtained were accurate.

________	Earned	ADD POINTS OF TASKS CHECKED
290	Points	TOTAL POINTS POSSIBLE
________	SCORE	DETERMINE SCORE (divide points earned by total points possible, multiply results by 100)

Actual Student Time Needed to Complete Procedure: ____________

Student's Initials: ____________ Instructor's Initials: ____________ Grade: ____________

Suggestions for Improvement: ____

Evaluator's Name (print) ____

Evaluator's Signature____

Comments ____

DOCUMENTATION

Chart the procedure in the patient's medical record.

Date: __________

Charting: ____

____

Student's Initials: ________

SKILLS COMPETENCY ASSESSMENT

Procedure 29–7: Administering an Intradermal Injection

Student's Name: ______________________________ Date: __________

Objective: To correctly administer a intradermal injection.

Conditions: The student demonstrates the ability to correctly administer an intradermal injection after receiving a physician's order, using the following equipment and supplies: medication as ordered by physician, with medicine card, appropriately sized needle-syringe unit, antiseptic wipe, disposable gloves, sharps container.

Time Requirements and Accuracy Standards: 5 minutes. Points assigned reflect importance of step to meeting objective: Important = (5) Essential = (10) Critical = (15). Automatic failure results if any of the **critical** tasks are omitted or performed incorrectly.

STANDARD PRECAUTIONS:

SKILLS ASSESSMENT CHECKLIST

Task Performed	Possible Points	TASKS
☐	5	Verifies the physician's order. Makes out a medicine card.
☐	15	Follows the "Six Rights."
☐	5	Performs medical asepsis hand wash. Adheres to OSHA guidelines.
☐	5	Works in a well-lighted, quiet, clean area.
☐	5	Obtains the appropriate equipment and supplies.
☐	15	Obtains the correct medication.
☐	15	Compares the medication label with the medicine card (first time). Checks expiration date.
☐	15	Calculates dosage, if necessary.
☐	15	Correctly prepares the parenteral medication.
☐	15	Compares medication label with the medicine card (second time).
☐	15	Replaces medication on appropriate shelf and compares medication label with medicine card (third time).
☐	10	Correctly transports the medicine to the patient.
☐	10	Identifies the patient. Explains the procedure.
☐	5	Assesses the patient. Puts on gloves.
☐	5	Prepares the patient for the injection (drapes, positions, allays apprehension).
☐	5	Selects a site on the anterior forearm, two to three inches below the antecubital fossa.
☐	5	Correctly cleanses the site using a circular motion and covering a two-inch diameter. Allows the skin to dry.
☐	5	Removes needle guard.

SKILLS COMPETENCY ASSESSMENT —continued

Procedure 29–7: Administering an Intradermal Injection

Task Performed	Possible Points	TASKS
☐	10	Pulls the skin tissue taut.
☐	15	Carefully inserts the needle at a 10- to 15-degree angle, beveled upward about ⅛ inch. **Does not aspirate.**
☐	15	Steadily injects the medicine. Produces a wheal, or slight elevation of the skin.
☐	5	Correctly removes the needle.
☐	5	Immediately disposes of needle and syringe in a sharps container.
☐	15	Covers site. Does not massage. Disposes of equipment. Removes gloves.
☐	5	Washes hands.
☐	5	Observes the patient for signs of difficulty.
☐	5	Provides for patient's safety.
☐	5	Documents the procedure.
☐	5	Completed the tasks within 5 minutes.
☐	15	Results obtained were accurate.

_______	Earned	ADD POINTS OF TASKS CHECKED
275	Points	TOTAL POINTS POSSIBLE
_______	SCORE	DETERMINE SCORE (divide points earned by total points possible, multiply results by 100)

Actual Student Time Needed to Complete Procedure: ____________

Student's Initials: ____________ Instructor's Initials: ____________ Grade: ____________

Suggestions for Improvement: ________________________________

Evaluator's Name (print) ________________________________

Evaluator's Signature________________________________

Comments ________________________________

DOCUMENTATION

Chart the procedure in the patient's medical record.

Date: ________

Charting: ________________________________

____

____

____

Student's Initials: _______

SKILLS COMPETENCY ASSESSMENT

Procedure 29–8: Reconstituting a Powder Medication for Administration

Student's Name: ______________________________ Date: __________

Objective: To reconstitute drugs supplied in a powdered (dry) form to a liquid for injection.

Conditions: The student demonstrates the ability to reconstitute drugs supplied in a powdered (dry) form to a liquid for injection using the following equipment and supplies: medication, as ordered by the physician, and medicine card, diluent, two appropriately sized needles and syringe units, antiseptic swabs, disposable gloves, sharps container.

Time Requirements and Accuracy Standards: 5 minutes. Points assigned reflect importance of step to meeting objective: Important = (5) Essential = (10) Critical = (15). Automatic failure results if any of the **critical** tasks are omitted or performed incorrectly.

STANDARD PRECAUTIONS:

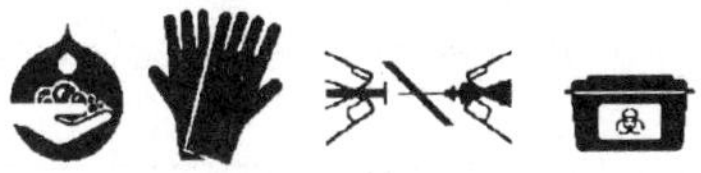

SKILLS ASSESSMENT CHECKLIST

Task Performed	Possible Points	TASKS
❑	5	Prepares the needle-syringe unit in preparation for reconstituting powder medication.
❑	10	Removes tops from diluent and powder medication containers and wipes with alcohol swabs.
❑	15	Inserts the needle of a sterile needle-syringe unit through the rubber stopper on the vial of diluent that has been cleansed with an antiseptic swab. The needle-syringe unit should have an amount of air in it equal to the amount of diluent to be withdrawn.
❑	15	Withdraws the appropriate amount of diluent to be added to the powder medication. Covers the sterile needle on the syringe containing appropriate amount of diluent.
❑	15	Adds this liquid to the powder medication that has been cleansed with an antiseptic swab.
❑	10	Removes needle and syringe from vial with powder medication and diluent and discards into sharps container.
❑	15	Rolls the vial between the palms of the hands to completely mix together the powder and diluent. Labels the multiple dose vial with the dilution or strength of the medication prepared, the date and time, and the expiration date, and initials.
❑	10	Withdraws the desired amount of medication with a second sterile needle and syringe.
❑	10	Flicks away any air bubbles that cling to side of syringe.
❑	10	Has the medicine tray with reconstituted medication ready for transport to the patient.
❑	5	Proceeds to administer an intramuscular injection to the patient (see Procedure 29–6).

SKILLS COMPETENCY ASSESSMENT — continued

Procedure 29–8: Reconstituting a Powder Medication for Administration

Task Performed	Possible Points	TASKS
❑	5	Documents the procedure.
❑	5	Completed the tasks within 5 minutes.
❑	15	Results obtained were accurate.

________	Earned	ADD POINTS OF TASKS CHECKED
145	Points	TOTAL POINTS POSSIBLE
________	SCORE	DETERMINE SCORE (divide points earned by total points possible, multiply results by 100)

Actual Student Time Needed to Complete Procedure: ____________

Student's Initials: ____________ Instructor's Initials: ____________ Grade: ____________

Suggestions for Improvement: ____

Evaluator's Name (print) ____

Evaluator's Signature ____

Comments ____

DOCUMENTATION

Record information included on the multiple dose vial of prepared reconstituted medication.

Date:____________

Label: ____

Document the intramuscular injection in the patient's medical record.

Date:____________

Charting: ____

____

____

Student's Initials: _______

SKILLS COMPETENCY ASSESSMENT

Procedure 29–9: "Z"-Track Intramuscular Injection Technique

Student's Name: ______________________________ Date: ____________

Objective: To correctly administer a "Z"-track intramuscular injection.

Conditions: The student demonstrates the ability to correctly administer a "Z"-track intramuscular injection after receiving a physician's order, using the following equipment and supplies: medication ordered by physician and medication card, appropriately sized needle-syringe unit, antiseptic wipe, disposable gloves, sharps container.

Time Requirements and Accuracy Standards: 5 minutes. Points assigned reflect importance of step to meeting objective: Important = (5) Essential = (10) Critical = (15). Automatic failure results if any of the **critical** tasks are omitted or performed incorrectly.

STANDARD PRECAUTIONS:

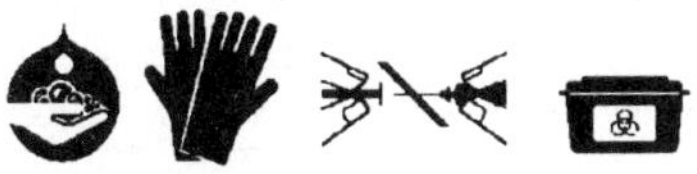

SKILLS ASSESSMENT CHECKLIST

Task Performed	Possible Points	TASKS
☐	10	Verifies the physician's order. Makes out a medicine card.
☐	15	Follows the "Six Rights."
☐	5	Performs medical asepsis hand wash. Adheres to OSHA guidelines.
☐	5	Works in a well-lighted, quiet, clean area.
☐	5	Obtains the appropriate equipment and supplies.
☐	15	Obtains the correct medication.
☐	10	Compares the medication label with the medicine card (first time).
☐	10	Checks expiration date.
☐	5	Calculates dosage, if necessary.
☐	15	Correctly prepares the parenteral medication.
☐	10	Compares medicine label with the medicine card (second time).
☐	10	Replaces medication on shelf and compares medication label with medicine card (third time).
☐	5	Correctly transports the medicine to the patient.
☐	5	Identifies the patient. Explains the procedure.
☐	5	Assesses the patient. Puts on gloves.
☐	5	Prepares the patient for the injection (drapes, positions, allays apprehension).
☐	10	Selects an appropriate injection site.
☐	10	Correctly cleanses the site using a circular motion and covering a two-inch diameter. Allows the skin to dry.
☐	5	Removes needle guard.

SKILLS COMPETENCY ASSESSMENT — continued

Procedure 29–9: "Z"-Track Intramuscular Injection Technique

Task Performed	Possible Points	TASKS
❑	10	Pulls the skin laterally 1½ inches away from the injection site.
❑	15	Inserts needle quickly, using a dartlike motion at a 90° angle. Maintains "Z" position.
❑	15	Aspirates to check for blood.
❑	10	Slowly injects medication.
❑	10	Waits ten seconds before removing needle to allow medication to begin to be absorbed.
❑	10	Removes needle and syringe at same angle of insertion.
❑	15	Releases traction of the "Z" position to seal off the needle track. Prevents medication from reaching the subcutaneous tissues and the surface of the skin.
❑	15	Immediately disposes of needle-syringe unit in a sharps container.
❑	5	Covers site. Does not massage. Removes gloves. Washes hands.
❑	5	Observes patient for signs of difficulty.
❑	5	Provides for the patient's safety.
❑	5	Documents the procedure.
❑	5	Completed the tasks within 5 minutes.
❑	15	Results obtained were accurate.

_______	Earned	ADD POINTS OF TASKS CHECKED
300	Points	TOTAL POINTS POSSIBLE
_______	SCORE	DETERMINE SCORE (divide points earned by total points possible, multiply results by 100)

Actual Student Time Needed to Complete Procedure: ____________

Student's Initials: ____________ Instructor's Initials: ____________ Grade: ____________

Suggestions for Improvement: ____

Evaluator's Name (print) ____

Evaluator's Signature ____

Comments ____

DOCUMENTATION

Chart the procedure in the patient's medical record.

Date: __________

Charting: ____

____

Student's Initials: _______

EVALUATION OF CHAPTER KNOWLEDGE

How has your instructor evaluated the knowledge you have achieved?

Knowledge	Instructor Evaluation *Good*	*Average*	*Poor*
Discusses legal and ethical implications of medication administration	_____	_____	_____
Describes medication order	_____	_____	_____
Describes the parts of a prescription	_____	_____	_____
Defines drug dosage	_____	_____	_____
States information contained on a medication label and can discuss the significance of the information	_____	_____	_____
Understands ratios and proportions	_____	_____	_____
Able to use metric, household, and apothecaries' systems of measurement and convert between metric and apothecary systems	_____	_____	_____
Understand units of medication dosage	_____	_____	_____
Correctly calculates adult and child dosages	_____	_____	_____
Lists guidelines to follow when preparing and administering medications	_____	_____	_____
Describes safe disposal of syringes, needles, and biohazardous materials	_____	_____	_____
Describes site selection for administration of injections	_____	_____	_____
Understands allergenic extracts	_____	_____	_____
Describes inhalation medication and its administration	_____	_____	_____
Exhibits therapeutic communication skills in administering medications to patients and attends to patients' emotional needs	_____	_____	_____
Documents accurately	_____	_____	_____
Complies with governmental regulations in the administration and disposal of controlled substances	_____	_____	_____
Possesses the ability to competently prepare and administer oral and parenteral medications as directed by a physician	_____	_____	_____

Student's Initials: ______ Instructor's Initials: ______

Grade: _______

CHAPTER 30

Medical Specialty Examinations and Procedures

PERFORMANCE OBJECTIVES

Patients with complaints specific to a particular body system or body part need specialized care. Medical assistants assist the physician with many clinical procedures that are an integral component of specialty examinations. Medical assistants who are employed in a specialist's office or a setting that treats a variety of patient problems will need additional skills and ongoing training to stay proficient in the most current, technologies and treatments used to provide quality care to patients. Medical assisting students should use this workbook chapter to become familiar with specialty and body system examinations and with the appropriate clinical procedures in pediatrics; the female reproductive system; the male reproductive system; urology; endoscopy; sensory; the respiratory system; the musculoskeletal, neurological, and circulatory systems; blood and lymph; and the integumentary system.

EXERCISES AND ACTIVITIES

Vocabulary Builder

Find the key vocabulary terms in the word search puzzle.

Akinesia
Alimentary canal
Alveoli
Aphasia
Appendicular skeleton
Aseptic
Auricle
Axial skeleton
Biopsy
Bronchi
Carbuncle
Choroid layer
Closed Fracture
Comedone
Demyelination
Dislocation
Equilibrium
Erythema
External respiration
Furuncle
Gait
Hydronephrosis
Ingestion
Internal respiration
Lesion
Malabsorption
Nebulizer
Obturator
Occluder
Ophthalmoscope
Optic nerve
Ossicle
Otoscope
Oval window
Peripheral nerve
Polycystic
Spirometry
Stratum corneum
Vesicle

N Q R I U P G U P I F P B I Y W Q W N N E B O V S E G B D I M C D C Z G S Q
R J N X E K B A O C V P I Y T X I H O N B R O J N E O G I K L I H I W A T C
F E O Z G I Q Y L O Q G M J P Z Y I Q G Q I T B Y G H W M O S F A T Y I R P
E E D P P M S O Y M P J W X U D S L S M X B J U T J J G V L P P V P X T A O
V L S U O Q W L C T V H R W R E V F K O A T P S V U H H O K U S F E D Y T E
M C C W L A D S Y W T J T O L J D A E L U K X A W O R C B F L X Y S I L U L
F I P N S C W J S J H H N H E V R E N C I T P O X I A A X L H F W A O B M B
K R V N U Q C K T V G E O U A E T W R I V C Q I E T T V T I Q F Z F G C C V
I U T Y Q B N O I S P Z A T C L N T B V O J W D I E A F P O P F G R H L O S
E A L Y Q F R S C H L F O R M X M R K R T C U O O N O X H Z R F N O O E R F
A L I M E N T A R Y C A N A L V D O R I Q S N S J V C R J P M Y R S P X N R
M D B D C D B O C V F N O T E L E K S R A L U C I D N E P P A O E V D T E H
U B U T H R S X R E J S N O U S O Z X C Y F V D P E J W M S I D D S P E U Q
B Z K R O I V E P P J O J U I B S D M R O F Z F C L A Y G D F T B L W R M Y
Y T C N S C Z O U B T C S B H W S M E J W P R M I B U L L R Z H U C M N S N
Y N C U J I C R X E I N Y V G V I P U Q U J E F M G I A A V C O C T F A W O
K H I O L S Z Z L A B I K N O M C G I T U G N H Q C Y C I F U R U N C L E I
I L P U O N X E B Y Z W Z K Q F L Y J R H I J T S E T V E X U E Y U V R F T
E W B T I E K S Z J S I S R C Y E V B R O K L E R U F I F Y U X S L M E W P
C E O N P S C J T S M C Z D O K Z W N D J M O I R H R U P X P Q W Y D S U R
N R B K L G F G K V D Q Y D M U N Z M O W T E E B G M V V Q E Z J T C P V O
V Q M A H C E V R E N L A R E H P I R E P G F T D R H K Q R Z U O C S I Y S
N O I T S E G N I P I Y M V D O K Q O N V V V D R J I X K Z O L N B J R Q B
I X Y F F S E V D L S R G T O R A H P J R T O J Q Y I U R B S Q M I B A M A
A H L L I T P T C B Y K G H N B B J V X E L C I S E V U M N Y H A K D T T L
E R Y T H E M A X F Y T A Z E W H A I S E N I K A D X Y A P H A S I A I S A
O V A L W I N D O W D E M Y E L I N A T I O N Z J B I Z Q L M B Y Y F O O M
I N T E R N A L R E S P I R A T I O N G M T M Y I L O E V L A C F B T N K I

Learning Review/Case Study

Mary O'Keefe has called for an emergency appointment for her 3-year-old son Chris for an examination with Dr. King because he awakened during the night with a high fever and severe pain in his right ear, which is draining.

1. Ellen Armstrong, CMA, must prepare the examination room for the patient. Based on Chris's symptoms, what equipment will Ellen want to assemble for Dr. King's physical examination of Chris? List the equipment in the order it will most likely be used in the examination.

____

____

____

____

2. When Mary O'Keefe arrives with her son, Ellen takes them to examination room #2 and prepares the patient for Dr. King's physical examination. Ellen tells Mary that Dr. King will be examining Chris's ear and may want to take some laboratory tests. Ellen takes and records the child's vital signs:

   T 102.1°F; P 115 (AP) bounding, sinus arrhythmia; R 28 rhonci; 76/42/0, rt. arm, sitting.

   A. Explain the meaning and significance of each vital sign measurement, including the method and equipment used.

Temperature: ____________________

Pulse: ____________________

Respiration: ____________________

Blood Pressure: ____________________

B. Chris is fussy and disagreeable, but not uncooperative, while Ellen takes his vital signs. What can a medical assistant do to facilitate the measurement of a fussy child's vital signs?

____

____

3. Ellen assists Dr. King with her physical examination of the patient. After assessing the vital sign measurements taken by the medical assistant, Dr. King examines Chris's ear and lungs. A swab of fluid discharge is taken from the patient's ear. What is the role of the medical assistant during the physician's examination of this patient?

____

____

____

____

4. Dr. King makes a clinical diagnosis of otitis media for this patient and orders laboratory testing to be performed on the patient's specimen.

A. What criteria are necessary for a physician to make a clinical diagnosis?

____

B. What is otitis media? Why are children more likely at risk for this condition? How is otitis media commonly treated? What patient education can the health care team offer? *Consult a medical reference or encyclopedia for help in answering this question.*

____

____

SUPPLEMENTARY RESOURCES

Study Guide Disk: Additional practice exercises for this chapter are available on the study guide disk found in the back of the textbook.

Medical Assisting Videos: Appropriate content is available on Delmar's Medical Assisting Videos, 2nd ed., for the following topics:

Tape 6: Take Vital Signs
Take and Record Rectal Temperature
Take and Record a Brachial Pulse (infant)
Use a Stethoscope to Take an Apical Pulse (infant)

Tape 7: Take and Record Blood Pressure
- Weigh and Measure an Infant
- Growth Chart As a Screening Procedure
- Vision Screen
- Using an Audiometer to Perform a Hearing Screen

Tape 8: Take an In-Depth Patient History
- Clean Examination Table and Countertops
- Assist Physician With Examination and Treatments
- Position and Drape the Patient
- Role of the Medical Assistant During the Examination
- Introduction to Health Promotion, Disease Prevention, and Self-Responsibility
- Testicular Self-Examination
- Breast Self-Examination

Tape 11: Prepare and Administer Medication As Directed By Physician
- Administer Eye Medications
- Administer Ear Medications
- Administer Sub-Lingual Medications
- Administer Rectal Suppositories
- Topical Applications
- Transdermal Patch Applications

SKILLS COMPETENCY ASSESSMENT

Procedure 30–1: Measuring the Infant: Weight, Height, Head, and Chest Circumference

Student's Name: ______________________________ Date: ____________

Objective: To obtain an accurate measurement of an infant's weight, height, head, and chest circumference.

Conditions: The student demonstrates the ability to obtain an accurate measurement of an infant's weight, height, head, and chest circumference for medical records and screen for growth abnormalities using the following equipment and supplies: infant scale, paper protector, flexible measuring tape, growth chart, patient's chart, pen, ruler, biohazard waste container.

Time Requirements and Accuracy Standards: 10 minutes for each measurement. Points assigned reflect importance of step to meeting objective: Important = (5) Essential = (10) Critical = (15). Automatic failure results if any of the **critical** tasks are omitted or performed incorrectly.

STANDARD PRECAUTIONS:

SKILLS ASSESSMENT CHECKLIST

Task Performed	Possible Points	TASKS
Measuring Infant's Weight		
☐	5	Washes hands. Explains procedure to parent(s).
☐	5	Undresses infant (including the diaper). Discards soiled diaper in biohazard waste container.
☐	10	Places all weights to left of scale to check balance.
☐	5	Places a clean utility towel on scale, checks balance scale for accuracy, being sure to compensate for the weight of the towel.
☐	5	*Rationale:* The paper helps protect against transmission of microorganisms and provides warmth for the infant, as the scale will be cool.
☐	10	Gently places infant on his or her back on the scale. Places own hand slightly above the infant's body to ensure safety.
☐	5	*Rationale:* Safeguards infant from falling.
☐	15	Places the bottom weight to its highest measurement that will not cause the balance to drop to the bottom edge.
☐	15	Slowly moves upper weight until the balance bar rests in the center of the indicator. A balanced scale will provide an accurate weight. Reads the infant's weight while he or she is lying still.
☐	15	Returns both weights to their resting position to the extreme left.
☐	10	Gently removes infant and applies fresh diaper. (Parent can help with diapering and holding infant.)
☐	5	Discards used protective paper towel per OSHA guidelines.
☐	5	Sanitizes scale.
☐	5	Washes hands.
☐	10	Documents results according to office policy (pounds and ounces or kilograms) on growth chart, patient's chart, and parent's booklet, if available. Connects dot from previous examination with a ruler to complete graph.

Task Performed	Possible Points	TASKS
❑	5	Completed the tasks within 10 minutes.
❑	15	Results obtained were accurate.

________		Earned	ADD POINTS OF TASKS CHECKED
	145	Points	TOTAL POINTS POSSIBLE
________		SCORE	DETERMINE SCORE (divide points earned by total points possible, multiply results by 100)

Measuring Infant's Length/Height

❑	5	Washes hands. Explains procedure to parent(s).
❑	5	Removes infant's shoes.
❑	15	Gently places infant on his or her back on the examination table. If the pediatric table has a headboard, asks parent to hold infant's head against (end) headboard of table at zero mark of ruler while medical assistant places infant's heels against footboard. Gently straightens infant's back and legs to line up along ruler. Uses right hand as a guide, if there is no footboard (to place infant's feet against). If necessary, gently places left hand over the infant's legs at the knees to secure the him or her in place and straightens legs so the recumbent length can be read from the head to the heel.
❑	5	*Rationale:* Sometimes it is difficult to straighten the infant's legs.
❑	15	Reads length in inches or centimeters from measuring device.
❑	5	Washes hands.
❑	10	Documents measurement on growth chart, patient's chart, and parent's booklet if available. Connects dot from previous examination with a ruler to complete graph.
❑	5	Completed the tasks within 10 minutes.
❑	15	Results obtained were accurate.

________		Earned	ADD POINTS OF TASKS CHECKED
	80	Points	TOTAL POINTS POSSIBLE
________		SCORE	DETERMINE SCORE (divide points earned by total points possible, multiply results by 100)

Measuring Infant's/Child's Head Circumference

❑	5	Washes hands and explains procedure to parent(s).
❑	5	Talks to infant to gain cooperation. Infant may be held by parent or may lie on examination table for procedure. Older children of two or three years may stand or sit if they will remain still.
❑	15	Places the measuring tape snugly around the head from the occipital protuberance to the supra-orbital prominence.
❑	15	Reads the measurement in either inches (to nearest $\frac{1}{2}$ inch) or centimeters (to nearest 0.01 cm).
❑	5	Washes hands.
❑	10	Documents results according to office policy on growth chart, patient's chart, and parent's booklet if available. Connects dot from previous examination with a ruler to complete graph.
❑	5	Completed the tasks within 10 minutes.
❑	15	Results obtained were accurate.

________		Earned	ADD POINTS OF TASKS CHECKED
	75	Points	TOTAL POINTS POSSIBLE
________		SCORE	DETERMINE SCORE (divide points earned by total points possible, multiply results by 100)

SKILLS COMPETENCY ASSESSMENT — continued

Procedure 30–1: Measuring the Infant: Weight, Height, Head, and Chest Circumference

Task Performed	Possible Points	TASKS
Measure Infant's Chest Circumference		
☐	5	Washes hands and explains procedure to parent(s).
☐	15	Uses one thumb to hold tape measure with zero mark against the infant's chest at the midsternal area. With the other hand, brings the tape around/under the back to meet the zero mark of the tape in front. Takes the measurement of the chest just above the nipples with the tape fitting around the infant's chest under the axillary region. Asks the parent or another medical assistant for assistance in holding the infant still, if necessary. Takes the measurement when the child is breathing normally and during the resting phase between respirations.
☐	15	Reads measurement to the nearest 0.01 cm or 1/16 inch.
☐	5	Washes hands.
☐	5	Documents results in patient's chart.
☐	5	Completed the tasks within 10 minutes.
☐	15	Results obtained were accurate.

_______	Earned	ADD POINTS OF TASKS CHECKED
65	Points	TOTAL POINTS POSSIBLE
_______	SCORE	DETERMINE SCORE (divide points earned by total points possible, multiply results by 100)

Actual Student Time Needed to Complete Procedure: ____________

Student's Initials: ____________ Instructor's Initials: ____________ Grade: ____________

Suggestions for Improvement: ____

Evaluator's Name (print) ____

Evaluator's Signature ____

Comments ____

DOCUMENTATION

Record the height, weight, head and chest circumference measurements in the patient's medical record.

Date: __________

Charting: ____

____

____

____

____

Student's Initials: _______

SKILLS COMPETENCY ASSESSMENT

Procedure 30–2: Taking an Infant's Rectal Temperature with a Mercury or Digital Thermometer

Student's Name: ______________________________ Date: ____________

Objective: To obtain a rectal temperature using a mercury or digital thermometer.

Conditions: The student demonstrates the ability to obtain a rectal temperature using the following equipment and supplies: mercury rectal thermometer (red tip) and sheath or digital thermometer (red probe) and probe cover, lubricating jelly, 4 × 4 gauze sponges, gloves, biohazard waste container.

Time Requirements and Accuracy Standards: 10 minutes. Points assigned reflect importance of step to meeting objective: Important = (5) Essential = (10) Critical = (15). Automatic failure results if any of the **critical** tasks are omitted or performed incorrectly.

STANDARD PRECAUTIONS:

SKILLS ASSESSMENT CHECKLIST

Task Performed	Possible Points	TASKS
		Using Mercury Thermometer
☐	5	Washes hands. Assembles equipment.
☐	5	Identifies patient. Explains procedure to parent(s) to gain assistance and cooperation.
☐	5	Removes infant's diaper and discards in biohazard waste container.
☐	10	Positions infant in a prone position having parent or another medical assistant safeguard infant.
☐	10	Places sheath on thermometer.
☐	5	*Rationale:* Sheath prevents microorganism cross-contamination.
☐	10	Places lubricant on a 4 × 4 gauze sponge and places tip of thermometer in lubricant.
☐	5	*Rationale:* Facilitates insertion of thermometer.
☐	5	Applies gloves.
☐	15	Spreads infant's buttocks, inserts thermometer gently into the rectum past the sphincter; for an infant, this is ½ inch.
☐	15	Holds buttocks together while holding the thermometer. If necessary, restrains infant movement by placing own arm across the infant's back. Parent can immobilize infant's legs.
☐	5	*Rationale:* Ensures infant's safety and comfort.
☐	15	Holds in place for five minutes. Does not let go of the thermometer.

SKILLS COMPETENCY ASSESSMENT — continued

Procedure 30–2: Taking an Infant's Rectal Temperature with a Mercury or Digital Thermometer

Task Performed	Possible Points	TASKS
❑	5	*Rationale:* Movement by infant can cause thermometer to move and can injure infant.
❑	5	Removes thermometer from rectum. Has parent attend to infant.
❑	5	Removes sheath and places in biohazard container.
❑	5	Reads thermometer.
❑	5	Washes, rinses, and dries thermometer. Places on clean paper towels.
❑	5	Removes gloves, discards in biohazard waste container. Washes hands.
❑	15	Places thermometer in a disinfectant solution for rectal thermometers.
❑	5	Assists parent in dressing infant if necessary.
❑	15	Records on the patient chart appropriately as a rectal temperature.
❑	5	Completed the tasks within 10 minutes.
❑	15	Results obtained were accurate.

______	Earned	ADD POINTS OF TASKS CHECKED
195	Points	TOTAL POINTS POSSIBLE
______	SCORE	DETERMINE SCORE (divide points earned by total points possible, multiply results by 100)

Using Digital Thermometer

Task Performed	Possible Points	TASKS
❑	5	Washes hands. Assembles equipment.
❑	5	Identifies patient. Explains procedure to parent(s) to gain assistance and cooperation.
❑	5	Removes infant's diaper and discards in biohazard waste container.
❑	10	Positions infant in a prone position having parent or another medical assistant safeguard infant.
❑	10	Places sheath on thermometer.
❑	5	*Rationale:* Sheath prevents microorganism cross-contamination.
❑	10	Places lubricant on a 4 × 4 gauze sponge and places tip of thermometer in lubricant.
❑	5	*Rationale:* Facilitates insertion of thermometer.
❑	5	Applies gloves.
❑	15	Spreads infant's buttocks, inserts thermometer gently into the rectum past the sphincter; for an infant, this is ½ inch.

Task Performed	Possible Points	TASKS
❑	15	Holds buttocks together while holding the thermometer. If necessary, restrains infant movement by placing own arm across the infant's back. Parent can immobilize infant's legs.
❑	5	*Rationale:* Ensures infant's safety and comfort.
❑	5	Holds digital thermometer in place until the beep is heard.
❑	5	Reads results on digital display window.
❑	5	Removes thermometer from rectum.
❑	5	Discards probe cover into biohazard waste container by pressing the eject button on probe end.
❑	5	Replaces thermometer on holder base.
❑	5	Removes gloves, discards in biohazard waste container, and washes hands.
❑	5	Assists patient in dressing and positions as necessary.
❑	15	Records on the patient chart appropriately as a rectal temperature.
❑	5	Washes hands.
❑	5	Completed the tasks within 10 minutes.
❑	15	Results obtained were accurate.

______	Earned	ADD POINTS OF TASKS CHECKED
175	Points	TOTAL POINTS POSSIBLE
______	SCORE	DETERMINE SCORE (divide points earned by total points possible, multiply results by 100)

Actual Student Time Needed to Complete Procedure: ____________

Student's Initials: ____________ Instructor's Initials: ____________ Grade: ____________

Suggestions for Improvement: ____

Evaluator's Name (print) ____

Evaluator's Signature ____

Comments ____

DOCUMENTATION

Record the rectal temperature in the patient's medical record.

Date: __________

Charting: ____

____

____

Student's Initials: ________

SKILLS COMPETENCY ASSESSMENT

Procedure 30–3: Taking an Apical Pulse on an Infant

Student's Name: ______________________________ Date: __________

Objective: To obtain an apical pulse rate.

Conditions: The student demonstrates the ability to obtain an apical pulse rate using the following equipment and supplies: stethoscope, watch with second hand, alcohol wipes.

Time Requirements and Accuracy Standards: 2 minutes. Points assigned reflect importance of step to meeting objective: Important = (5) Essential = (10) Critical = (15). Automatic failure results if any of the **critical** tasks are omitted or performed incorrectly.

STANDARD PRECAUTIONS:

SKILLS ASSESSMENT CHECKLIST

Task Performed	Possible Points	TASKS
❑	5	Washes hands. Assembles equipment.
❑	5	Identifies patient. Explains procedure to parent.
❑	5	Assists in disrobing infant, if necessary.
❑	10	Provides a drape for infant's warmth, if necessary.
❑	5	Positions the infant in a supine position or seated in the parent's lap.
❑	5	*Rationale:* Understands the supine position may offer easier access to apex of heart if the child is calm.
❑	15	Locates the fifth intercostal space, midclavicular line, left of sternum.
❑	10	Places warmed stethoscope on the site and listens for the lub-dup sound of the heart.
❑	15	Counts the pulse for one minute; each lub-dup equals one heartbeat or pulse.
❑	5	Washes hands.
❑	5	Records the pulse in the infant's chart with the designation of (AP) to denote method of obtaining the pulse.
❑	10	Notes any arrhythmias.
❑	5	Assists patient, and parents, as needed.
❑	5	Cleans earpieces and diaphragm of stethoscope with alcohol wipes.
❑	5	*Rationale:* Prevents cross-contamination of microbes between patients.

Task Performed	Possible Points	TASKS
☐	5	Washes hands again.
☐	5	Completed the tasks within 2 minutes.
☐	15	Results obtained were accurate.

________	Earned	ADD POINTS OF TASKS CHECKED
135	Points	TOTAL POINTS POSSIBLE
________	SCORE	DETERMINE SCORE (divide points earned by total points possible, multiply results by 100)

Actual Student Time Needed to Complete Procedure: ____________

Student's Initials: ____________ Instructor's Initials: ____________ Grade: ____________

Suggestions for Improvement: ____

Evaluator's Name (print) ____

Evaluator's Signature ____

Comments ____

DOCUMENTATION

Record the apical pulse in the patient's medical record. This patient also has a rectal temperature of 37.5°C.

Date: __________

Charting: ____

____

____

____

____

____

Student's Initials: _______

SKILLS COMPETENCY ASSESSMENT

Procedure 30–4: Measuring Infant's Respiration Rate

Student's Name: ______________________________ Date: __________

Objective: To measure the infant's respiration rate.

Conditions: The student demonstrates the ability to measure the infant's respiratory rate using the following equipment and supplies: watch with second hand. The most accurate respiration rate is taken immediately before or after the pulse rate.

Time Requirements and Accuracy Standards: 2 minutes. Points assigned reflect importance of step to meeting objective: Important = (5) Essential = (10) Critical = (15). Automatic failure results if any of the **critical** tasks are omitted or performed incorrectly.

STANDARD PRECAUTIONS:

SKILLS ASSESSMENT CHECKLIST

Task Performed	Possible Points	TASKS
❑	5	Washes hands. Identifies the patient.
❑	5	Positions infant in a supine position.
❑	15	Places own hand on the infant's chest to feel the rise and fall of the chest wall for one minute.
❑	15	Notes depth, rhythm, and breath sounds while counting.
❑	5	Washes hands.
❑	10	Records respiration rate in patient chart, noting any irregularities and sounds.
❑	5	Completed the tasks within 2 minutes.
❑	15	Results obtained were accurate.

________	Earned	ADD POINTS OF TASKS CHECKED
75	Points	TOTAL POINTS POSSIBLE
________	SCORE	DETERMINE SCORE (divide points earned by total points possible, multiply results by 100)

Actual Student Time Needed to Complete Procedure: ____________

Student's Initials: ____________ Instructor's Initials: ____________ Grade: ____________

Suggestions for Improvement: ____

Evaluator's Name (print) ____

Evaluator's Signature ____

Comments ____

DOCUMENTATION

Record the respiration rate in the patient's medical record. This patient has a rectal temperature of 99°F and an apical pulse of 114 beats per minute with no arrhythmias.

Date: __________

Charting: ____

____

____

Student's Initials: ________

SKILLS COMPETENCY ASSESSMENT

Procedure 30–5: Obtaining a Urine Specimen From an Infant or a Young Child

Student's Name: ______________________________ Date: ____________

Objective: To obtain a specimen of urine from an infant or a young child.

Conditions: The student demonstrates the ability to obtain a specimen of urine from an infant or a young child by using the following equipment and supplies: urine collection bag, laboratory request form, gloves, washcloth, soap, water, towel, biohazard waste container.

Time Requirements and Accuracy Standards: 10 minutes. Points assigned reflect importance of step to meeting objective: Important = (5) Essential = (10) Critical = (15). Automatic failure results if any of the **critical** tasks are omitted or performed incorrectly.

STANDARD PRECAUTIONS:

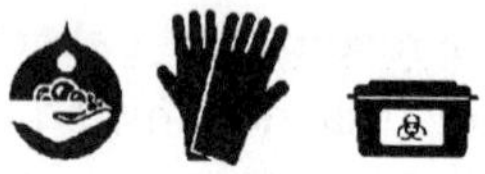

SKILLS ASSESSMENT CHECKLIST

Task Performed	Possible Points	TASKS
☐	5	Washes and gloves hands following standard precautions. Assembles equipment.
☐	5	Identifies patient and explains procedure to parent(s).
☐	5	Instructs parent to remove diaper.
☐	10	Washes and dries perineal area.
☐	5	*Rationale:* Understands that cleaning the area reduces the microorganism level and provides a better-quality urine specimen.
☐	15	Applies collection bag, secures with adhesive tabs. • Females: spreads perineum, places bag over labia • Males: places bag over penis and scrotum
☐	5	Replaces diaper carefully.
☐	5	Frequently checks bag for urine.
☐	5	Removes bag carefully after specimen has been collected.
☐	15	Prepares specimen as required. Sends to laboratory in a specimen container with a requisition or processes the specimen in the POL.
☐	5	Removes gloves and discards in biohazard waste container. Washes hands.
☐	5	Records collection in patient's chart.

Task Performed	Possible Points	TASKS
❑	5	Completed the tasks within 10 minutes.
❑	15	Results obtained were accurate.

_______	Earned	ADD POINTS OF TASKS CHECKED
105	Points	TOTAL POINTS POSSIBLE
_______	SCORE	DETERMINE SCORE (divide points earned by total points possible, multiply results by 100)

Actual Student Time Needed to Complete Procedure: __________

Student's Initials: __________ Instructor's Initials: __________ Grade: __________

Suggestions for Improvement: ______________________________

Evaluator's Name (print) ______________________________

Evaluator's Signature ______________________________

Comments ______________________________

DOCUMENTATION

Record the urine collection in the patient's medical record.

Date: ____________________

Charting: ______________________________

____

____

Student's Initials: ______________

SKILLS COMPETENCY ASSESSMENT

Procedure 30–6: Instructing Patient in Breast Self-Examination

Student's Name: ______________________________ Date: ____________

Objective: To properly instruct a woman in the procedure for performing a breast self-examination.

Conditions: The student demonstrates the ability to properly instruct a woman in the procedure for performing a breast self-examination using the following equipment and supplies: breast model, breast self-exam pamphlets.

Time Requirements and Accuracy Standards: 5 minutes. Points assigned reflect importance of step to meeting objective: Important = (5) Essential = (10) Critical = (15). Automatic failure results if any of the **critical** tasks are omitted or performed incorrectly.

SKILLS ASSESSMENT CHECKLIST

Task Performed	Possible Points	TASKS
		Medical assistant instructs the patient in the following steps involved in breast self-examination while in a warm bath or shower
❑	5	Examine breasts in a warm bath or shower.
❑	5	*Rationale:* Warm water softens skin and hands glide easily.
❑	10	Using the flat pads of the three middle fingers and moving in a circular motion, use the right hand to examine the left breast and the left hand to examine the right breast. Begin at the top outside edge using a circular, clockwise motion, examining every part of each breast, ending at the nipple.
❑	15	Check for lumps, thickening, and anything that is different from previous exams.
		Medical assistant instructs the patient in the following steps involved in breast self-examination in front of a mirror
❑	5	Inspect the breasts with arms at sides.
❑	5	Raise arms high overhead.
❑	5	Look for any change in contour of each breast.
❑	15	Observe for swelling, hard lump(s), dimpling of skin (orange skin), or changes in nipple (retracting, swelling, or discharge).
❑	5	Rest both hands on hips and press down while flexing chest muscles.
		Medical assistant instructs the patient in the following steps involved in breast self-examination while lying down
❑	5	Place a pillow or towel under right shoulder with the right hand behind the head to examine the right breast.

Task Performed	Possible Points	TASKS
❑	15	With left hand and fingers flat, press gently in small circular motions, starting at the top of the breast and moving toward the nipple. Examine every part of the right breast tissue.
❑	5	Repeat the procedure on the left breast, using a pillow or towel under the left shoulder and examine using the right hand.
❑	5	Squeeze the nipple of each breast gently between thumb and index finger.
❑	10	Report any abnormalities to the physician.
❑	15	Medical assistant answers any questions the patient has about breast self-examination during instructions. Any questions the medical assistant cannot answer are referred to the physician.
❑	5	Medical assistant checks that patient has received a breast self-examination pamphlet.
❑	5	Completed the tasks within 5 minutes.
❑	15	Results obtained were accurate.

______	Earned	ADD POINTS OF TASKS CHECKED
150	Points	TOTAL POINTS POSSIBLE
______	SCORE	DETERMINE SCORE (divide points earned by total points possible, multiply results by 100)

Actual Student Time Needed to Complete Procedure: ____________

Student's Initials: ____________ Instructor's Initials: ____________ Grade: ____________

Suggestions for Improvement: ____________________________________

Evaluator's Name (print) ____________________________________

Evaluator's Signature ____________________________________

Comments ____________________________________

DOCUMENTATION

Chart the procedure in the patient's medical record.

Date: ____________________

Charting: ____________________________________

____

____

Student's Initials: ____________

SKILLS COMPETENCY ASSESSMENT

Procedure 30–7: Assisting with Gynecologic or Pelvic Examination and a Papanicolaou (Pap) Test

Student's Name: ______________________________ Date: __________

Objective: To assist the physician in collecting cervical cells for laboratory analysis for early detection of malignant cells of the cervix, assess the health of the reproductive organs, and to detect diseases leading to early diagnosis and treatment.

Conditions: The student demonstrates the ability to assist the physician in collecting cervical cells for laboratory analysis using the following equipment and supplies: two pairs of nonsterile gloves, two to three frosted end glass slides, vaginal speculum (plastic or metal), basin of warm water, long cotton-tipped applicator or cytology brush, cervical scrapers, fixative, light source, drape sheet, marking pencil, lubricant, slide holder, lab requisition, urine specimen container, tissues, biohazard waste container.

Time Requirements and Accuracy Standards: 10 minutes. Points assigned reflect importance of step to meeting objective: Important = (5) Essential = (10) Critical = (15). Automatic failure results if any of the **critical** tasks are omitted or performed incorrectly.

STANDARD PRECAUTIONS:

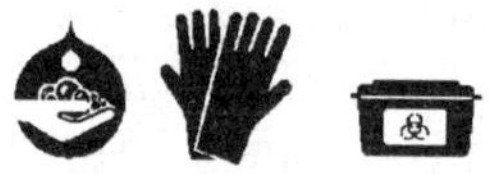

SKILLS ASSESSMENT CHECKLIST

Task Performed	Possible Points	TASKS
☐	5	Washes hands and assembles necessary supplies near patient.
☐	10	Requests that patient empty her bladder. (Instructs patient to save urine specimen and provide specimen container if ordered by physician.)
☐	5	*Rationale:* Understands that an empty bladder facilitates examination of the uterus and provides a specimen for urinalysis.
☐	5	Provides patient with gown and requests her to completely undress.
☐	5	Explains procedure to patient.
☐	15	Instructs patient to sit at end of table when ready. Drapes patient for privacy. Correctly labels the frosted end of the slide with a marking pencil to include patient's name and cite of specimen collection.
☐	5	Encourages patient to breathe slowly and deeply through the mouth during exam.
☐	5	*Rationale:* Understands that slow, deep breathing allows for relaxation of the pelvic muscles and for easier insertion of vaginal speculum.
☐	5	Warms stainless steel vaginal speculum with warm water or places on a heating pad. Does not lubricate speculum.

Task Performed	Possible Points	TASKS
❑	5	*Rationale:* Understands that lubricant would obscure exfoliated cervical cells when Pap test is performed.
❑	5	Hands speculum and spatula or cytology brush to physician.
❑	5	Applies gloves.
❑	10	Holds slides for physician to apply smear of exfoliated cells, one for vaginal (v), one for cervical (c), and one for endocervical (e), in that order.
❑	10	Sprays fixative over each slide within ten seconds at a distance of about six inches. Allows to dry for at least ten minutes.
❑	5	*Rationale:* Fixing slides preserves cell appearance and avoids contamination of cells. Understands that slides must be fixed before they dry to maintain cell appearance and that getting too close with the spray may destroy or damage cells.
❑	10	Places lubricant on physician's gloved fingers without touching gloves, for bimanual and rectal exams. The physician will insert the index and middle fingers into the vagina. The other hand is placed on the lower abdomen. The size, shape, and position of the uterus and ovaries are palpated.
❑	5	The physician will insert one gloved finger into the rectum to check the tone of the rectal and pelvic muscles. Hemorrhoids, rectal fissures, or other lesions may be palpated.
❑	5	Assists patient to wipe genitalia and rectum.
❑	15	Helps patient to a seated position, allowing her to rest awhile. Checks her pulse and skin color.
❑	5	*Rationale:* Understands that some patients, especially the elderly, can experience orthostatic hypotension.
❑	5	Discards disposable supplies per OSHA guidelines. If stainless steel speculum was used, soaks in cool water. Sanitizes and sterilizes as soon as it is convenient.
❑	5	Removes gloves and washes hands.
❑	5	Assists patient down and off the table if necessary.
❑	5	Instructs patient to dress. Informs patient of how and when test results will be reported to her.
❑	15	Prepares laboratory requisition (cytology request) form. Includes physician name and address, date, source of specimen, patient's name, address, date of last menstrual period (LMP), and hormone therapy. Places slides in slide container, attaches requisition to container, and sends to laboratory.
❑	5	Documents that test is performed and slide has been sent to reference laboratory in the patient's chart.

SKILLS COMPETENCY ASSESSMENT — continued

Procedure 30–7: Assisting with Gynecologic or Pelvic Examination and a Papanicolaou (Pap) Test

Task Performed	Possible Points	TASKS
☐	5	Completed the tasks within 10 minutes.
☐	15	Results obtained were accurate.

_______	Earned	ADD POINTS OF TASKS CHECKED
200	Points	TOTAL POINTS POSSIBLE
_______	SCORE	DETERMINE SCORE (divide points earned by total points possible, multiply results by 100)

Actual Student Time Needed to Complete Procedure: ____________

Student's Initials: ____________ Instructor's Initials: ____________ Grade: ____________

Suggestions for Improvement: ______________________________

Evaluator's Name (print) ______________________________

Evaluator's Signature ______________________________

Comments ______________________________

DOCUMENTATION

Chart the procedure in the patient's medical record.

Date: ____________________

Charting: ______________________________

____

____

Student's Initials: ____________

SKILLS COMPETENCY ASSESSMENT

Procedure 30–8: Instructing Patient in Testicular Self-Examination

Student's Name: ________________________ Date: __________

Objective: To provide a patient with the correct procedure for performing testicular self-examinations.

Conditions: The student demonstrates the ability to provide a patient with information concerning testicular self-screening for the presence of a painless mass in the scrotum using the following equipment and supplies: testicular self-examination card.

Time Requirements and Accuracy Standards: 5 minutes. Points assigned reflect importance of step to meeting objective: Important = (5) Essential = (10) Critical = (15). Automatic failure results if any of the **critical** tasks are omitted or performed incorrectly.

SKILLS ASSESSMENT CHECKLIST

Task Performed	Possible Points	TASKS
		Medical assistant instructs the patient in the following steps involved in testicular self-examination
❑	5	Patient should examine his testicles in a warm shower.
❑	5	*Rationale:* Warmth causes the scrotal skin to relax.
❑	10	Examine each testicle separately with both hands.
❑	15	Place the index and middle fingers underneath the testicle and the thumbs on top. Roll the testicle gently between the fingers.
❑	10	Locate the epididymis. Look for swelling or changes in the scrotal area.
❑	5	*Rationale:* Understands that patient must be instructed in the location and size of the epididymis, as a lump can be similar in size and patient must be able to distinguish the two.
❑	15	Provides a chart to the patient that illustrates the testes and epididymis. Medical assistant also provides the patient with a testicular self-examination card and encourages the patient to report anything unusual to the physician.
❑	5	Completed the tasks within 5 minutes.
❑	15	Results obtained were accurate.

______	Earned	ADD POINTS OF TASKS CHECKED
85	Points	TOTAL POINTS POSSIBLE
______	SCORE	DETERMINE SCORE (divide points earned by total points possible, multiply results by 100)

Actual Student Time Needed to Complete Procedure: __________

Student's Initials: __________ Instructor's Initials: __________ Grade: __________

Suggestions for Improvement: ______________________________

Evaluator's Name (print) ______________________________

Evaluator's Signature ______________________________

Comments ______________________________

SKILLS COMPETENCY ASSESSMENT

Procedure 30–9: Performing a Urinary Catheterization on a Female Patient

Student's Name: ______________________________ Date: __________

Objective: To perform urinary catheterization to obtain a sterile urine specimen for analysis or to relieve urinary retention.

Conditions: The student demonstrates the ability to obtain a sterile urine specimen for analysis or to relieve urinary retention using the following equipment and supplies: catheter kit (commercially available), sterile gloves, antiseptic solution, waxed paper bag, lubricant, sterile cotton balls, sterile urine container with label, sterile 2 × 2 gauze sponges, forceps, sterile absorbent plastic pad, sterile catheter (size and type as ordered by physician), biohazard waste container, laboratory requisition form.

Time Requirements and Accuracy Standards: 10 minutes. Points assigned reflect importance of step to meeting objective: Important = (5) Essential = (10) Critical = (15). Automatic failure results if any of the **critical** tasks are omitted or performed incorrectly.

STANDARD PRECAUTIONS:

SKILLS ASSESSMENT CHECKLIST

Task Performed	Possible Points	TASKS
❑	5	Instructs patient to breathe slowly and deeply during procedure.
❑	5	*Rationale:* Understands that slow, deep breathing helps the patient relax the abdominal and pelvic muscles and facilitates easier insertion of catheter.
❑	5	Washes hands and assembles supplies.
❑	5	Identifies the patient and explains the procedure. Places catheter kit on Mayo stand near the patient.
❑	5	Provides adequate lighting. Has patient disrobe below the waist; provides a drape.
❑	5	Positions patient into a dorsal recumbent position on an exam table.
❑	5	*Rationale:* Understands that dorsal recumbent position allows for access to the urinary meatus.
❑	10	Drapes patient with sheet exposing only external genitalia.
❑	5	Opens outer wrapping of sterile kit.
❑	10	Places sterile absorbent plastic pad under patient's buttocks. Places catheter tray between patient's legs.
❑	5	Asks patient to keep knees apart.
❑	5	*Rationale:* This position provides a good view of the urinary meatus.

Task Performed	Possible Points	TASKS
❑	5	Washes hands and puts on sterile gloves.
❑	5	Pours antiseptic solution over three cotton balls in an appropriate compartment of the kit.
❑	5	Opens urine specimen container.
❑	15	Applies sterile lubricant to a gauze sponge and places tip of catheter in lubricant and other end of catheter in sterile basin.
❑	15	Reminds patient to breathe slowly. Spreads labia with nondominant hand. Dominant hand remains sterile. With dominant hand and sterile forceps, wipes genitalia with each of the three antiseptic-soaked cotton balls, with a front-to-back motion. First, wipes the right labia using front-to-back motion. Discards cotton ball into waxed paper bag that is placed away from sterile area. Second, wipes the left labia, repeating procedure, and last, wipes down the center, discarding cotton ball after each wipe. Discards forceps. Continues to hold labia apart until catheter is inserted.
❑	5	*Rationale:* Knows that holding labia open will keep urinary meatus from becoming contaminated from labia while inserting catheter.
❑	15	Using sterile gloved hand, picks up catheter and holds it about three to four inches from lubricated end.
❑	15	Gently inserts lubricated tip of catheter into urinary meatus approximately six inches or until urine begins to flow. Moves nondominant hand to hold catheter in place.
❑	10	Interrupts urine flow by clamping off.
❑	5	*Rationale:* Understands that this will stop the flow of urine while the specimen container is positioned.
❑	10	Positions end of catheter into urine specimen container.
❑	10	Collects specimen by releasing clamp and collecting approximately 60 mL of urine.
❑	5	Allows remaining urine to flow into basin until flow ceases. Pinches catheter closed.
❑	5	Removes catheter gently and slowly.
❑	5	Dries area with remaining cotton balls.
❑	5	Tightens lid on the urine specimen container.
❑	5	Removes procedure items.
❑	5	Positions patient for comfort. Assists patient in sitting up or relaxing in a horizontal recumbent position. After a rest period, helps patient sit on edge of table. Checks patient's color and pulse.
❑	5	Discards disposable items per OSHA guidelines.

SKILLS COMPETENCY ASSESSMENT — continued

Procedure 30-9: Performing a Urinary Catheterization on a Female Patient

Task Performed	Possible Points	TASKS
❑	15	Labels specimen container and attaches to completed laboratory requisition form if collecting specimen for analysis.
❑	5	Assists patient from exam table.
❑	5	Cleans room and table. Removes gloves and discards in biohazard waste container. Washes hands.
❑	15	Documents procedure in patient's chart, including the amount of urine collected. Documents that specimen was sent to outside laboratory (if appropriate).
❑	5	Completed the tasks within 10 minutes.
❑	15	Results obtained were accurate.

________	Earned	ADD POINTS OF TASKS CHECKED
280	Points	TOTAL POINTS POSSIBLE
________	SCORE	DETERMINE SCORE (divide points earned by total points possible, multiply results by 100)

Actual Student Time Needed to Complete Procedure: ____________

Student's Initials: ____________ Instructor's Initials: ____________ Grade: ____________

Suggestions for Improvement: ______________________________

Evaluator's Name (print) ______________________________

Evaluator's Signature ______________________________

Comments ______________________________

DOCUMENTATION

Chart the procedure in the patient's medical record, including the amount of urine collected.

Date: ______________________________

Charting: ______________________________

____

____

Student's Initials: ____________

SKILLS COMPETENCY ASSESSMENT

Procedure 30–10: Performing a Urine Drug Screening

Student's Name: ______________________________ Date: __________

Objective: To accurately obtain a urine specimen from a patient to screen for traces of drugs.

Conditions: The student demonstrates the ability to accurately obtain a urine specimen from a patient to screen for traces of drugs using the following equipment and supplies: Urine Drug Kit (provide at least two choices), gloves, biohazard waste container.

Time Requirements and Accuracy Standards: 5 minutes. Points assigned reflect importance of step to meeting objective: Important = (5) Essential = (10) Critical = (15). Automatic failure results if any of the **critical** tasks are omitted or performed incorrectly.

STANDARD PRECAUTIONS:

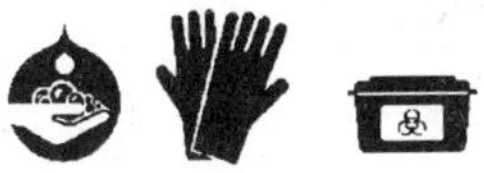

SKILLS ASSESSMENT CHECKLIST

Task Performed	Possible Points	TASKS
☐	15	Asks patient to show a photo ID and has patient sign a consent form, keeping copies for the patient file.
☐	5	*Rationale:* Only the person scheduled to take the test will be able to do so.
☐	5	Washes hands and explains procedures to the patient.
☐	10	Supplies at least two collection kits and allows the patient to choose one of them.
☐	15	Has patient remove unnecessary outer garments, empty pockets, and wash and dry hands.
☐	5	*Rationale:* Patient is not given the opportunity to substitute another specimen.
☐	15	Instructs patient to collect at least 40 mL of urine in the collection container.
☐	5	Puts on gloves. Records temperature of specimen, volume, and any contamination.
☐	5	*Rationale:* Understands that a fresh urine specimen will have a temperature of at least 98.6° F.
☐	15	Labels specimen and has patient initial specimen lid.
☐	15	Seals tamper-proof specimen kit bag and has patient initial.
☐	15	Secures sample in a locked container until pickup.
☐	15	Has collector and donor sign off on the test collection procedure to document that all procedural steps were followed.

SKILLS COMPETENCY ASSESSMENT — continued

Procedure 30–10: Performing a Urine Drug Screening

Task Performed	Possible Points	TASKS
❑	5	Removes gloves and disposes in biohazard waste container. Washes hands.
❑	5	Documents procedure in patient's chart.
❑	5	Completed the tasks within 5 minutes.
❑	15	Results obtained were accurate.

________	Earned	ADD POINTS OF TASKS CHECKED
170	Points	TOTAL POINTS POSSIBLE
________	SCORE	DETERMINE SCORE (divide points earned by total points possible, multiply results by 100)

Actual Student Time Needed to Complete Procedure: ____________

Student's Initials: ____________ Instructor's Initials: ____________ Grade: ____________

Suggestions for Improvement: ____

Evaluator's Name (print) ____

Evaluator's Signature ____

Comments ____

DOCUMENTATION

Chart the procedure in the patient's medical record.

Date: ________________________

Charting: ____

____

____

Student's Initials: ________________

SKILLS COMPETENCY ASSESSMENT

Procedure 30–11: Assisting with Proctosigmoidoscopy

Student's Name: ______________________________ Date: ____________

Objective: To assist the physician in assessing the status of the sigmoid colon and the rectum for signs of disease such as tumors, polyps, ulcerations, hemorrhoids, or rectal bleeding.

Conditions: The student demonstrates the ability to assist the physician with proctosigmoidoscopy using the following equipment and supplies: sigmoidoscope with obturator (either a flexible fiberoptic sigmoidoscope or a rigid sigmoidoscope), sterile biopsy forceps, patient gown, sterile specimen container with preservative, laboratory requisition form, tissues, biohazard waste container, patient drape, small pillow, anoscope, rectal speculum, insufflator, suction machine and tip, probe with bulb tip, gloves, finger cots, long cotton applicators, lubricating jelly, basin of water, 4 × 4 gauze sponges.

Time Requirements and Accuracy Standards: 15 minutes. Points assigned reflect importance of step to meeting objective: Important = (5) Essential = (10) Critical = (15). Automatic failure results if any of the **critical** tasks are omitted or performed incorrectly.

STANDARD PRECAUTIONS:

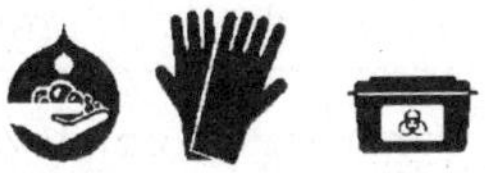

SKILLS ASSESSMENT CHECKLIST

Task Performed	Possible Points	TASKS
☐	5	Washes hands and prepares equipment and supplies.
☐	15	Checks the lights on the illuminated instruments for loose bulbs by turning the bulb clockwise. Turns the switch to the "on" position to verify the light is working, then turns light off.
☐	10	Labels specimen container with patient's name, address, date, and source.
☐	5	Checks to see that obturators are correctly positioned.
☐	5	Has a basin ready to receive used instruments.
☐	5	Prepares a basin of water to rinse out suction pump.
☐	15	Tests suction machine.
☐	15	Prepares patient. Makes sure patient has been properly prepared; that is, necessary laxative taken, enema administered, and adequate results obtained from enema.
☐	15	Identifies patient. Verifies consent form has been signed. Explains procedure to the patient to promote relaxation and reduce apprehension.
☐	5	Asks patient to empty bladder and saves specimen (if required).
☐	5	*Rationale:* Understands that an empty bladder facilitates examination and is more comfortable for the patient.
☐	5	Asks patient to disrobe and put on gown.

SKILLS COMPETENCY ASSESSMENT — continued

Procedure 30–11: Assisting with Proctosigmoidoscopy

Task Performed	Possible Points	TASKS
❑	5	Assists patient into the knee-chest position or the Sims' lateral position, which assures accessibility to the rectum and sigmoid colon. Some physicians use proctologic tables that tilt the patient into the knee-chest position.
❑	5	*Rationale:* Understands that the abdominal contents tip forward and away from the pelvic area, making it easier to insert the sigmoidoscope.
❑	10	Drapes the patient and places small towel directly over the anus and under the perineal area or uses a fenestrated drape over the anus.
❑	5	Applies gloves and assists the physician during examination.
❑	5	Places lubricant on physician's gloves for digital examination.
❑	5	Warms metal scope by placing in warm water for a few minutes.
❑	10	Lubricates scope tip.
❑	10	Plugs in scope when physician is ready to use.
❑	5	*Rationale:* Understands that plugging the scope in too soon allows the light source to get too hot, which may harm the patient.
❑	5	Reminds the patient to take slow deep breaths to promote relaxation of muscles to facilitate insertion of the sigmoidoscope.
❑	10	Attaches inflation bulb; attaches light source.
❑	5	Observes patient throughout procedure. Provides support and reassurance.
❑	5	Takes instruments from physician as needed.
❑	5	Passes long cotton-tipped applicators to the physician and assists with suction equipment.
❑	5	Places suction tubing in basin of water.
❑	5	Places instruments in basin.
❑	10	Assists with collection of biopsy by handing biopsy forceps to the physician. Does not touch inside of specimen container. Receives and cares for specimen; labels properly.
❑	5	*Rationale:* Sterile container will become contaminated if the inside is touched and may cause inaccurate results.
❑	5	Cleans patient's anus with tissue.
❑	5	Removes gloves, washes hands.
❑	15	Assists patient to supine position after examination. Does not let patient rise too rapidly because of the possibility of dizziness. Checks patient's blood pressure.

Task Performed	Possible Points	TASKS
❑	5	*Rationale:* Understands that vagal nerve stimulation may cause shocklike symptoms, or that orthostatic hypotension can occur from lying flat for an extended period.
❑	5	Assists patient to dress if needed.
❑	5	Applies gloves. Transports specimen with completed lab requisition form.
❑	15	Cleans room and equipment following OSHA guidelines. Flexible sigmoidoscope should be sanitized and subjected to cold sterilization according to manufacturer's directions. Metal (rigid) sigmoidoscope must be sanitized and sterilized in the autoclave.
❑	5	Removes gloves and washes hands.
❑	5	Documents procedure in patient's chart. If specimen is taken, documents that it has been sent to the laboratory. Also documents the patient's blood pressure reading and any unusual circumstances or patient reactions.
❑	5	Completed the tasks within 15 minutes.
❑	15	Results obtained were accurate.

______	Earned	ADD POINTS OF TASKS CHECKED
305	Points	TOTAL POINTS POSSIBLE
______	SCORE	DETERMINE SCORE (divide points earned by total points possible, multiply results by 100)

Actual Student Time Needed to Complete Procedure: ____________

Student's Initials: ____________ Instructor's Initials: ____________ Grade: ____________

Suggestions for Improvement: ____

Evaluator's Name (print) ____

Evaluator's Signature ____

Comments ____

DOCUMENTATION

Chart the procedure in the patient's medical record.

Date: ____________________________

Charting: ____

____

____

Student's Initials: ________________

SKILLS COMPETENCY ASSESSMENT

Procedure 30–12: Fecal Occult Blood Test

Student's Name: ______________________________ Date: ____________

Objective: To test feces for occult blood.

Conditions: The student demonstrates the ability to test feces for occult blood using the following equipment and supplies: three guaiac slide test kits, prepared fecal slides from patient, occult blood developer, kit reference card, gloves, biohazard waste container.

Time Requirements and Accuracy Standards: 5 minutes. Points assigned reflect importance of step to meeting objective: Important = (5) Essential = (10) Critical = (15). Automatic failure results if any of the **critical** tasks are omitted or performed incorrectly.

STANDARD PRECAUTIONS:

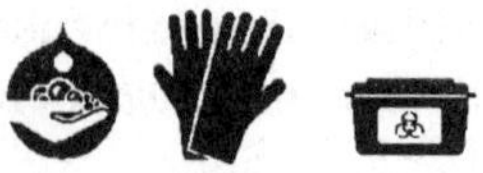

SKILLS ASSESSMENT CHECKLIST

Task Performed	Possible Points	TASKS
❑	10	Checks expiration dates on occult slides.
❑	5	*Rationale:* Understands that outdated slides can give an inaccurate reading.
❑	5	Identifies the patient.
❑	5	Fills out all information on the front flap of all three slides.
❑	15	Explains stool collection process to patient: • Keep slides at room temperature away from sunlight, which destroys the effectiveness of the guaiac paper and may give inaccurate results. • Open the front flap of the first slide. • Use one end of the wooden applicator to apply a thin smear of the stool sample from the toilet to Box " A." (Patient should not collect sample during menstrual period or if hemorrhoids are present.) • Repeat the procedure using the other end of the applicator, taking a specimen from a different section of the same stool and applying a thin smear to Box " B." (Occult blood may be distributed differently throughout the bowel movement.) • Dispose of the applicator in a waste container. • Close the cover after air-drying slide overnight. • Date the front flap. • Repeat the process with the next two bowel movements, on subsequent days.
❑	5	Provides the patient with an envelope to return the slides to the physician's office.
❑	5	Documents that the test kit and instructions were given to the patient.

Developing the fecal occult slide

The medical assistant will be responsible for developing the slides to determine the results when the patient returns the fecal occult samples to the office. The medical assistant should develop the results as soon as possible. Although most slides may be stored for up to fourteen days before developing, the patient may have already stored them for several days. Test results are important to ensure prompt treatment should a problem be discovered.

Task Performed	Possible Points	TASKS
❑	5	Checks the expiration date on the developer.
❑	5	Applies gloves.
❑	5	Opens the window flap on the back of the slide.
❑	15	Applies two drops of the developer to each Box "A" and "B", directly over each smear.
❑	15	Interprets the results within thirty to sixty seconds. Records the results.
❑	5	Looks for a blue halo appearing around the perimeter of the specimen, indicating a positive reaction.
❑	15	Performs the quality control procedure by processing the positive and negative monitor strip on each slide to confirm the test system is functional. If quality control is not functional, rechecks expiration dates on slide and developer. Repeats test, if necessary.
❑	5	Disposes of all supplies according to OSHA guidelines.
❑	5	Removes gloves and disposes in biohazard waste container. Washes hands.
❑	5	Documents results in patient's chart.
❑	5	Completed the tasks within 5 minutes.
❑	15	Results obtained were accurate.

______	Earned	ADD POINTS OF TASKS CHECKED
150	Points	TOTAL POINTS POSSIBLE
______	SCORE	DETERMINE SCORE (divide points earned by total points possible, multiply results by 100)

Actual Student Time Needed to Complete Procedure: __________

Student's Initials: __________ Instructor's Initials: __________ Grade: __________

Suggestions for Improvement: ______________________________

Evaluator's Name (print) ______________________________

Evaluator's Signature ______________________________

Comments ______________________________

DOCUMENTATION

Record the results of the fecal occult blood test in the patient's medical record.

Date: ______________________

Charting: ______________________________

____

____

Student's Initials: ______________

SKILLS COMPETENCY ASSESSMENT

Procedure 30–13: Performing Visual Acuity Testing Using a Snellen Chart

Student's Name: ______________________________ Date: ____________

Objective: To perform a visual screening test to determine a patient's distance visual acuity.

Conditions: The student demonstrates the ability to perform a visual screening test to determine a patient's distance visual acuity using the following equipment and supplies: Snellen eye chart placed at eye level (appropriate for age and reading ability of patient), pointer, occluder, alcohol wipes.

Time Requirements and Accuracy Standards: 10 minutes. Points assigned reflect importance of step to meeting objective: Important = (5) Essential = (10) Critical = (15). Automatic failure results if any of the **critical** tasks are omitted or performed incorrectly.

STANDARD PRECAUTIONS:

SKILLS ASSESSMENT CHECKLIST

Task Performed	Possible Points	TASKS
❑	5	Washes hands and assembles equipment.
❑	10	Prepares a well-lighted room, free from distractions and with a distance mark twenty feet from the eye chart.
❑	5	Explains the procedure to the patient. Tests patients with their glasses on or contact lenses in, unless otherwise indicated by the physician.
❑	10	Instructs the patient to stand behind the mark and cover the left eye with the occluder. Instructs the patient to keep the left eye open under the occluder and not to apply pressure to the eyeball.
❑	5	*Rationale:* Keeps patient from squinting when reading the chart.
❑	15	Stands next to the chart and points to row 3, instructing the patient to read each letter with the right eye, verbally identifying each letter read. Goes to line 2 or line 1 if patient is unable to read line 3.
❑	5	*Rationale:* Pointing helps patient focus on one row of letters at a time.
❑	15	Records the results at the smallest line the patient can read with two or less errors. Allows the patient to repeat the line to verify accuracy. Records vision as right eye, left eye, both eyes (Examples: OD 20/25; OS 20/20; OU 20/20).
❑	5	*Rationale:* Can state that visual acuity is recorded as a fraction, with the top number indicating the distance the patient stands from the chart and the bottom number indicating the distance from which a person with normal vision can read that row of letters.

Task Performed	Possible Points	TASKS
☐	5	Records the patient's reaction during the test, such as leaning forward, squinting or straining, or tearing eyes.
☐	5	*Rationale:* These patient reactions may indicate an eye problem.
☐	5	Uses the same procedure to test the left eye.
☐	5	Wipes occluder with alcohol. Washes hands. Records the results.
☐	5	Completed the tasks within 10 minutes.
☐	15	Results obtained were accurate.

_______	Earned	ADD POINTS OF TASKS CHECKED
115	Points	TOTAL POINTS POSSIBLE
_______	SCORE	DETERMINE SCORE (divide points earned by total points possible, multiply results by 100)

Actual Student Time Needed to Complete Procedure: ____________

Student's Initials: ____________ Instructor's Initials: ____________ Grade: ____________

Suggestions for Improvement: ____________

Evaluator's Name (print) ____________

Evaluator's Signature ____________

Comments ____________

DOCUMENTATION

Record results in the patient's medical record.

Date: ____________

Charting: ____________

____

____

____

Student's Initials: ____________

SKILLS COMPETENCY ASSESSMENT

Procedure 30–14: Measuring Near Visual Acuity

Student's Name: ______________________________ Date: ____________

Objective: To obtain the near vision of the patient.

Conditions: The student demonstrates the ability to obtain the near vision of the patient using the following equipment and supplies: appropriate near visual acuity chart, 3 × 5 cards or occluder.

Time Requirements and Accuracy Standards: 15 minutes. Points assigned reflect importance of step to meeting objective: Important = (5) Essential = (10) Critical = (15). Automatic failure results if any of the **critical** tasks are omitted or performed incorrectly.

STANDARD PRECAUTIONS:

SKILLS ASSESSMENT CHECKLIST

Task Performed	Possible Points	TASKS
❑	5	Washes hands.
❑	10	Identifies patient. Explains procedure to patient; provides occluder. Positions patient in a comfortable position.
❑	15	Positions the near visual acuity fourteen inches from the patient by measuring with a tape measure.
❑	5	*Rationale:* Measuring the distance with a tape measure ensures accurate results.
❑	5	Has patient lightly (no pressure) cover the left eye with the occluder.
❑	5	*Rationale:* Understands that applying pressure will cause blurring of the eye to be tested next.
❑	15	Has patient read the paragraphs printed on the card.
❑	15	Notes the visual acuity for that eye when the patient has reached a line where more than two mistakes are made (allows the patient to repeat the line to verify acuity).
❑	5	Repeats the process to measure the left eye.
❑	5	Repeats the process to measure both eyes.
❑	5	Records the result in the patient chart.
❑	5	Discards the 3 × 5 card or disinfects the occluder to prevent microorganism cross-contamination.
❑	5	Washes hands.

Task Performed	Possible Points	TASKS
☐	5	Records results.
☐	5	Completed the tasks within 15 minutes.
☐	15	Results obtained were accurate.

______	Earned	ADD POINTS OF TASKS CHECKED
125	Points	TOTAL POINTS POSSIBLE
______	SCORE	DETERMINE SCORE (divide points earned by total points possible, multiply results by 100)

Actual Student Time Needed to Complete Procedure: ______________

Student's Initials: ______________ Instructor's Initials: ______________ Grade: ______________

Suggestions for Improvement: ______________________________

Evaluator's Name (print) ______________________________

Evaluator's Signature ______________________________

Comments ______________________________

DOCUMENTATION

Record near visual acuity test results in the patient's medical record.

Date: ______________________________

Charting: ______________________________

____

____

Student's Initials: ______________

SKILLS COMPETENCY ASSESSMENT

Procedure 30–15: Performing Color Vision Test Using the Ishihara Plates

Student's Name: ______________________________ Date: ____________

Objective: To assess a patient's ability to distinguish between the colors red and green.

Conditions: The student demonstrates the ability to assess a patient's ability to distinguish between the colors red and green using the following equipment and supplies: Ishihara plates (1–12).

Time Requirements and Accuracy Standards: 10 minutes. Points assigned reflect importance of step to meeting objective: Important = (5) Essential = (10) Critical = (15). Automatic failure results if any of the **critical** tasks are omitted or performed incorrectly.

STANDARD PRECAUTIONS:

SKILL ASSESSMENT CHECKLIST

Task Performed	Possible Points	TASKS
☐	5	Explains that the purpose of the test is to determine if the patient has a color vision deficiency.
☐	5	Shows patient plate number 12 as an example of the test process.
☐	5	*Rationale:* With normal vision, plate number 12 can be easily identified.
☐	5	Washes hands and assembles the equipment in a room lighted by daylight.
☐	5	*Rationale:* Understands that direct sunlight or electric light may produce errors in the results because of an alteration in the appearance of shades of color.
☐	15	Holds each plate 75 cm or 30 inches from the patient and tilts each so the plane of each plate is at right angles to the line of the patient's vision.
☐	15	Records the number given by the patient on each plate.
☐	10	Assesses the patient's readings and records.
☐	5	*Rationale:* Knows that ten or more plates read correctly indicates normal color vision.
☐	15	Keeps test plates covered when not in use to avoided fading of color plates from exposure to sunlight, which can lead to inaccurate test interpretation.
☐	5	Completed the tasks within 10 minutes.
☐	15	Results obtained were accurate.

________	Earned	ADD POINTS OF TASKS CHECKED
105	Points	TOTAL POINTS POSSIBLE
________	SCORE	DETERMINE SCORE (divide points earned by total points possible, multiply results by 100)

Actual Student Time Needed to Complete Procedure: ____________

Student's Initials: ____________ Instructor's Initials: ____________ Grade: ____________

Suggestions for Improvement: ____

Evaluator's Name (print) ____

Evaluator's Signature ____

Comments ____

DOCUMENTATION

Chart the procedure in the patient's medical record.

Date: ____________________________

Charting: ____

____

____

Student's Initials: ________________

SKILLS COMPETENCY ASSESSMENT

Procedure 30–16: Performing Eye Instillation

Student's Name: ______________________________ Date: ____________

Objective: To treat eye infections, soothe irritation, anesthetize, and dilate pupils.

Conditions: The student demonstrates the ability to treat eye infections, soothe irritation, anesthetize, and dilate pupils using the following equipment and supplies: sterile eye dropper, sterile ophthalmic medication as ordered by the physician (either drops or ointment), sterile cotton balls, sterile water or sterile normal saline, sterile gloves. Use separate medication for each eye, if both are affected.

Time Requirements and Accuracy Standards: 5 minutes. Points assigned reflect importance of step to meeting objective: Important = (5) Essential = (10) Critical = (15). Automatic failure results if any of the **critical** tasks are omitted or performed incorrectly.

STANDARD PRECAUTIONS:

SKILLS ASSESSMENT CHECKLIST

Task Performed	Possible Points	TASKS
❑	5	Washes hands. Assembles supplies.
❑	15	Checks medication carefully as ordered by the physician, including expiration date. Reads label three times.
❑	10	Identifies patient. Explains procedure to the patient and informs the patient that instillation may temporarily blur vision.
❑	10	Positions the patient in a seated or lying down position. Instructs the patient to stare at a fixed spot during instillation of the drops.
❑	15	Puts on sterile gloves, moistens two to three sterile cotton balls with sterile water or sterile normal saline.
❑	5	Wipes the affected eye from the inner to outer canthus to remove any exudate that may be present.
❑	5	Prepares medication using either drops or ointment.
❑	10	Has the patient look up to the ceiling and expose the lower conjunctival sac of the affected eye by using fingers over a tissue to pull down.
❑	15	Places the number of drops ordered in the center of the lower conjunctival sac or a thin line of ointment in the lower surface of the eyelid, being careful not to touch the eyelid, eyeball, or eyelashes with the tip of the medication applicator. Replaces dropper in bottle to avoid contamination.
❑	5	Has the patient close the eye and roll the eyeball.

Task Performed	Possible Points	TASKS
❑	5	*Rationale:* Understands that rolling the eyeball helps distribute medication evenly.
❑	5	Blots excess medication from eyelids with cotton ball from inner to outer canthus.
❑	5	Disposes of supplies. Washes hands.
❑	5	Records procedure in patient's chart.
❑	5	Completed the tasks within 5 minutes.
❑	15	Results obtained were accurate.

________	Earned	ADD POINTS OF TASKS CHECKED
135	Points	TOTAL POINTS POSSIBLE
________	SCORE	DETERMINE SCORE (divide points earned by total points possible, multiply results by 100)

Actual Student Time Needed to Complete Procedure: ____________

Student's Initials: ____________ Instructor's Initials: ____________ Grade: ____________

Suggestions for Improvement: ____

Evaluator's Name (print) ____

Evaluator's Signature ____

Comments ____

DOCUMENTATION

Chart the procedure in the patient's medical record.

Date:____________________________

Charting: ____

____

____

____

Student's Initials:________________

SKILLS COMPETENCY ASSESSMENT

Procedure 30–17: Performing Eye Patch Dressing Application

Student's Name: ______________________________ Date: __________

Objective: To apply a sterile eye patch.

Conditions: The student demonstrates the ability to apply a sterile eye patch using the following equipment and supplies: tape, sterile eye patch, sterile gloves.

Time Requirements and Accuracy Standards: 10 minutes. Points assigned reflect importance of step to meeting objective: Important = (5) Essential = (10) Critical = (15). Automatic failure results if any of the **critical** tasks are omitted or performed incorrectly.

STANDARD PRECAUTIONS: 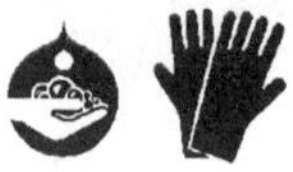

SKILLS ASSESSMENT CHECKLIST

Task Performed	Possible Points	TASKS
☐	5	Washes hands and assembles supplies.
☐	5	Identifies patient. Explains the procedure. Positions the patient in a seated position.
☐	15	Instructs the patient to close both eyes during the application of the patch. Prepares sterile area by opening the sterile package and using the inside of the package as a sterile field. Applies sterile gloves.
☐	15	Places the patch over the affected eye using sterile gloves.
☐	10	Secures the patch with three to four strips of transparent tape diagonally from mid-forehead to below the ear.
☐	5	Removes gloves. Washes hands.
☐	5	Documents the procedure and provides verbal and written care instructions to the patient.
☐	5	Completed the tasks within 10 minutes.
☐	15	Results obtained were accurate.

________	Earned	ADD POINTS OF TASKS CHECKED
80	Points	TOTAL POINTS POSSIBLE
________	SCORE	DETERMINE SCORE (divide points earned by total points possible, multiply results by 100)

Actual Student Time Needed to Complete Procedure: ____________

Student's Initials: ____________ Instructor's Initials: ____________ Grade: ____________

Suggestions for Improvement: ____________

Evaluator's Name (print) ____________

Evaluator's Signature ____________

Comments ____________

DOCUMENTATION

Chart the procedure in the patient's medical record.

Date: ____________

Charting: ____________

____

____

____

Student's Initials: ____________

SKILLS COMPETENCY ASSESSMENT

Procedure 30–18: Performing Eye Irrigation

Student's Name: ______________________________ Date: ____________

Objective: To irrigate the patient's affected eye for any of the following reasons: a. to cleanse a foreign object; b. to cleanse a discharge; c. to cleanse chemicals; d. to apply antiseptic; e. to apply heat.

Conditions: The student demonstrates the ability to irrigate the patient's affected eye using the following equipment and supplies: sterile irrigation solution as ordered by the physician, sterile bulb syringe (rubber), kidney-shaped basin to catch irrigation solution, sterile cotton balls, sterile gloves, biohazard waste container, towel, pillow. Use separate medication for each eye if both eyes are irrigated.

Time Requirements and Accuracy Standards: 10 minutes. Points assigned reflect importance of step to meeting objective: Important = (5) Essential = (10) Critical = (15). Automatic failure results if any of the **critical** tasks are omitted or performed incorrectly.

STANDARD PRECAUTIONS:

SKILLS ASSESSMENT CHECKLIST

Task Performed	Possible Points	TASKS
☐	5	Washes hands and assembles supplies.
☐	5	Identifies patient. Explains the procedure to the patient. Positions the patient in the supine position.
☐	15	Checks expiration date on solution bottle. Checks medication label three times. Warms solution to body temperature (98.6° F).
☐	10	Tilts head toward affected eye. Places towel on patient's shoulder. Places basin beside the affected eye.
☐	5	*Rationale:* Understands that tilting head toward affected eye allows solution to flow from affected eye into basin without causing cross-contamination of the unaffected eye. Basin acts as a catch receptacle for solution.
☐	15	Pours sterile solution into a sterile container.
☐	15	Puts on sterile gloves.
☐	5	Moistens two to three cotton balls with irrigation solution and cleans the eyelids and eyelashes of the affected eye from inner to outer canthus. Discards after each wipe.
☐	5	Exposes the lower conjunctiva by separating the eyelid with index finger and thumb.
☐	5	Has the patient stare at a fixed spot.

Task Performed	Possible Points	TASKS
☐	15	Irrigates the affected eye with sterile solution by resting the sterile bulb syringe on the bridge of the patient's nose, being careful not to touch the eye or conjunctival sac with the syringe tip. Allows the stream to flow from the inside canthus to the outer corner of the eye.
☐	5	*Rationale:* This avoids cross-contamination of the unaffected eye from the flow of solution.
☐	5	Dries the eyelid and eyelashes with sterile cotton balls following the irrigation.
☐	5	Discards supplies in biohazard waste container if discharge or exudate is present.
☐	5	Removes gloves. Washes hands. Documents procedure.
☐	5	Completed the tasks within 10 minutes.
☐	15	Results obtained were accurate.

______	Earned	ADD POINTS OF TASKS CHECKED
140	Points	TOTAL POINTS POSSIBLE
______	SCORE	DETERMINE SCORE (divide points earned by total points possible, multiply results by 100)

Actual Student Time Needed to Complete Procedure: ____________

Student's Initials: ____________ Instructor's Initials: ____________ Grade: ____________

Suggestions for Improvement: ____

Evaluator's Name (print) ____

Evaluator's Signature ____

Comments ____

DOCUMENTATION

Chart the procedure in the patient's medical record.

Date: ______________________

Charting: ____

____

____

____

Student's Initials: ______________

SKILLS COMPETENCY ASSESSMENT

Procedure 30–19: Assisting with Audiometry

Student's Name: ______________________________ Date: __________

Objective: To assist in testing patient for hearing loss.

Conditions: The student demonstrates the ability to assist in testing patient for hearing loss using the following equipment and supplies: audiometer with headphones, quiet room.

Time Requirements and Accuracy Standards: 15 minutes. Points assigned reflect importance of step to meeting objective: Important = (5) Essential = (10) Critical = (15). Automatic failure results if any of the **critical** tasks are omitted or performed incorrectly.

STANDARD PRECAUTIONS:

SKILLS ASSESSMENT CHECKLIST

Task Performed	Possible Points	TASKS
❑	5	Washes hands and assembles equipment and supplies.
❑	5	Prepares room. Holds test in a room without outside noises.
❑	5	*Rationale:* Understands that outside interference can cause inaccurate test results, especially in the lower frequencies, which are more difficult to hear.
❑	15	Explains procedure to patient. • Explains the use and purpose of the audiometer and explains that the test measures the frequency of sound waves and the ability of the patient to hear various frequencies of sound waves (one frequency at a time). • Explains that when the patient hears a new frequency, the tester is signaled.
❑	5	Positions patient in a comfortable sitting position. Has patient put on headphones. Does the procedure on each ear separately.
❑	15	If the medical assistant has been thoroughly trained to do the procedure, the physician will allow the medical assistant to perform the audiometry. Starts the audiometer at low frequency. Has patient indicate when the sound is heard and plots it on the audiogram.
❑	15	Increases the frequencies gradually, until completed.
❑	5	Checks the other ear in the same manner.
❑	15	Gives the results to the physician for interpretation.
❑	5	Cleans equipment following manufacturer's instructions. Washes hands.
❑	5	Documents procedure on patient's chart.

Task Performed	Possible Points	TASKS
☐	5	Completed the tasks within 15 minutes.
☐	15	Results obtained were accurate.
______	Earned	ADD POINTS OF TASKS CHECKED
115	Points	TOTAL POINTS POSSIBLE
______	SCORE	DETERMINE SCORE (divide points earned by total points possible, multiply results by 100)

Actual Student Time Needed to Complete Procedure: ____________

Student's Initials: ____________ Instructor's Initials: ____________ Grade: ____________

Suggestions for Improvement: ____________

Evaluator's Name (print) ____________

Evaluator's Signature ____________

Comments ____________

DOCUMENTATION

Chart the procedure in the patient's medical record.

Date: ____________

Charting: ____________

____

____

____

Student's Initials: ____________

SKILLS COMPETENCY ASSESSMENT

Procedure 30–20: Performing Ear Irrigation

Student's Name: ______________________________ Date: __________

Objective: To perform an ear irrigation to relieve inflammation, to remove cerumen, discharge, or foreign materials from the ear canal as directed by the physician.

Conditions: The student demonstrates the ability to perform ear irrigation as directed by the physician using the following equipment and supplies: irrigation solution, as ordered by the physician, warmed to body temperature (98.6° F), ear syringe or bulb, ear basin or emesis basin, basin for warmed solution, towel, cotton balls, otoscope.

Time Requirements and Accuracy Standards: 10 minutes. Points assigned reflect importance of step to meeting objective: Important = (5) Essential = (10) Critical = (15). Automatic failure results if any of the **critical** tasks are omitted or performed incorrectly.

STANDARD PRECAUTIONS:

SKILLS ASSESSMENT CHECKLIST

Task Performed	Possible Points	TASKS
☐	5	Washes hands and assembles equipment.
☐	5	Identifies patient. Explains the procedure and informs the patient that during the procedure a minimal amount of discomfort and dizziness may be experienced, caused by solution coming into contact with the tympanic membrane.
☐	5	Places the patient in a sitting position and uses an otoscope to visualize the affected ear.
☐	10	Cleanses the outer ear with a wet cotton ball moistened with irrigation solution.
☐	5	Tilts the head toward the affected ear.
☐	10	Gently pulls the auricle upward and back to straighten the ear canal.
☐	10	Tilts the patient's head slightly forward and to the affected side to allow solution to flow into basin by force of gravity.
☐	5	Places towel on the patient's shoulder on the affected side.
☐	5	Places the ear basin under the affected ear and has the patient hold the basin in place.
☐	15	Checks label of solution three times for correctness and also checks the expiration date of the solution.
☐	15	Pours the solution into a basin and fills the syringe with the warmed irrigation solution as prescribed by the physician. Uses about 30 cc to 50 cc of solution at a time.
☐	5	Once again cleanses the outer ear with a cotton ball moistened with irrigation solution.
☐	10	Straightens the external auditory canal by pulling back and upward on the auricle for adults.
☐	15	Expels air from syringe and gently inserts the syringe tip into the affected ear, being careful not to insert too deeply. Does not occlude external auditory canal. Directs the flow of the solution upward toward roof of canal.

Task Performed	Possible Points	TASKS
❑	5	*Rationale:* Understands that this will avoid injury to the tympanic membrane, prevent occlusion of external auditory canal, and allow solution to drain out.
❑	5	Repeats the irrigation, allowing the solution to drain from the ear, noting the return. Allows for free flow of return each time.
❑	5	Dries the outer ear and views the inner ear with the otoscope to verify the procedure has removed or dislodged the foreign body.
❑	5	Notifies the physician that the procedure has been completed. Removes the ear basin and towel.
❑	10	Has patient lie on affected side on exam table for ear to continue draining.
❑	5	Provides dry cotton balls to the patient to catch any further drainage, if directed by the physician.
❑	5	Disposes of supplies. Washes hands.
❑	5	Documents the procedure, noting return and amount.
❑	5	Provides post-care instructions to patient: Report any pain or dizziness to the physician. Do not insert any foreign object (i.e., cotton applicator) into the ear canal.
❑	5	Completed the tasks within 10 minutes.
❑	15	Results obtained were accurate.
______		Earned ADD POINTS OF TASKS CHECKED
190		Points TOTAL POINTS POSSIBLE
______		SCORE DETERMINE SCORE (divide points earned by total points possible, multiply results by 100)

Actual Student Time Needed to Complete Procedure: ____________

Student's Initials: ____________ Instructor's Initials: ____________ Grade: ____________

Suggestions for Improvement: ____

Evaluator's Name (print) ____

Evaluator's Signature ____

Comments ____

DOCUMENTATION

Chart the procedure in the patient's medical record.

Date: ____________________

Charting: ____

____

____

Student's Initials: ____________

SKILLS COMPETENCY ASSESSMENT

Procedure 30–21: Performing Ear Instillation

Student's Name: ______________________________ Date: ____________

Objective: To perform ear instillation to soften impacted cerumen, fight infection with antibiotics, or relieve pain.

Conditions: The student demonstrates the ability to perform ear instillation using the following equipment and supplies: otic medication, as prescribed by the physician, sterile ear dropper, cotton balls, gloves.

Time Requirements and Accuracy Standards: 5 minutes. Points assigned reflect importance of step to meeting objective: Important = (5) Essential = (10) Critical = (15). Automatic failure results if any of the **critical** tasks are omitted or performed incorrectly.

STANDARD PRECAUTIONS:

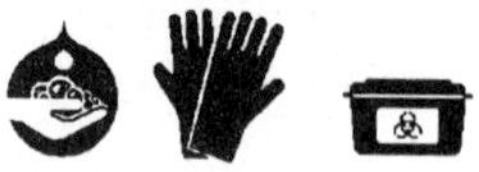

SKILLS ASSESSMENT CHECKLIST

Task Performed	Possible Points	TASKS
☐	5	Washes hands and assembles supplies.
☐	15	Identifies patient. Explains procedure to the patient. Positions patient to either lie on unaffected side or in seated position with head tilted toward unaffected ear to facilitate flow of medication.
☐	15	Checks otic medication three times against the physician's order and checks the expiration date of the medication.
☐	5	*Rationale:* Understands that only otic medication can be used in the ear.
☐	10	Draws up the prescribed amount of medication.
☐	15	Gently pulls the top of the ear upward and back for adults, or pulls earlobe downward and backward for children.
☐	10	Instills prescribed dose of medication (number of drops) by squeezing rubber bulb on dropper into the affected ear.
☐	10	Has the patient maintain the position for about five minutes to retain medication.
☐	5	Inserts moistened cotton ball into external ear canal for fifteen minutes, when instructed by the physician.
☐	5	*Rationale:* Understands that a moistened cotton ball will not absorb medication and will help retain medication in the ear.
☐	5	Disposes of supplies. Washes hands. Documents procedure.
☐	5	Completed the tasks within 5 minutes.

Task Performed	Possible Points	TASKS
❑	15	Results obtained were accurate.

________	Earned	ADD POINTS OF TASKS CHECKED
120	Points	TOTAL POINTS POSSIBLE
________	SCORE	DETERMINE SCORE (divide points earned by total points possible, multiply results by 100)

Actual Student Time Needed to Complete Procedure: ____________

Student's Initials: ____________ Instructor's Initials: ____________ Grade: ____________

Suggestions for Improvement: ____

Evaluator's Name (print) ____

Evaluator's Signature ____

Comments ____

DOCUMENTATION

Chart the procedure in the patient's medical record.

Date: ____________________

Charting: ____

____

____

____

Student's Initials: ____________

SKILLS COMPETENCY ASSESSMENT

Procedure 30–22: Assisting with Nasal Examination

Student's Name: ______________________________ Date: ____________

Objective: To assist the physician with the nasal examination when looking for polyps, engorged superficial blood vessels, and the possible removal of a foreign body.

Conditions: The student demonstrates the ability to assist the physician with the nasal examination using the following equipment and supplies: nasal speculum, light source, gloves, bayonet forceps, kidney basin.

Time Requirements and Accuracy Standards: 15 minutes. Points assigned reflect importance of step to meeting objective: Important = (5) Essential = (10) Critical = (15). Automatic failure results if any of the **critical** tasks are omitted or performed incorrectly.

STANDARD PRECAUTIONS:

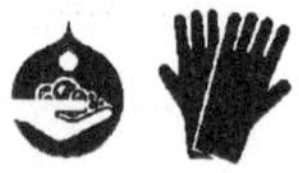

SKILLS ASSESSMENT CHECKLIST

Task Performed	Possible Points	TASKS
❑	5	Washes hands and assembles supplies.
❑	15	Identifies patient. Explains the procedure to the patient. • When a foreign object is involved, instructs the patient not to blow the nose or to attempt to remove the object because this could cause tissue damage or push the object deeper into the nasal passage.
❑	5	Places the patient in a seated position. Reassures the patient.
❑	5	Hands the physician equipment and supplies as needed.
❑	5	Cleans equipment and disposes of supplies per OSHA guidelines. Washes hands.
❑	5	Documents procedure noting foreign object, if applicable.
❑	5	Completed the tasks within 15 minutes.
❑	15	Results obtained were accurate.

______	Earned	ADD POINTS OF TASKS CHECKED
60	Points	TOTAL POINTS POSSIBLE
______	SCORE	DETERMINE SCORE (divide points earned by total points possible, multiply results by 100)

Actual Student Time Needed to Complete Procedure: ____________

Student's Initials: ____________ Instructor's Initials: ____________ Grade: ____________

Suggestions for Improvement: ______________________________

Evaluator's Name (print) ______________________________

Evaluator's Signature ______________________________

Comments ______________________________

SKILLS COMPETENCY ASSESSMENT

Procedure 30–23: Procedure for Obtaining a Throat Culture

Student's Name: ______________________________ Date: __________

Objective: To obtain secretions from the nasopharnyx and tonsillar area in order to incubate for means of identifying a pathogenic microorganism.

Conditions: The student demonstrates the ability to obtain a throat culture using the following equipment and supplies: tongue depressor, culture tube with applicator stick or commercially prepared culture collection system, label and requisition form, gloves and mask.

Time Requirements and Accuracy Standards: 5 minutes. Points assigned reflect importance of step to meeting objective: Important = (5) Essential = (10) Critical = (15). Automatic failure results if any of the **critical** tasks are omitted or performed incorrectly.

STANDARD PRECAUTIONS:

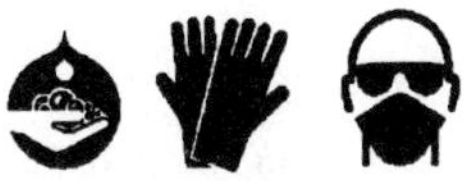

SKILLS ASSESSMENT CHECKLIST

Task Performed	Possible Points	TASKS
☐	10	Identifies patient and explains procedure. Has patient in a seated position. Adjusts good light source.
☐	5	Washes hands. Gathers equipment. Applies mask and gloves.
☐	5	Removes sterile applicator from culture tube.
☐	5	Asks patient to open mouth widely. Depresses tongue with tongue depressor.
☐	15	Swabs the back of the throat and the tonsillar area.
☐	5	*Rationale:* Is certain to obtain a good sample of secretions or exudate from the very back of the throat, paying special attention to redness, rawness, or pustules.
☐	5	Takes separate culture from each side of the throat, if directed by the physician.
☐	10	Removes applicator stick and places in culture tube(s).
☐	5	Removes tongue blade and discards in biohazard waste container.
☐	15	Pushes the applicator stick into the culture medium until the medium compartment is punctured and growth medium is released.
☐	5	*Rationale:* Understands that this keeps the sample alive, because the medium contains nutrients similar to human tissues.
☐	5	Assures patient comfort.
☐	15	Labels culture tube(s) and sends to outside laboratory or processes the specimen according to agency policy.

SKILLS COMPETENCY ASSESSMENT — continued

Procedure 30–23: Procedure for Obtaining a Throat Culture

Task Performed	Possible Points	TASKS
❑	5	Removes gloves and masks. Washes hands.
❑	5	Documents procedure.
❑	5	Completed the tasks within 5 minutes.
❑	15	Results obtained were accurate.

______	Earned	ADD POINTS OF TASKS CHECKED
135	Points	TOTAL POINTS POSSIBLE
______	SCORE	DETERMINE SCORE (divide points earned by total points possible, multiply results by 100)

Actual Student Time Needed to Complete Procedure: ____________

Student's Initials: ____________ Instructor's Initials: ____________ Grade: ____________

Suggestions for Improvement: ____

Evaluator's Name (print) ____

Evaluator's Signature ____

Comments ____

DOCUMENTATION

Chart the procedure in the patient's medical record.

Date: ______________________

Charting: ____

____

Student's Initials: ______________

SKILLS COMPETENCY ASSESSMENT

Procedure 30–24: Performing Nasal Irrigation

Student's Name: ______________________________ Date: ____________

Objective: To perform nasal irrigation to remove a foreign body, relieve inflammation, or increase drainage.

Conditions: The student demonstrates the ability to perform nasal irrigation using the following equipment and supplies: bulb-tip syringe, emesis basin, basins for irrigation solution, towels, nonsterile gloves.

Time Requirements and Accuracy Standards: 10 minutes. Points assigned reflect importance of step to meeting objective: Important = (5) Essential = (10) Critical = (15). Automatic failure results if any of the **critical** tasks are omitted or performed incorrectly.

STANDARD PRECAUTIONS:

SKILLS ASSESSMENT CHECKLIST

Task Performed	Possible Points	TASKS
☐	5	Washes hands and assembles supplies.
☐	5	Identifies patient. Explains the procedure to the patient.
☐	10	Warms irrigation solution to 98.6° F.
☐	10	Positions patient in a seated position with head slightly tilted to facilitate nasal drainage.
☐	5	Places towel across patient's chest and shoulders to absorb solution that may splash.
☐	5	Has the patient hold the emesis basin under the nose.
☐	5	Pours warmed irrigation solution into a basin and withdraws the irrigating solution into the bulb syringe.
☐	15	Inserts the tip of the syringe into the affected nostril and gently squeezes the bulb. Does not occlude nostril.
☐	5	Repeats until the required amount of solution has been used.
☐	5	Assists the patient when complete. Gives the patient a towel to wipe the face.
☐	15	Instructs the patient not to blow the nose for five minutes after the procedure, as blowing the nose could force solution into the sinuses or ears.
☐	5	Disposes of supplies per OSHA guidelines. Washes hands.
☐	5	Documents the procedure.
☐	5	Completed the tasks within 10 minutes.

SKILLS COMPETENCY ASSESSMENT — continued

Procedure 30–24: Performing Nasal Irrigation

Task Performed	Possible Points	TASKS
☐	15	Results obtained were accurate.

______	Earned	ADD POINTS OF TASKS CHECKED
115	Points	TOTAL POINTS POSSIBLE
______	SCORE	DETERMINE SCORE (divide points earned by total points possible, multiply results by 100)

Actual Student Time Needed to Complete Procedure: ____________

Student's Initials: ____________ Instructor's Initials: ____________ Grade: ____________

Suggestions for Improvement: ____________

Evaluator's Name (print) ____________

Evaluator's Signature ____________

Comments ____________

DOCUMENTATION

Chart the procedure in the patient's medical record.

Date: ____________

Charting: ____________

____

____

____

Student's Initials: ____________

SKILLS COMPETENCY ASSESSMENT

Procedure 30-25: Performing Nasal Instillation

Student's Name: ______________________________ Date: ____________

Objective: To provide medication to the nose as ordered by the physician.

Conditions: To perform nasal instillation as ordered by the physician, using the following equipment and supplies: medication as ordered by physician, medicine dropper, cotton balls or 2 × 2 gauze sponges.

Time Requirements and Accuracy Standards: 5 minutes. Points assigned reflect importance of step to meeting objective: Important = (5) Essential = (10) Critical = (15). Automatic failure results if any of the **critical** tasks are omitted or performed incorrectly.

STANDARD PRECAUTIONS:

SKILLS ASSESSMENT CHECKLIST

Task Performed	Possible Points	TASKS
❑	5	Washes hands and assembles equipment.
❑	10	Identifies patient and explains procedure. Positions the patient with the head lower than the shoulders.
❑	5	Instructs patient to keep head tilted back during the procedure to allow medication to cover the nasal tissues.
❑	15	Draws medication into dropper after checking medication three times and checking expiration date.
❑	15	Places the dropper over the center of the affected nostril. Takes care not to touch the inside of the nostril.
❑	5	*Rationale:* Understands that touching the inside of the nostril will lead to contamination of the dropper and possible injury to the patient's mucosa.
❑	5	Repeats the procedure for the other nostril, if required.
❑	5	Instructs patient to remain in position for five minutes.
❑	5	Provides cotton balls or gauze sponges to the patient when the patient returns to seated position. Instructs patient to not blow nose.
❑	5	*Rationale:* Medication may still drain from the nostrils.
❑	5	Disposes of supplies per OSHA guidelines; washes hands; documents procedure.
❑	5	Completed the tasks within 5 minutes.

SKILLS COMPETENCY ASSESSMENT — continued

Procedure 30–25: Performing Nasal Instillation

Task Performed	Possible Points	TASKS
❑	15	Results obtained were accurate.

______	Earned	ADD POINTS OF TASKS CHECKED
100	Points	TOTAL POINTS POSSIBLE
______	SCORE	DETERMINE SCORE (divide points earned by total points possible, multiply results by 100)

Actual Student Time Needed to Complete Procedure: ____________

Student's Initials: ____________ Instructor's Initials: ____________ Grade: ____________

Suggestions for Improvement: ____________

Evaluator's Name (print) ____________

Evaluator's Signature ____________

Comments ____________

DOCUMENTATION

Chart the procedure in the patient's medical record.

Date: ____________

Charting: ____________

____

____

____

Student's Initials: ____________

SKILLS COMPETENCY ASSESSMENT

Procedure 30–26: Obtaining a Sputum Specimen

Student's Name: ______________________________ Date: ____________

Objective: To collect a quality sputum specimen for laboratory analysis to assist in diagnosing disease.

Conditions: The student demonstrates the ability to collect a quality sputum specimen for laboratory analysis using the following equipment and supplies: tissues, small plastic bag to deliver specimen to laboratory, sterile sputum container and label, laboratory requisition, nonsterile gloves, goggles, gown, biohazard waste container.

Time Requirements and Accuracy Standards: 5 minutes. Points assigned reflect importance of step to meeting objective: Important = (5) Essential = (10) Critical = (15). Automatic failure results if any of the **critical** tasks are omitted or performed incorrectly.

STANDARD PRECAUTIONS:

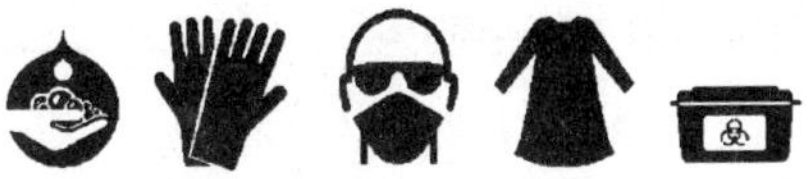

SKILLS ASSESSMENT CHECKLIST

Task Performed	Possible Points	TASKS
☐	5	Washes hands, assembles supplies, and labels container.
☐	15	Identifies patient. Explains procedure to the patient. Instructs patient that if specimen must be collected at home, the container must be closed, labeled with date, time, and patient's name. Tells patient to collect three specimens on three different days if specimen is to be collected for AFB (acid-fast bacillus). Encourages patient to drink plenty of fluids.
☐	5	*Rationale:* Increased fluid intake keeps mucus moist.
☐	10	Puts on gloves, goggles, and gown.
☐	15	Instructs patient to cough deeply and to expectorate directly into the sterile container. Tells patient to take several deep breaths in order to cough up sputum and not saliva.
☐	5	*Rationale:* Understands that cough must be deep because this will bring up secretions from the lungs and bronchial tubes.
☐	15	Secures the top of the container. Fills out laboratory requisition and secures it to the specimen container. Delivers to laboratory within thirty minutes after collection.
☐	5	Disposes of supplies per OSHA guidelines. Washes hands.
☐	5	Documents the procedure.
☐	5	Completed the tasks within 5 minutes.

SKILLS COMPETENCY ASSESSMENT — continued

Procedure 30–26: Obtaining a Sputum Specimen

Task Performed	Possible Points	TASKS
❑	15	Results obtained were accurate.

________	Earned	ADD POINTS OF TASKS CHECKED
100	Points	TOTAL POINTS POSSIBLE
________	SCORE	DETERMINE SCORE (divide points earned by total points possible, multiply results by 100)

Actual Student Time Needed to Complete Procedure: ____________

Student's Initials: ____________ Instructor's Initials: ____________ Grade: ____________

Suggestions for Improvement: ______________________________

Evaluator's Name (print) ______________________________

Evaluator's Signature ______________________________

Comments ______________________________

DOCUMENTATION

Chart the procedure in the patient's medical record.

Date: ____________________

Charting: ______________________________

____

____

____

Student's Initials: ____________

SKILLS COMPETENCY ASSESSMENT

Procedure 30–27: Administer Oxygen By Nasal Cannula for Minor Respiratory Distress

Student's Name: ______________________________ Date: ____________

Objective: To provide a low dose of concentrated oxygen to a patient during periods of respiratory distress (e.g., chronic obstructive pulmonary disease).

Conditions: The student demonstrates the ability to administer oxygen by nasal cannula for minor respiratory distress using the following equipment and supplies: portable oxygen tank with stand, disposable nasal cannula with connecting tube, flowmeter, pressure regulator.

Time Requirements and Accuracy Standards: 5 minutes. Points assigned reflect importance of step to meeting objective: Important = (5) Essential = (10) Critical = (15). Automatic failure results if any of the **critical** tasks are omitted or performed incorrectly.

STANDARD PRECAUTIONS:

SKILLS ASSESSMENT CHECKLIST

Task Performed	Possible Points	TASKS
☐	5	Washes hands.
☐	15	Identifies patient. Explains procedure to patient. • Demonstrates the position of the nasal prongs of the cannula into the nose. Shows how they face upward and the tab rests above the upper lip. • Describes how to clear the oxygen cylinder valve by turning it counterclockwise. • Explains that oxygen supports combustion and that a fire can start with oxygen in use. Instructs that friction, static electricity, or a lighted cigarette or cigar can cause ignition.
☐	15	Opens the cylinder one full turn, counterclockwise. Checks the pressure gauge.
☐	5	*Rationale:* Understands that this will determine the amount of pressure in the cylinder.
☐	10	Attaches the nasal cannula to the tubing and then to the flowmeter.
☐	15	Adjusts the flow rate according to the physician's order.
☐	10	Checks for oxygen flow through the cannula.
☐	5	Places the tips of the cannula into the nares no more than one inch.
☐	5	Adjusts the tubing around the patient's ears and secures it under the chin.
☐	5	Answers patient's questions.
☐	5	Washes hands.
☐	5	Documents the procedure.

SKILLS COMPETENCY ASSESSMENT — continued

Procedure 30–27: Administer Oxygen By Nasal Cannula for Minor Respiratory Distress

Task Performed	Possible Points	TASKS
❑	5	Completed the tasks within 5 minutes.
❑	15	Results obtained were accurate.

_______	Earned	ADD POINTS OF TASKS CHECKED
120	Points	TOTAL POINTS POSSIBLE
_______	SCORE	DETERMINE SCORE (divide points earned by total points possible, multiply results by 100)

Actual Student Time Needed to Complete Procedure: ____________

Student's Initials: ____________ Instructor's Initials: ____________ Grade: ____________

Suggestions for Improvement: ________________________________

Evaluator's Name (print) ________________________________

Evaluator's Signature ________________________________

Comments ________________________________

DOCUMENTATION

Chart the procedure in the patient's medical record.

Date: ____________________

Charting: ________________________________

____

____

____

Student's Initials: ____________

SKILLS COMPETENCY ASSESSMENT

Procedure 30–28: Instructing Patient in Use of Metered Dose Nebulizer

Student's Name: ______________________________ Date: ____________

Objective: To instruct a patient in the correct use of a handheld nebulizer, a device that delivers a fine mist of medication, with or without the use of oxygen, to the respiratory tract, including the lungs.

Conditions: The student demonstrates the ability to instruct a patient in the correct use of a handheld nebulizer using the following equipment and supplies: handheld nebulizer containing medication ordered by the physician.

Time Requirements and Accuracy Standards: 10 minutes. Points assigned reflect importance of step to meeting objective: Important = (5) Essential = (10) Critical = (15). Automatic failure results if any of the **critical** tasks are omitted or performed incorrectly.

STANDARD PRECAUTIONS:

SKILLS ASSESSMENT CHECKLIST

Task Performed	Possible Points	TASKS
❑	5	Washes hands and assembles equipment.
❑	10	Identifies patient.
❑	15	Demonstrates the use of the equipment to the patient, then has the patient repeat the demonstration.
❑	5	Instructs the patient to exhale fully.
❑	10	Instructs the patient to hold the nebulizer upside down and close the mouth, lips, and teeth around the mouthpiece.
❑	10	Instructs the patient to tilt the head back, take a deep breath and at the same time push the bottle against the mouthpiece.
❑	10	Instructs the patient to continue to inhale until the lungs are full.
❑	5	Has patient remove the mouthpiece and slowly exhale.
❑	5	Repeats procedure if the physician has ordered more than one dose.
❑	5	Washes hands.
❑	15	Documents that patient is given written instructions for use and maintenance (clean the inhaler by rinsing mouthpiece in warm water) and that use of the nebulizer has been demonstrated.
❑	5	Completed the tasks within 10 minutes.

SKILLS COMPETENCY ASSESSMENT — continued

Procedure 30–28: Instructing Patient in Use of Metered Dose Nebulizer

Task Performed	Possible Points	TASKS
❑	15	Results obtained were accurate.

________	Earned	ADD POINTS OF TASKS CHECKED
115	Points	TOTAL POINTS POSSIBLE
________	SCORE	DETERMINE SCORE (divide points earned by total points possible, multiply results by 100)

Actual Student Time Needed to Complete Procedure: ____________

Student's Initials: ____________ Instructor's Initials: ____________ Grade: ____________

Suggestions for Improvement: ____________

Evaluator's Name (print) ____________

Evaluator's Signature ____________

Comments ____________

DOCUMENTATION

Chart the procedure in the patient's medical record.

Date: ____________

Charting: ____________

____

____

____

Student's Initials: ____________

SKILLS COMPETENCY ASSESSMENT

Procedure 30–29: Assisting With Spirometry

Student's Name: ______________________________ Date: ____________

Objective: To prepare a patient for spirometry to obtain optimum test results.

Conditions: The student demonstrates the ability to prepare a patient for spirometry to obtain optimum test results using the following equipment and supplies: spirometer, disposable mouthpiece.

Time Requirements and Accuracy Standards: 10 minutes. Points assigned reflect importance of step to meeting objective: Important = (5) Essential = (10) Critical = (15). Automatic failure results if any of the **critical** tasks are omitted or performed incorrectly.

STANDARD PRECAUTIONS:

SKILLS ASSESSMENT CHECKLIST

Task Performed	Possible Points	TASKS
❑	5	Washes hands and assembles equipment.
❑	15	Identifies the patient. Explains the parameters needed for successful completion of the test. • Instructs patient to refrain from the use of bronchodilators for 24 hours prior to test. • Explains that patient must inhale deeply and quickly and exhale quickly and forcibly until no air can be expelled. • Explains to the patient that maximum effort is required for accurate test results.
❑	15	Explains the procedure and equipment to the patient. • Allows the patient to breathe into the machine to become acquainted with the equipment. • Reinforces the importance of good posture during the process. • Explains that when blowing into the mouthpiece, the lips must seal tightly around it.
❑	5	Places the patient in a comfortable position (seated/standing).
❑	10	Instructs the patient not to bend at the waist when blowing into the mouthpiece.
❑	10	Reinforces the inhalation process (deep breaths to fill the lungs to maximum capacity).
❑	10	Instructs the patient to continue to blow into the mouthpiece until instructed to stop.
❑	5	Is supportive and encouraging throughout the test.
❑	5	Washes hands.
❑	5	Attends to patient's needs.

SKILLS COMPETENCY ASSESSMENT — continued

Procedure 30–29: Assisting with Spirometry

Task Performed	Possible Points	TASKS
❑	15	Places the test results on the patient's chart, after review by the physician.
❑	5	Completed the tasks within 10 minutes.
❑	15	Results obtained were accurate.

________	Earned	ADD POINTS OF TASKS CHECKED
120	Points	TOTAL POINTS POSSIBLE
________	SCORE	DETERMINE SCORE (divide points earned by total points possible, multiply results by 100)

Actual Student Time Needed to Complete Procedure: ____________

Student's Initials: ____________ Instructor's Initials: ____________ Grade: ____________

Suggestions for Improvement: ____

Evaluator's Name (print) ____

Evaluator's Signature ____

Comments ____

DOCUMENTATION

Chart the procedure in the patient's medical record.

Date:____________________

Charting:____

____

____

____

Student's Initials:________________

SKILLS COMPETENCY ASSESSMENT

Procedure 30–30: Assisting With Plaster-of-Paris Cast Application

Student's Name: ______________________________ Date: ____________

Objective: To assist physician in cast application.

Conditions: The student demonstrates the ability to assist the physician in cast application using the following equipment and supplies: plaster bandage roll or synthetic tape, container of 75° F water, which is lined with plastic or cloth to catch loose plaster, water, stockinette (3-inch width for arms, 4-inch for leg casts), webril (sheet wadding), bandage, scissors, rubber gloves, sponge rubber for padding.

Time Requirements and Accuracy Standards: 15 minutes. Points assigned reflect importance of step to meeting objective: Important = (5) Essential = (10) Critical = (15). Automatic failure results if any of the **critical** tasks are omitted or performed incorrectly.

STANDARD PRECAUTIONS: 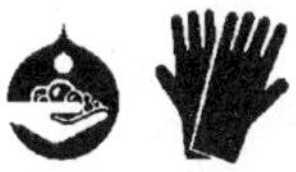

SKILLS ASSESSMENT CHECKLIST

Task Performed	Possible Points	TASKS
☐	5	Provides the patient with an explanation of the procedure.
☐	5	Answers any questions about the injury or cast application within the scope of the medical assistant's training.
☐	5	Washes hands and assembles the equipment and supplies.
☐	5	Positions the patient in a seated position or as required by the physician.
☐	5	Puts on gloves.
☐	10	Cleans and dries the area to be casted, as directed by the physician. Charts any areas of bruising, redness, or open areas.
☐	5	*Rationale:* Knows that appropriate documentation of skin condition is needed to assist in the evaluation of the extremity at a later time.
☐	10	Pads bony prominence with sponge rubber to protect from pressure.
☐	5	Provides the correct width of stockinette for the area on which cast is being applied.
☐	5	*Rationale:* Knows that if stockinette is too large it will form creases, creating possible injury to tissues.
☐	5	Provides physician with correct width of webril.
☐	5	*Rationale:* Knows that webril provides protection to the patient's skin preventing pressure sores, and that folds in the padding could lead to irritation of the skin.
☐	10	Places the bandage in the container of warm water for five seconds. Removes from water and gently squeezes to remove excess water. Does not wring.
☐	5	Assists with the application of cast material as requested by the physician.
☐	5	Reassures patient, as needed.

SKILLS COMPETENCY ASSESSMENT — continued

Procedure 30–30: Assisting With Plaster-of-Paris Cast Application

Task Performed	Possible Points	TASKS
❑	15	After cast application, reviews cast care instructions and provides written instructions for cast care and isometric exercises (if prescribed by the physician). Reinforces any precautions given by the physician. Instructs patient in how to cover cast when bathing. Provides patient with dietary information for bone healing.
❑	5	*Rationale:* Understands that reviewing possible complications with the patient enhances the immediate reporting of circulatory impairment and infection.
❑	5	Discards water down the sink drain, being cautious to keep plaster on the plastic or cloth. Discards plaster in trash receptacle.
❑	5	Cleans work area. Removes gloves and washes hands.
❑	10	Schedules patient for next appointment to have cast checked.
❑	15	Documents the procedure, including skin condition prior to cast application.
❑	5	Completed the tasks within 15 minutes.
❑	15	Results obtained were accurate.

______	Earned	ADD POINTS OF TASKS CHECKED
165	Points	TOTAL POINTS POSSIBLE
______	SCORE	DETERMINE SCORE (divide points earned by total points possible, multiply results by 100)

Actual Student Time Needed to Complete Procedure: ____________

Student's Initials: ____________ Instructor's Initials: ____________ Grade: ____________

Suggestions for Improvement: ____________

Evaluator's Name (print) ____________

Evaluator's Signature ____________

Comments ____________

DOCUMENTATION

Chart the procedure in the patient's medical record.

Date: ____________

Charting: ____________

____

____

Student's Initials: ____________

SKILLS COMPETENCY ASSESSMENT

Procedure 30–31: Assisting With Cast Removal

Student's Name: ______________________________ Date: ____________

Objective: To assist the physician with the removal of a cast.

Conditions: The student demonstrates the ability to assist the physician with the removal of a cast using the following equipment and supplies: cast cutter, cast spreader, bandage scissors, bag for disposal of cast materials.

Time Requirements and Accuracy Standards: 10 minutes. Points assigned reflect importance of step to meeting objective: Important = (5) Essential = (10) Critical = (15). Automatic failure results if any of the **critical** tasks are omitted or performed incorrectly.

STANDARD PRECAUTIONS:

SKILLS ASSESSMENT CHECKLIST

Task Performed	Possible Points	TASKS
☐	5	Washes hands.
☐	10	Explains the cast removal process to the patient. Explains that the cutter vibrates and does not spin and that some pressure and warmth may be experienced.
☐	5	*Rationale:* Explaining procedure allays patient's fears about being cut with the blade.
☐	5	Reassures the patient that skin color and muscle tone will improve with therapy.
☐	5	Hands the physician the equipment, as requested.
☐	15	After procedure, provides patient with written instructions for post-care.
☐	5	Cleans equipment. Washes hands.
☐	15	Documents cast removal and appearance of body part from which cast was removed.
☐	5	Completed the tasks within 10 minutes.
☐	15	Results obtained were accurate.

________	Earned	ADD POINTS OF TASKS CHECKED
85	Points	TOTAL POINTS POSSIBLE
________	SCORE	DETERMINE SCORE (divide points earned by total points possible, multiply results by 100)

SKILLS COMPETENCY ASSESSMENT — continued

Procedure 30–31: Assisting With Cast Removal

Actual Student Time Needed to Complete Procedure: ____________

Student's Initials: ____________ Instructor's Initials: ____________ Grade: ____________

Suggestions for Improvement: ____

Evaluator's Name (print) ____

Evaluator's Signature ____

Comments ____

DOCUMENTATION

Chart the procedure in the patient's medical record.

Date: ____________________

Charting: ____

____

____

____

Student's Initials: ______________

SKILLS COMPETENCY ASSESSMENT

Procedure 30–32: Assisting the Physician During a Lumbar Puncture

Student's Name: ______________________________ Date: ____________

Objective: To assemble supplies and position the patient for removal of cerebrospinal fluid from the lumbar area, which will be sent to the laboratory for analysis.

Conditions: The student demonstrates the ability to assist the physician during a lumbar puncture using the following equipment and supplies: drape, xylocaine 1%–2%, sterile syringe and needle for anesthetic, sterile gloves, disposable sterile lumbar puncture tray to include skin antiseptic with applicator, Band-Aid, spinal puncture needle, three test tubes with corks or tops, drape, manometer, laboratory requisition, examination light.

Time Requirements and Accuracy Standards: 15 minutes. Points assigned reflect importance of step to meeting objective: Important = (5) Essential = (10) Critical = (15). Automatic failure results if any of the **critical** tasks are omitted or performed incorrectly.

STANDARD PRECAUTIONS:

SKILLS ASSESSMENT CHECKLIST

Task Performed	Possible Points	TASKS
☐	15	Reinforces physician's explanation of the procedure and answers questions. Reviews post-spinal tap instructions, including: • The patient should remain in a prone position for two to three hours to allow tissues to close over the puncture site and to minimize cerebrospinal fluid leakage. • Reinforce the need to increase fluid intake, as this helps replace fluid loss. • Report any severe headaches or alterations in neurological status (paralysis, numbness, tingling, and so on).
☐	15	Verifies that the patient has signed a consent form.
☐	5	Instructs the patient to empty the bladder and bowel.
☐	15	Washes hands and sets up sterile field for the physician.
☐	10	Cleans the puncture site with antiseptic soap and water. Rinses.
☐	10	Positions the patient in a lateral recumbent position with the back at the edge of the exam table and a small pillow under the head.
☐	5	*Rationale:* Understands that patient's alignment of the spine is best achieved in a horizontal position.
☐	5	Drapes patient for warmth and privacy.
☐	10	Has the patient draw the knees up to the abdomen and grasp onto knees, flexing chin on chest.

SKILLS COMPETENCY ASSESSMENT — continued

Procedure 30–32: Assisting the Physician During a Lumbar Puncture

Task Performed	Possible Points	TASKS
❑	5	*Rationale:* Understands that this position allows for easier needle insertion into the subarachnoid space of the spinal cord, because this position widens the space between the lumbar vertebrae.
❑	15	The physician will swab the puncture site with an antiseptic such as Betadine.
❑	5	The physician drapes the area with a fenestrated drape.
❑	15	Assists physician to aspirate anesthetic.
❑	10	Helps the patient maintain this position until the needle has reached the subarachnoid space.
❑	5	*Rationale:* Understands that patient movement could produce trauma to the spinal cord area.
❑	15	Reminds patient to breathe evenly, not to hold breath or talk, since this may interfere with the pressure reading.
❑	5	At the physician's direction, has the patient straighten the legs.
❑	5	*Rationale:* Understands that muscle tension can give false pressure reading.
❑	5	The physician will apply a Band-Aid to the puncture site after the procedure is completed. Assists patient into a prone position to rest for two to three hours, or as directed by the physician.
❑	5	Applies gloves. Caps specimens tightly. Labels samples with date and numbers CSF #1, #2, #3.
❑	5	Sends the specimen to the laboratory with the appropriate laboratory requisition. Stores in incubator.
❑	5	Cleans area using standard precautions. Removes gloves. Washes hands.
❑	10	Documents procedure in patient's chart, noting that specimen will be sent to a reference laboratory, and notes any patient problems or unusual occurrences.
❑	5	Completed the tasks within 15 minutes.
❑	15	Results obtained were accurate.

_______	Earned	ADD POINTS OF TASKS CHECKED
220	Points	TOTAL POINTS POSSIBLE
_______	SCORE	DETERMINE SCORE (divide points earned by total points possible, multiply results by 100)

Actual Student Time Needed to Complete Procedure: ____________

Student's Initials: ____________ Instructor's Initials: ____________ Grade: ____________

Suggestions for Improvement: ____________

Evaluator's Name (print) ____________

Evaluator's Signature ____________

Comments ____________

DOCUMENTATION

Chart the procedure in the patient's medical record.

Date: ____________

Charting: ____________

____

____

____

Student's Initials: ____________

SKILLS COMPETENCY ASSESSMENT

Procedure 30–33: Assisting the Physician With a Neurological Screening Examination

Student's Name: ______________________________ Date: __________

Objective: To determine a patient's neurological status.

Conditions: The student demonstrates the ability to assist in determining a patient's neurological status using the following equipment and supplies: percussion hammer, safety pin, material for odor identification, cotton ball, tuning fork, flashlight, tongue blade, ophthalmoscope.

Time Requirements and Accuracy Standards: 10 minutes. Points assigned reflect importance of step to meeting objective: Important = (5) Essential = (10) Critical = (15). Automatic failure results if any of the **critical** tasks are omitted or performed incorrectly.

STANDARD PRECAUTIONS:

SKILLS ASSESSMENT CHECKLIST

Task Performed	Possible Points	TASKS
❑	5	Washes hands and assembles equipment.
❑	15	Identifies patient. Informs the patient that the purpose of the exam is to assess the response to pain and touch reflexes and other neurological functions. Explains that the physician will use several supplies to test the function of each cranial nerve and to test the reflexes and coordination of the patient.
❑	15	Performs a mental status examination when taking the patient's medical history by observing the following: when taking patient's history, pays special attention to level of awareness, memory, cognition, and mood; notes if behavior is appropriate for the circumstances when the patient answers questions during the history-taking.
❑	10	The physician will evaluate the cranial nerve functions by using the results of the visual acuity tests, as well as results of other tests.
❑	5	Assists the patient as needed during the exam.
❑	5	Cleans equipment per standard precautions and washes hands.
❑	10	Documents patient problems, such as disorientation, confusion, or forgetfulness that are evident when taking the patient's history.
❑	5	Completed the tasks within 10 minutes.

Task Performed	Possible Points	TASKS
❑	15	Results obtained were accurate.

_______		Earned	ADD POINTS OF TASKS CHECKED
	85	Points	TOTAL POINTS POSSIBLE
_______		SCORE	DETERMINE SCORE (divide points earned by total points possible, multiply results by 100)

Actual Student Time Needed to Complete Procedure: ___________

Student's Initials: ___________ Instructor's Initials: ___________ Grade: ___________

Suggestions for Improvement: ___________

Evaluator's Name (print) ___________

Evaluator's Signature ___________

Comments ___________

DOCUMENTATION

Chart the procedure in the patient's medical record.

Date: ___________

Charting: ___________

____

____

____

Student's Initials: ___________

EVALUATION OF CHAPTER KNOWLEDGE

How has your instructor evaluated the knowledge you have achieved?

Knowledge	Instructor Evaluation *Good*	*Average*	*Poor*
Describes pediatric care, including measuring height, weight, head, chest circumference, and vital signs	_____	_____	_____
Lists supplies needed for a gynecological examination with and without a Pap test	_____	_____	_____
Discusses the importance of self-breast and self-testicular examinations and describes how each is performed	_____	_____	_____
Describes how to perform urinary catheterization on a female patient	_____	_____	_____
States proper protocol when collecting urine for drug screening	_____	_____	_____
Describes patient preparation for occult blood testing	_____	_____	_____
Discusses patient instructions for the upper GI series, a barium enema, and a cholescystogram	_____	_____	_____
Differentiates between an instillation and an irrigation	_____	_____	_____
Discusses the different types of visual acuity tests and how to use each appropriately	_____	_____	_____
Explains the medical assistant's role when assisting with audiometry	_____	_____	_____
Describes how to perform a nasal irrigation	_____	_____	_____
Describes the proper use of a metered dose nebulizer	_____	_____	_____
Discusses the role of the medical assistant during spirometry	_____	_____	_____
Explains the medical assistant's role in cast application and cast removal and the guidelines for cast care	_____	_____	_____
Lists items required by the physician for a neurological exam and explains the medical assistant's role in assisting in the exam	_____	_____	_____
Identifies patient education information for sputum collections	_____	_____	_____
Explains oxygen administration using a nasal cannula	_____	_____	_____
Applies principles of aseptic technique and observes standard precautions for infection control	_____	_____	_____
Properly prepares patients for procedures	_____	_____	_____
Performs selected tests that assist the physician with diagnosis and treatment	_____	_____	_____
Properly prepares and administers medications as directed by the physician	_____	_____	_____
Maintains medical records and documents accurately	_____	_____	_____
Exhibits therapeutic communications skills in interaction with patients and attends to patients' emotional needs	_____	_____	_____
Communicates at the level proper for the receiver's ability to understand	_____	_____	_____

Student's Initials: ______ Instructor's Initials: ______

Grade: _______

CHAPTER 31

Electrocardiography

PERFORMANCE OBJECTIVES

Electrocardiography is a noninvasive, safe, and painless procedure many physicians include as part of a complete physical examination. An electrocardiogram (ECG) measures the amount of electrical activity produced by the heart and the time it takes for the electrical impulses to travel through the heart during each heartbeat. The ECG is used in conjunction with other laboratory and diagnostic tests to assess total cardiac health. During an electrocardiogram, the medical assistant is responsible for patient preparation; patient education; operation of the electrocardiograph; elimination of artifacts; mounting, labeling, and placing the ECG reading in the patient's medical record; and proper maintenance and care of the equipment. It is important that the medical assistant perform electrocardiograms skillfully and accurately.

EXERCISES AND ACTIVITIES

Vocabulary Builder

Across

2. A series of X-rays of a blood vessel(s) following injection of a radiopaque substance.
5. The part of the heart cycle in which the heart is in contraction.
6. The flat, horizontal line that separates the various waves of the ECG cycle.
10. Chemical substance that enhances the conduction of electrical activity.
11. Conversion of a pathological cardiac rhythm (arrhythmia) to normal sinus rhythm.
12. Local and temporary lack of blood to an organ or a part due to obstruction of circulation.
16. Procedure used to obtain cardiac blood samples, detect abnormalities, and determine intracardiac pressure.
23. Heated slender wire of the electrocardiograph that melts the wax off the ECG paper during the recording.
24. Graphic record usually of an event that changes with time, as with the electrical activity of the heart.

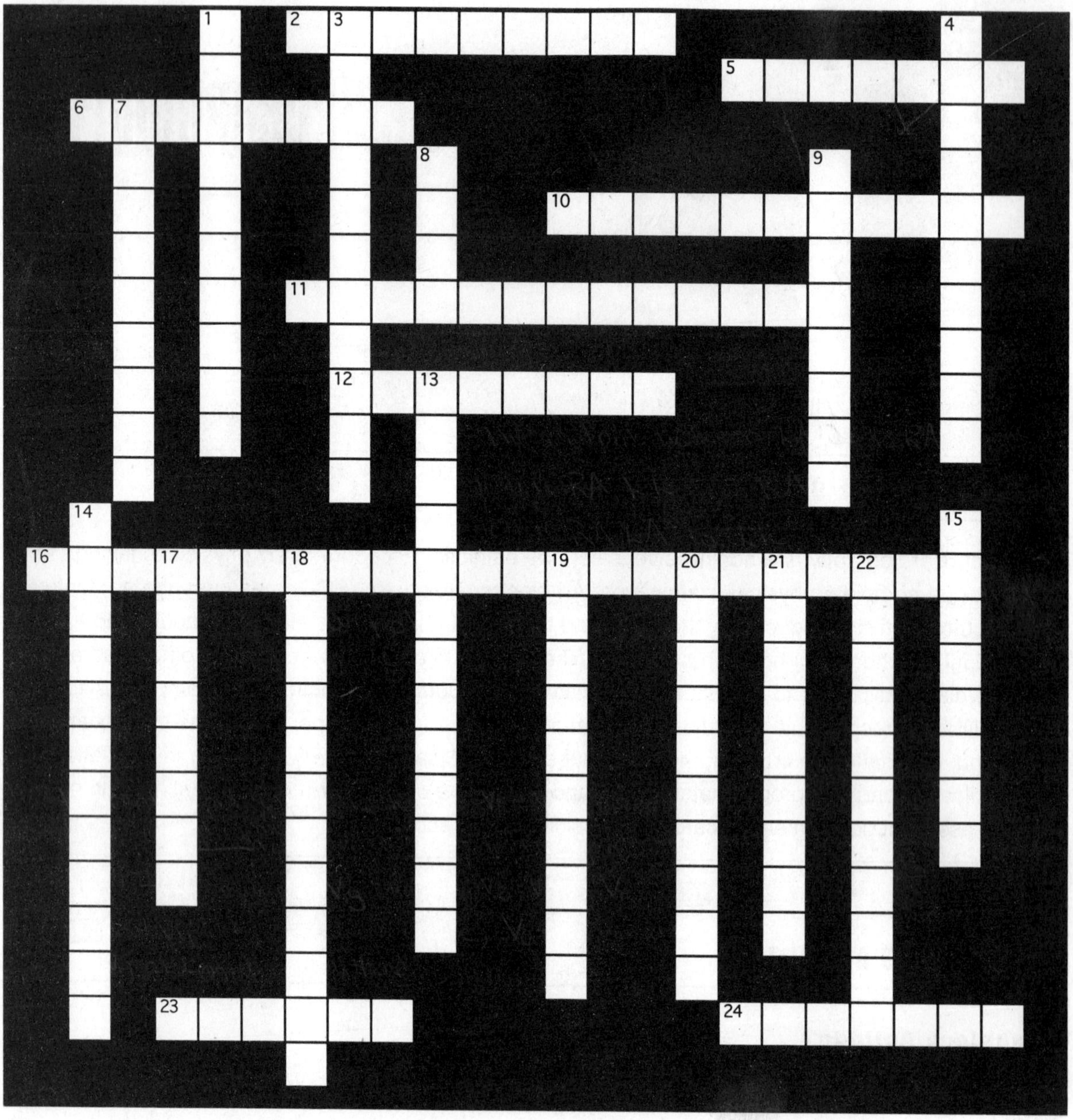

Down

1. Pertaining to the area on the anterior surface of the body overlying the heart.
3. Procedures that do not require entering the body or puncturing the skin.
4. Sensor used to conduct electricity from the body to the electrocardiograph.
7. To add or increase.
8. An electrocardiograph record. Consists of limb and chest.
9. Process of applying in sequence a portion of each of the twelve leads of the ECG recording onto a document placed in the patient's chart.
13. Applications of electric current to the heart, directly or indirectly, to alter a disturbance in cardiac rhythm.
14. Mechanism in the electrocardiograph that changes the voltage into a mechanical motion for recording purposes.

SKILLS COMPETENCY ASSESSMENT

Procedure 31–1: Perform Twelve-Lead Electrocardiogram, Single Channel

Student's Name: ______________________________ Date: ____________

Objective: To perform a twelve-lead electrocardiogram, single channel.

Conditions: The student demonstrates the ability to obtain an accurate, graphic, artifact-free reading of the electrical activity of the patient's heart so that the physician may identify arrhythmias; estimate damage caused by MI; assess effects of cardiac medication; determine if electrolyte imbalance is present; identify cardiac ischemia; and determine the effects of hypertension or other disorders on the heart. The student uses the following equipment and supplies: examination or ECG table with pillow and sheet or blanket, patient gown, single-channel electrocardiograph with patient cable wires, electrolyte (gel, lotion, paste, or presaturated pads), ECG tracing paper, metal electrodes, rubber straps, gauze squares, and a mounting form.

Time Requirements and Accuracy Standards: 15 minutes. Points assigned reflect importance of step to meeting objective: Important = (5) Essential = (10) Critical = (15). Automatic failure results if any of the **critical** tasks are omitted or performed incorrectly.

STANDARD PRECAUTIONS:

SKILLS ASSESSMENT CHECKLIST

Task Performed	Possible Points	TASKS
❑	5	Performs tracing in a quiet, warm, and comfortable room away from electrical equipment that may cause artifacts.
❑	5	*Rationale:* Patient is less apprehensive in a quiet atmosphere. Alternating current (AC) interference is minimized when ECG is performed away from electrical equipment.
❑	10	Washes hands, gathers equipment, identifies the patient, and explains the procedure to the patient.
❑	5	*Rationale:* Following these universal steps minimizes transmission of microorganisms and reassures patient.
❑	5	Has the patient remove clothing from the waist up and uncover lower legs (stockings must be removed but socks may be worn); provides a sheet or blanket for privacy and warmth. Places the patient in a supine position on the examination table with arms and legs supported.
❑	5	*Rationale:* All four limbs and chest must be uncovered for proper electrode placement. Electrodes must be placed on bare skin for optimum conductivity of electricity.
❑	5	Explains that the procedure is painless and explains why it is necessary not to move or talk during the procedure.
❑	5	*Rationale:* Patient cooperation ensures good quality tracing.

SKILLS COMPETENCY ASSESSMENT — continued

Procedure 31–1: Perform Twelve-Lead Electrocardiogram, Single Channel

Task Performed	Possible Points	TASKS
❑	10	Places the electrocardiograph with the power cord pointing away from the patient. Does not allow the cable to go underneath the table.
❑	5	*Rationale:* This helps reduce AC interference.
❑	15	Applies the limb electrodes by first connecting the rubber straps to the tabs on the electrodes; applies a pea-size dab of electrolyte to the electrode; applies the electrodes to the fleshy parts of the four limbs; rubs the electrolytes into the patient's skin; makes sure the lead connectors of the electrodes are pointing toward the feet; pulls the rubber straps around the limb until they just meet, then pulls tighter one more hole and secures.
❑	5	*Rationale:* A more stable connection with the lead wires is possible when the lead connectors point to the feet. Electrolyte rubbed into the patient's skin helps ensure a good contact between the electrode and the skin. Straps applied too tightly or too loosely can cause artifacts. By applying electrodes to the fleshy part of the limbs, artifacts are minimized.
❑	10	Welch cup chest electrode • Applies electrolyte to chest position. Rubs the edge of each cup in the electrolyte, securing the cups in position by squeezing the bulb end of the cup to create suction on the skin of the chest wall.
❑	15	Welch cup chest electrode with a single channel non-automatic machine • Places chest lead V-1 in position, along with the first 6 leads: I, II, III, aVR, aVL, and aVF, and records. • Turns machine to "AMP OFF" and positions next V lead. Adjusts stylus. Turns machine to "AMP ON" and records six to eight inches of the V lead. Turns machine to "AMP OFF." • Repeats procedure until each V lead is manually positioned and recorded.
❑	10	Tightly connects the lead wires to the electrodes; makes sure to connect the correct lead wires to the correct electrodes; makes sure the lead wires follow the patient's body contour.
❑	5	*Rationale:* Following body contour minimizes artifacts.
❑	5	Makes sure the patient cable is supported either on the table or the patient's abdomen; plugs the patient cable into the electrocardiograph.
❑	5	Turns instrument to ON position.

Task Performed	Possible Points	TASKS
❑	10	Makes sure the lead selector switch is on STD; centers the stylus; makes sure the record switch is on Run. Checks the standardization for the instrument by quickly pressing the standardization button; makes sure the standardization mark is 10 mm or 10 small squares high.
❑	5	*Rationale:* Standardization ensures a dependable and accurate tracing.
❑	15	Centers the stylus and runs about four to five inches of each lead I, II, and III by placing the record switch on Run and turning the lead selector switch appropriately. • Makes sure the stylus and recording are near the center of the paper while recording. Adjusts using position control knob, if necessary. • Watches for artifacts and corrects if present. • Determines if a change in standard or stylus position is needed by observing the amplitude of the R wave.
❑	10	Continues with leads aVR, aVL, aVF, and records about four to five inches of each lead by turning the lead selector to the appropriate position.
❑	15	Records six to eight complexes of each of the V leads by turning the lead selector control to the appropriate position.
❑	10	Places another standardization at the end of the tracing by putting the lead selector on STD and depressing the button; runs the tracing through the instrument and turns the machine to the OFF position; removes the tracing from the instrument and immediately labels with patient's name, date, and time of day; initials; unplugs power cord.
❑	5	Disconnects the lead wires and removes the rubber straps and electrodes from the patient.
❑	5	Cleans patient's skin to remove paste or gel electrolyte.
❑	5	Assists patient as needed.
❑	5	Provides physician with uncut tracing.
❑	5	Cleans and returns equipment per OSHA guidelines.
❑	5	Washes hands.
❑	5	Documents procedure.
❑	5	Cuts and mounts the tracing, remembering to handle it correctly; labels appropriately and places in patient's record.
❑	5	Completed the tasks within 15 minutes.

SKILLS COMPETENCY ASSESSMENT — continued

Procedure 31–1: Perform Twelve-Lead Electrocardiogram, Single Channel

Task Performed	Possible Points	TASKS
❑	15	Results obtained were accurate.

_______	Earned	ADD POINTS OF TASKS CHECKED
225	Points	TOTAL POINTS POSSIBLE
_______	SCORE	DETERMINE SCORE (divide points earned by total points possible, multiply results by 100)

Actual Student Time Needed to Complete Procedure: ____________

Student's Initials: ____________ Instructor's Initials: ____________ Grade: ____________

Suggestions for Improvement: ____

Evaluator's Name (print) ____

Evaluator's Signature ____

Comments ____

DOCUMENTATION

Chart the procedure in the patient's medical record.

Date: ____________________

Charting: ____

____

____

Student's Initials: ____________________

SKILLS COMPETENCY ASSESSMENT

Procedure 31–2: Perform Twelve-Lead Electrocardiogram, Three Channel

Student's Name: ______________________________ Date: ____________

Objective: To perform a twelve-lead electrocardiogram, three channel

Conditions: The student demonstrate the ability to obtain an accurate, graphic, artifact-free reading of the electrical activity of the patient's heart so that the physician may identify arrhythmias, estimate damage caused by MI, assess effects of cardiac medication, determine if electrolyte imbalance is present, identify cardiac ischemia, and determine the effects of hypertension on or other disorders of the heart. The student uses the following equipment and supplies: examination or ECG table with pillow and sheet or blanket, patient gown, three-channel automatic electrocardiograph with patient cable wires, disposable electrodes, ECG tracing paper, gauze squares, and mounting form.

Time Requirements and Accuracy Standards: 10 minutes. Points assigned reflect importance of step to meeting objective: Important = (5) Essential = (10) Critical = (15). Automatic failure results if any of the **critical** tasks are omitted or performed incorrectly.

STANDARD PRECAUTIONS:

SKILLS ASSESSMENT CHECKLIST

Task Performed	Possible Points	TASKS
☐	10	Washes hands; gathers equipment; identifies patient and explains procedure.
☐	5	Has patient remove clothing from the waist up and uncover lower legs. Places patient in supine position on examination table with arms and legs supported.
☐	5	Explains that procedure is painless and why the patient must not talk or move during the procedure. Places electrocardiograph appropriately.
☐	10	Prepares patient's skin for disposable electrode attachment; if patient's skin is oily, wipes electrode area with alcohol and lets dry.
☐	15	Applies electrodes firmly to fleshy parts of limbs; points tabs of electrodes attached to arms in a downward position, tears off electrodes attached to legs in an upward position.
☐	5	*Rationale:* Tab position allows for better connection and keeps lead wire pulling to a minimum.
☐	10	Locates chest sites and applies electrodes with tabs pointing in a downward position.
☐	10	Connects lead wires to the electrodes with alligator clips.
☐	10	Plugs patient cable into machine; supports patient cable to avoid pulling or tangling.
☐	10	Turns on the ECG; enters patient data by keying it into machine.
☐	5	Presses AUTO for automatic and runs the ECG to obtain the tracing; watches for artifacts and takes the appropriate steps to eliminate them, should they occur.
☐	5	Disconnects the lead wires and removes the electrodes from the patient; disposes of the electrodes.

SKILLS COMPETENCY ASSESSMENT — continued

Procedure 31–2: Perform Twelve-Lead Electrocardiogram, Three Channel

Task Performed	Possible Points	TASKS
❑	5	Assists patient as needed.
❑	5	Provides physician with uncut tracing.
❑	5	Cleans and returns equipment per OSHA guidelines.
❑	5	Washes hands.
❑	5	Documents procedure.
❑	15	Cuts and mounts the tracing, remembering to handle carefully. Labels appropriately and places in patient's record.
❑	5	Completed the tasks within 10 minutes.
❑	15	Results obtained were accurate.

________	Earned	ADD POINTS OF TASKS CHECKED
160	Points	TOTAL POINTS POSSIBLE
________	SCORE	DETERMINE SCORE (divide points earned by total points possible, multiply results by 100)

Actual Student Time Needed to Complete Procedure: ____________

Student's Initials: ____________ Instructor's Initials: ____________ Grade: ____________

Suggestions for Improvement: ____________

Evaluator's Name (print) ____________

Evaluator's Signature ____________

Comments ____________

DOCUMENTATION

Chart the procedure in the patient's medical record.

Date: ____________

Charting: ____________

____

____

Student's Initials: ____________

SKILLS COMPETENCY ASSESSMENT

Procedure 31–3: Perform Holter Monitor Application

Student's Name: ______________________________ Date: __________

Objective: To perform a Holter monitor application.

Conditions: The student demonstrates the ability to perform a Holter monitor application using the following equipment and supplies: Holter monitor, patient activity diary, blank magnetic tape, disposable electrodes, razor, alcohol swabs, gauze, tape, carrying case, belt or shoulder strap.

Time Requirements and Accuracy Standards: 15 minutes. Points assigned reflect importance of step to meeting objective: Important = (5) Essential = (10) Critical = (15). Automatic failure results if any of the **critical** tasks are omitted or performed incorrectly.

STANDARD PRECAUTIONS:

SKILLS ASSESSMENT CHECKLIST

Task Performed	Possible Points	TASKS
☐	5	Washes hands and assembles equipment.
☐	10	Prepares the equipment by removing old (used) battery from the monitor and replacing it with a new battery; inserts a blank magnetic tape into the monitor.
☐	5	*Rationale:* Installing a new battery each 24-hour period will ensure that the monitor will function because it will have sufficient power.
☐	5	Washes hands.
☐	10	Identifies the patient and explains the procedure.
☐	5	*Rationale:* Adherence to patient guidelines helps ensure an accurate tracing.
☐	5	Has patient remove clothing from the waist up.
☐	5	Has patient sit on the examination table or chair.
☐	5	*Rationale:* This allows for patient comfort and relaxation and for the medical assistant to appropriately place the electrodes.
☐	15	Locates the correct electrode placement on the chest wall; prepares the skin in the following way: • Dry shaves the patient's chest at each electrode site, if chest is hairy. • Rubs the shaved area with an alcohol swab; lets area dry. • Abrades the skin slightly with a dry 4 × 4 gauze. Areas should be red.
☐	5	*Rationale:* Shaved site and abraded skin help electrodes adhere better to the skin and facilitate easier removal.

SKILLS COMPETENCY ASSESSMENT — continued

Procedure 31–3: Perform Holter Monitor Application

Task Performed	Possible Points	TASKS
❑	5	Takes the electrodes from the package and peels away the backing from one of them; continues to remove electrodes one by one and attach correctly.
❑	10	Applies adhesive-backed electrodes to the appropriate sites by applying firm pressure at the center of the electrode and moving outward toward the edges; runs fingers along the outer rim to ensure attachment. Avoids moving from one side of electrode to the other to keep gel from being forced out, causing interference.
❑	5	*Rationale:* Firmly attached electrodes ensure a good-quality tracing.
❑	5	Attaches the lead wires to the electrodes; connects them to the patient cable.
❑	5	Secures each electrode with adhesive tape.
❑	5	*Rationale:* The tape secures the electrodes by reducing the tugging and pulling on them.
❑	10	Plugs the monitor into an electrocardiograph with the test cable; runs a baseline tracing.
❑	5	*Rationale:* Running a baseline tracing will validate proper setup of electrodes and confirm that there is no malfunction of the leads or cable.
❑	5	Places the electrode cable so it extends from between the buttons of the patient's shirt or from below the bottom of the shirt.
❑	15	Places the recorder into its carrying case and either attaches it to the patient's belt or over the patient's shoulder; makes sure there is no pulling on the lead wires.
❑	5	*Rationale:* Pulling on electrodes could cause them to become detached.
❑	10	Plugs the electrode cable into the monitor; records the starting time in the patient's activity log.
❑	5	*Rationale:* The beginning time is noted is order to correlate cardiac activity with the patient's activity log.
❑	15	Gives the activity log to the patient, being certain the patient information is completed.
❑	5	*Rationale:* The activity log helps correlate cardiac activity with the patient's symptoms.
❑	5	Informs the patient what time the following day the monitor will be removed; reminds the patient to bring along the activity log.
❑	5	Washes hands.
❑	5	Documents the procedure in the patient's record.
❑	5	Completed the tasks within 15 minutes.

Task Performed	Possible Points	TASKS
☐	15	Results obtained were accurate.

_______	Earned	ADD POINTS OF TASKS CHECKED
220	Points	TOTAL POINTS POSSIBLE
_______	SCORE	DETERMINE SCORE (divide points earned by total points possible, multiply results by 100)

Actual Student Time Needed to Complete Procedure: ___________

Student's Initials: ___________ Instructor's Initials: ___________ Grade: ___________

Suggestions for Improvement: ___________

Evaluator's Name (print) ___________

Evaluator's Signature ___________

Comments ___________

DOCUMENTATION

Chart the procedure in the patient's medical record.

Date: ___________

Charting: ___________

____

____

Student's Initials: ___________

EVALUATION OF CHAPTER KNOWLEDGE

How has your instructor evaluated the knowledge you have achieved?

Knowledge	Instructor Evaluation *Good*	*Average*	*Poor*
Follows the circulation of blood through the heart, starting at the vena cava	_____	_____	_____
Describes the electrical conduction system of the heart	_____	_____	_____
Identifies reasons a patient requires an electrocardiogram	_____	_____	_____
Identifies the various positive and negative deflections and describes what each represents in the cardiac cycle	_____	_____	_____
Explains the purpose of standardization of the electrocardiograph	_____	_____	_____
Identifies the twelve leads of an ECG and describes what area of the heart each lead represents	_____	_____	_____
States the function of ECG graph paper, electrodes (sensors), and electrolyte	_____	_____	_____
Describes various types of ECGs and describes their capabilities	_____	_____	_____
Explains each type of artifact and how each can be eliminated	_____	_____	_____
Names and describes the purposes of the various cardiac diagnostic tests	_____	_____	_____
Identifies the placement of Holter monitor electrodes	_____	_____	_____
Describes the reason for a patient activity diary during ambulatory cardiography	_____	_____	_____
Identifies common arrhythmias and explains the causes of each	_____	_____	_____
Explains how to calculate heart rates from an ECG tracing	_____	_____	_____
Identifies a common coding system used to code each lead on an ECG tracing	_____	_____	_____
Describes the procedure for mounting an ECG tracing	_____	_____	_____
Documents accurately	_____	_____	_____
Prepares patient for procedures and attends to his or her emotional needs	_____	_____	_____

Student's Initials: _____ Instructor's Initials: _____

Grade: _______

CHAPTER 32

Introduction to the Medical Laboratory

PERFORMANCE OBJECTIVES

Along with clinical laboratory personnel, medical assistants perform a key role in laboratory testing. Medical assistants may be responsible for patient preparation and instruction, obtaining specimens, and testing or sending specimens to a laboratory. It is important that medical assistants have a knowledge of laboratory procedures, perform quality controls, and observe standard precautions for infection control to ensure accurate testing and to safeguard the health of patients and health care personnel. When collecting, processing, or analyzing specimens, medical assistants are aiding in the physician's diagnosis and treatment of conditions and illnesses. Attention to detail and accuracy are essential skills for the medical assistant to possess in performing duties in the medical laboratory.

EXERCISES AND ACTIVITIES

Vocabulary Builder

A. *Insert the proper key vocabulary terms into the sentences below. Each sentence describes a situation you might find in a physician's office laboratory, or in a reference laboratory.*

assay	normal flora	baseline
objective	biopsy	glucose
quantitative tests	condenser	serum
diagnosis	invasive	clinical diagnosis
profile	control test	diaphragm
reagents	qualitative tests	requisition
differential diagnosis	electrolytes	asymptomatic

1. Wanda Slawson, CMA, is examining a specimen in the lab using a compound microscope. The objective is the lense system closest to the specimen she is viewing.

2. Dr. Mark Woo orders laboratory tests for a female emergency patient suffering severe abdominal cramps to make a differential diagnosis that will distinguish between a diagnoses of appendicitis or an ovarian cyst.
3. Ralph Samson receives a job offer from a construction company that requires all employees to be tested for misuse or abuse of legal or illegal drugs before they can work on the site. Bruce Goldman, CMA, performs Ralph's blood test under the direction of Dr. Whitney; his test comes back clean. The results of Ralph's test can be used in the future as a ______________________ measurement, a record of healthy normal results.
4. Dr. King needs a red blood cell count, a white blood cell count, and a platelet count for Maria Jover. Joe Guerrero, CMA, performs a venipuncture on Maria and sends a tube of her blood to the lab, along with a written ______________________ containing specific information and instructions about what tests to perform on the specimens.
5. Bruce Goldman, CMA, is examining a specimen under a compound microscope. Because he is having difficulty seeing clearly, Bruce opens the microscope's______________________ to increase the amount of light on the specimen.
6. Dr. Lewis asks Audrey Jones, CMA, to send a tube of Herb Fowler's blood to the laboratory for analysis. Dr. Lewis wants to determine the constituents and relative proportion of each of the enzymes in Herb's serum; this type of analysis is called an ______________________.
7. Jim Marshall comes to see Dr. Lewis complaining that he has been constantly tired for the past two or three months. Because Jim's symptoms are so vague, Dr. Lewis orders a blood ______________________ to help narrow the diagnosis possibilities.
8. Bruce Goldman, CMA, always follows standard precautions and washes his hands before touching a patient. Although everyone's body contains many natural microorganisms, called ______________________, aseptic handwashing lessens the potential for exposure to or transmission of pathogens.
9. Hematology laboratories count the white blood cells (WBC) or red blood cells (RBC) in a sample of a patient's blood. In general, these type of counting tests are known as ______________________.
10. As a method of quality control, a ______________________ sample is tested along with a patient's sample as a method of ensuring the accuracy of test results.
11. Joe Guerrero, CMA, asks Abigail Johnson, whom he knows is diagnosed with diabetes mellitus, whether she regularly tests her blood at home to measure her ______________________ level.
12. The hematology laboratory performs tests that measure characteristics of blood such as size, shape, and maturity of cells. These types of tests are known in general as________________.
13. Histology is the study of tissue samples to determine disease. In most cases, a frozen tissue sample or ________________ is sliced, stained, and microscopically examined for anomalies.

SKILLS COMPETENCY ASSESSMENT

Procedure 32-1: Using the Microscope

Student's Name: ______________________________ Date: ____________

Objective: To properly use a microscope.

Conditions: The student demonstrates the ability to use a microscope properly to view microscopic organisms using the coarse and fine adjustments as well as the low- and high-power and oil objectives. The student uses the following equipment and supplies: hand disinfectant, microscope (monocular or binocular), lens paper, prepared slides, immersion oil, surface disinfectant. Note: Procedure will vary slightly according to microscope design. Consult the operating procedure in the microscope manual for specific instructions.

Time Requirements and Accuracy Standards: 20 minutes. Points assigned reflect importance of step to meeting objective: Important = (5) Essential = (10) Critical = (15). Automatic failure results if any of the **critical** tasks are omitted or performed incorrectly.

STANDARD PRECAUTIONS:

SKILLS ASSESSMENT CHECKLIST

Task Performed	Possible Points	TASKS
☐	5	Washes hands.
☐	5	Assembles equipment and materials.
☐	5	Cleans the ocular(s) and objectives with lens paper.
☐	10	Uses the coarse adjustment to raise the nosepiece unit.
☐	5	Raises the condenser knob as far as possible by turning the condenser knob.
☐	5	Rotates the 10× objective into position, so it is directly over the opening in the stage.
☐	5	Turns on the microscope light.
☐	5	Opens the diaphragm until maximum light comes up through the condenser.
☐	5	Places the slide on the stage, specimen side up, and secures with clips.
☐	5	Condenser is positioned so it is almost touching the bottom of the slide.
☐	5	Locates the coarse adjustment.
☐	5	Looks directly at the stage and 10× objective and turns the coarse objective until the objective is as close to the slide as it will go.
☐	5	Stops turning when the objective no longer moves.
☐	5	*Rationale:* Understands not to lower any objective toward a slide while looking through the ocular(s).

SKILLS COMPETENCY ASSESSMENT — continued

Procedure 32-1: Using the Microscope

Task Performed	Possible Points	TASKS
❑	15	Looks into the ocular(s) and slowly turns the coarse adjustment in the direction to raise the objective (or lower the stage) until the object on the slide comes into view.
❑	5	Locates the fine adjustment.
❑	10	Turns the fine adjustment to sharpen the image.
		Adjusts oculars for each individual's eyes if a binocular microscope is used:
	❑ 5	• Adjusts the distance between the oculars so one image is seen.
	❑ 5	• Uses the coarse and fine adjustments to bring the object into focus while looking through the right ocular with the right eye.
	❑ 5	• Closes the right eye, looks into the left ocular with the left eye, and uses the knurled collar on the left ocular to bring the object into sharp focus. Does not turn the coarse or fine adjustment at this time.
	❑ 5	• Looks into the oculars with both eyes to observe that the object is in clear focus. If not, repeats procedure.
	20 Points	(subtotal for adjusting oculars with binocular microscope)
❑	10	• Uses the stage knobs the move the slide left and right and backward and forward while looking through the ocular(s), or • Moves the slide with the fingers while looking through the ocular(s) (for a microscope without a movable stage).
❑	10	Rotates the 40× objective into position while observing the objective and slide to see that the objective does not strike the slide.
❑	5	Looks through the ocular(s) to view the object on the slide.
❑	5	Locates the fine adjustment.
❑	15	Looks through the ocular(s) and turns the fine adjustment until the object in focus. Does not use coarse adjustment.
❑	5	Scans the slide, using the fine adjustment to keep the object is in focus if necessary.
❑	5	Rotates the oil-immersion objective to the side slightly (so that no objective is in position).
❑	10	Places one drop of immersion oil on the portion of the slide that is directly over the condenser.
❑	5	Rotates the oil-immersion objective into position and is careful not to rotate the 45× objective through the oil.

Task Performed	Possible Points	TASKS
❑	15	Looks to see that the oil-immersion objective is touching the drop of oil.
❑	5	Looks through the ocular(s) and slowly turns the fine adjustment until the image is clear. Uses only the fine adjustment to focus the oil-immersion objective.
❑	5	Scans the slide.
❑	10	Rotates the 10× objective into position. Does not allow the 45× objective to touch the oil.
❑	15	Removes the slide from the microscope stage and gently cleans the oil from the objective with clean lens paper.
❑	10	Cleans the oculars, 10× objective and 45× objective with clean lens paper.
❑	15	Cleans the 100× objective with lens paper to remove all oil.
❑	15	Cleans any oil from the microscope stage and condenser.
❑	5	Turns off the microscope light and disconnects.
❑	5	Positions the nosepiece in the lowest position, using the coarse adjustment.
❑	5	Centers the stage so it does not project from either side of the microscope.
❑	5	Covers the microscope and returns it to storage.
❑	5	Cleans the work area; returns slides to storage.
❑	5	Washes hands.
❑	5	Completed the tasks within 20 minutes.
❑	15	Results obtained were accurate.

________	Earned	ADD POINTS OF TASKS CHECKED
335	Points	TOTAL POINTS POSSIBLE (Binocular +20)
________	SCORE	DETERMINE SCORE (divide points earned by total points possible, multiply results by 100)

Actual Student Time Needed to Complete Procedure: ____________

Student's Initials: ____________ Instructor's Initials: ____________ Grade: ____________

Suggestions for Improvement: ____

Evaluator's Name (print) ____

Evaluator's Signature ____

Comments ____

EVALUATION OF CHAPTER KNOWLEDGE

Knowledge	Instructor Evaluation *Good*	*Average*	*Poor*
Explains the purposes of laboratory testing	_____	_____	_____
Understands the differences and similarities between independent laboratories and physician's office laboratories	_____	_____	_____
Identifies departments within the medical laboratory and lists the types of testing performed within each department	_____	_____	_____
Knows nine of the most common laboratory profiles and the body system that each covers	_____	_____	_____
Understands quality control programs in the medical laboratory	_____	_____	_____
Knows the general safety rules within the medical laboratory	_____	_____	_____
Knows how to fill out a laboratory requisition form	_____	_____	_____
Understands the information required on a written laboratory requisition form	_____	_____	_____
Can explain the function of and identify the parts of a compound microscope	_____	_____	_____
Understands how to properly use and care for a compound microscope	_____	_____	_____
Follows all standard precautions	_____	_____	_____

Student's Initials: ______ Instructor's Initials: ______

Grade: _______

Task Performed	Possible Points	TASKS
❑	5	*Rationale:* Understands that hand veins have a greater tendency to roll.
❑	5	Completed the tasks within 10-20 minutes.
❑	15	Results obtained were accurate.
	_______	Earned ADD POINTS OF TASKS CHECKED
	130	Points TOTAL POINTS POSSIBLE
	_______	SCORE DETERMINE SCORE (divide points earned by total points possible, multiply results by 100)

Actual Student Time Needed to Complete Procedure: _______

Student's Initials: _______ Instructor's Initials: _______ Grade: _______

Suggestions for Improvement: _______

Evaluator's Name (print) _______

Evaluator's Signature _______

Comments _______

SKILLS COMPETENCY ASSESSMENT

Procedure 33-2: Venipuncture by Syringe Procedure

Student's Name: ______________________________ Date: ____________

Objective: To obtain venous blood acceptable for laboratory testing, as required by a physician. To aliquot venous blood collected into evacuated tubes and/or special collection containers.

Conditions: Students demonstrate the ability to obtain and aliquot venous blood using the following equipment: gloves, goggles and mask, syringes, disposable needle for syringe (21- or 22-gauge needle), evacuated tubes(s) or special collection tube(s), tourniquet, 70 percent isopropyl alcohol swab, gauze or cotton balls, adhesive bandage or tape, and sharps and biohazard waste containers.

Time Requirements and Accuracy Standards: 15 minutes. Points assigned reflect importance of step to meeting objective: Important = (5) Essential = (10) Critical = (15). Automatic failure results if any of the **critical** tasks are omitted or performed incorrectly.

STANDARD PRECAUTIONS:

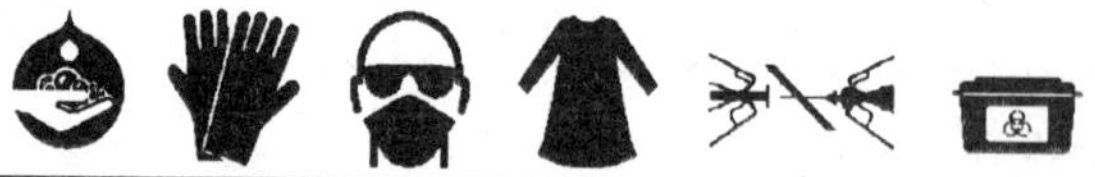

SKILLS ASSESSMENT CHECKLIST

Task Performed	Possible Points	TASKS
☐	15	Positions and identifies the patient, asking patient's name and verifying it with the computer label or identification number.
☐	10	Verifies compliance with fasting instructions, if appropriate.
☐	5	Washes hands.
☐	5	Puts on gloves and, if potential for blood spatter is present, puts on goggles and mask.
☐	5	Opens the sterile needle and syringe packages, attaching the needle if necessary.
☐	10	Prevents the plunger from sticking by pulling it halfway out and pushing it all the way in one time.
☐	10	Selects the proper tube(s) to transfer the blood after collection.
☐	10	Finds the vein and applies the tourniquet.
☐	5	Instructs patient to close hand.
☐	5	*Rationale:* Patient should not pump hand, as this action will change the values of the laboratory tests.
☐	10	Places patient's hand in a downward position.
☐	10	Selects a vein, noting location and direction of the vein.
☐	10	Cleans the venipuncture site with a 70 percent isopropyl alcohol swab in a circular motion from the center outward.

Task Performed	Possible Points	TASKS
❑	15	Does not touch venipuncture site.
❑	10	Draws patient's skin taut with thumb, placing thumb one to two inches below the puncture site.
❑	10	Positions the bevel of the needle up and lines up the needle with the vein.
❑	10	Enters the vein approximately ¼ inch below the vein location at the point where the vein was palpated.
❑	5	Pushes needle into the skin.
❑	5	Feels the "pop" (sense of resistance followed by easy penetration), stops, and does not move.
❑	10	Takes the opposite hand and pulls gently on the plunger of syringe. Pulls only as fast as the syringe will fill with blood.
❑	5	*Rationale:* Pulling too hard or too fast will cause the vein to collapse temporarily. If the vein collapses, stops pulling on plunger and lets the vein refill with blood.
❑	5	Pulls plunger back until the desired amount of blood is obtained.
❑	5	Asks patient to open hand.
❑	5	Releases tourniquet.
❑	5	Lightly places sterile gauze or cotton ball above the venipuncture site.
❑	5	Removes needle from the patient's arm.
❑	5	Applies pressure to site for three to five minutes. May ask patient to assist by elevating arm above heart level.
❑	15	Aliquots blood into appropriate tube(s). Punctures the stopper of the evacuated tube with the syringe needle and allows the blood to enter the tube freely until the flow stops. Does not push on plunger. Mixes if any anticoagulant is present.
❑	5	Immediately discards the syringe and needle in the appropriate waste containers.
❑	5	*Rationale:* All sharps must be discarded in a sharps container.
❑	5	Discards the gauze and other waste in biohazard containers.
❑	15	Labels all tubes before leaving the examination room.
❑	5	Applies adhesive bandage.
❑	5	Removes and discards gloves, goggles, and mask in biohazard container.
❑	5	Washes hands.
❑	5	Documents procedure.

SKILLS COMPETENCY ASSESSMENT — continued

Procedure 33-2: Venipuncture by Syringe Procedure

Task Performed	Possible Points	TASKS
❑	5	Completed the tasks within 15 minutes.
❑	15	Results obtained were accurate.

________		Earned	ADD POINTS OF TASKS CHECKED
	295	Points	TOTAL POINTS POSSIBLE
________		SCORE	DETERMINE SCORE (divide points earned by total points possible, multiply results by 100)

Actual Student Time Needed to Complete Procedure: ____________

Student's Initials: ____________ Instructor's Initials: ____________ Grade: ____________

Suggestions for Improvement: ____

Evaluator's Name (print) ____

Evaluator's Signature ____

Comments____

DOCUMENTATION

Chart the procedure in the patient's medical record.

Date:____________________________

Charting: ____

____

____

Student's Initials:________________

SKILLS COMPETENCY ASSESSMENT

Procedure 33-3: Venipuncture by Evacuated Tube System

Student's Name: ______________________________ Date: ____________

Objective: To obtain venous blood acceptable for laboratory testing, as required by a physician.

Conditions: Students demonstrate the ability to obtain venous blood using the following equipment: gloves, goggles and mask, evacuated tube holder, disposable needle for evacuated system (20-, 21-, or 22-gauge needle), evacuated tube(s) or special collection tube(s), tourniquet, 70 percent isopropyl alcohol swab, gauze or cotton balls, adhesive bandage or tape, and sharps and biohazard waste containers.

Time Requirements and Accuracy Standards: 15 minutes. Points assigned reflect importance of step to meeting objective: Important = (5) Essential = (10) Critical = (15). Automatic failure results if any of the **critical** tasks are omitted or performed incorrectly.

STANDARD PRECAUTIONS:

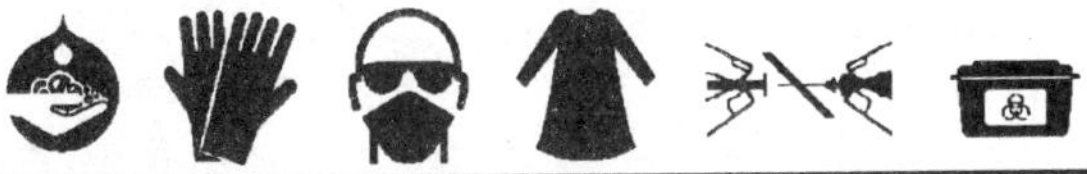

SKILLS ASSESSMENT CHECKLIST

Task Performed	Possible Points	TASKS
☐	5	Positions and identifies the patient, asking patient's name and verifying it with the computer label or identification number. Verifies compliance with fasting instructions, if appropriate.
☐	5	Washes hands and puts on gloves. Puts on goggles and mask if potential for blood spatter is present.
☐	5	Assembles equipment. Assembles tubes in correct order of draw and keeps extra tubes on hand.
☐	5	*Rationale:* Access to extra tubes is important in the event of a faulty vacuum.
☐	5	Breaks needle seal. Threads the appropriate needle into the holder using the needle sheath as a wrench.
☐	10	Before using, taps all tubes containing additives to ensure that all additive is dislodged from the stopper and wall of the tube.
☐	5	Inserts the tube into the holder until the needle slightly enters the stopper.
☐	5	*Rationale:* Avoids pushing the needle beyond the recessed guideline, because a loss of vacuum may result.
☐	5	If tube retracts slightly, leaves it in the retracted position to avoid prematurely puncturing the rubber stopper.
☐	5	Applies tourniquet.
☐	5	Instructs patient to close hand.

SKILLS COMPETENCY ASSESSMENT — continued

Procedure 33-3: Venipuncture by Evacuated Tube System

Task Performed	Possible Points	TASKS
❑	5	*Rationale:* Patient must not be allowed to pump the hand, as this action will change the values of the laboratory tests.
❑	10	Places patient's arm in a downward position.
❑	10	Selects a vein, noting its location and direction.
❑	10	Cleans the venipuncture site with a 70 percent isopropyl alcohol swab.
❑	15	Does not touch venipuncture site.
❑	10	Draws patient's skin taut with thumb, placing thumb one to two inches below the puncture site.
❑	15	Positions the bevel of the needle up and lines up the needle with the vein.
❑	10	Punctures the vein. Removes hand from drawing skin taut. Grasps the flange of the evacuated tube holder and pushes the tube forward until the butt end of the needle punctures the stopper.
❑	15	Does not change hands while performing venipuncture. The hand performing the venipuncture is the hand that holds the evacuated tube holder; the other hand manipulates the tubes.
❑	5	Fills the tube until the vacuum is exhausted and blood flow into the tube ceases.
❑	5	*Rationale:* Ensures the proper blood-to-anticoagulant ratio.
❑	10	When blood flow ceases, removes the tube from the holder. Grasps the evacuated tube holder securely with one hand and changes the tubes with the other hand. The shutoff valve recovers the point, stopping the flow of blood until the next tube of blood is inserted.
❑	10	Immediately mixes each tube containing an additive by inverting the tube five to ten times to provide adequate mixing without causing hemolysis.
❑	10	Asks patient to open hand. Releases the tourniquet. Lightly places sterile gauze or cotton ball above the venipuncture site.
❑	15	Removes needle from the arm. Checks to make sure that the last tube drawn was removed from the holder before removing the needle.
❑	5	*Rationale:* This prevents blood from dripping off the tip of the needle.
❑	5	Applies pressure to site for three to five minutes. May ask patient to assist by elevating arm above heart level to reduce blood flow.

Task Performed	Possible Points	TASKS
❑	15	Immediately discards the needle and disposable tube holders in the appropriate waste containers.
❑	5	*Rationale:* All sharps must be discarded in a sharps container.
❑	15	Labels all tubes at the patient's side before leaving the examination room.
❑	5	Applies adhesive bandage.
❑	5	Removes and discards gloves, goggles, and mask in a biohazard container.
❑	5	Washes hands.
❑	5	Documents the procedure.
❑	5	Completed the tasks within 15 minutes.
❑	15	Results obtained were accurate.

________	Earned	ADD POINTS OF TASKS CHECKED
300	Points	TOTAL POINTS POSSIBLE
________	SCORE	DETERMINE SCORE (divide points earned by total points possible, multiply results by 100)

Actual Student Time Needed to Complete Procedure: ____________

Student's Initials: ____________ Instructor's Initials: ____________ Grade: ____________

Suggestions for Improvement: ________________________________

Evaluator's Name (print) ________________________________

Evaluator's Signature ________________________________

Comments ________________________________

DOCUMENTATION

Chart the procedure in the patient's medical record.

Date:________________________

Charting: ________________________________

____

____

Student's Initials:______________

SKILLS COMPETENCY ASSESSMENT

Procedure 33-4: Venipuncture by Butterfly Needle System

Student's Name: ______________________________ Date: ____________

Objective: To obtain venous blood acceptable for laboratory testing, as required by a physician.

Conditions: Students demonstrate the ability to obtain venous blood using the following equipment: gloves, goggles and mask, evacuated tube holder, disposable needle for evacuated system (21-, 23-, or 25-gauge needle with or without leur adapter), evacuated tube(s) or special collection tube(s), tourniquet, 70 percent isopropyl alcohol swab, gauze or cotton balls, adhesive bandage or tape, and sharps and biohazard waste containers.

Time Requirements and Accuracy Standards: 15 minutes. Points assigned reflect importance of step to meeting objective: Important = (5) Essential = (10) Critical = (15). Automatic failure results if any of the **critical** tasks are omitted or performed incorrectly.

STANDARD PRECAUTIONS:

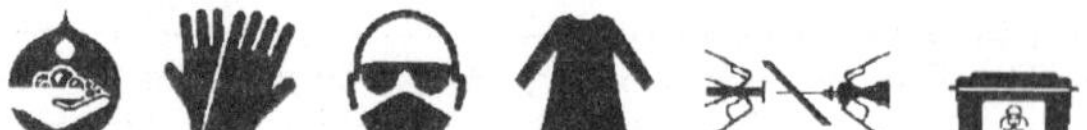

SKILLS ASSESSMENT CHECKLIST

Task Performed	Possible Points	TASKS
With Evacuated Tube Leur Adapter		
☐	10	Positions and identifies the patient, asking the patient's name and verifying it with the computer label or identification number. Verifies compliance with fasting instructions, if appropriate.
☐	5	Washes hands and puts on gloves. Puts on goggles and mask if potential for blood spatter is present.
☐	5	Assembles equipment.
☐	5	Opens the butterfly needle system package with evacuated tube leur adapter. Screws leur into the evacuated tube holder. Threads the leur needle into the holder.
☐	5	Before using, taps all tubes that contain additives to ensure that all additive is dislodged from the stopper and wall of the tube.
☐	10	Inserts the tube into the holder until the needle slightly enters the stopper. Avoids pushing the needle beyond the recessed guideline.
☐	5	*Rationale:* Understands that pushing beyond the recessed guideline may result in a loss of vacuum.
☐	5	If tube retracts slightly, leaves in the retracted position.
☐	5	Applies the tourniquet.
☐	5	Asks patient to close the hand and places the patient's arm in a downward position.
☐	5	*Rationale:* Does not allow patient to pump hand, as pumping the hand will change the values of laboratory tests.
☐	10	Selects a vein, noting its location and direction.
☐	10	Cleans the venipuncture site with a 70 percent isopropyl alcohol swab.
☐	15	Does not touch the venipuncture site.
☐	10	Draws the patient's skin taut with the thumb; places the thumb one to two inches below the puncture site.
☐	10	Holds the wings of the butterfly with the bevel up. Lines up with needle with the vein and performs the venipuncture. Removes hand from drawing the skin taut.
☐	5	Grasps the flange of the evacuated tube holder and pushes the tube forward until the butt end of the needle punctures the stopper.
☐	10	Fills the tube until the vacuum is exhausted and blood flow into the tube ceases.

Task Performed	Possible Points	TASKS
❑	5	*Rationale:* Understands that this will assure the proper blood-to-anticoagulant ratio. Due to air in the tubing, a loss of approximately 0.5 mL will result when collecting the initial evacuated tube.
❑	5	When the blood flow ceases, removes the tube from the holder. While securely grasping the evacuated tube holder with one hand, uses the other hand to change the tubes.
❑	5	*Rationale:* The shutoff valve recovers the point, stopping the flow of blood until the next tube of blood is inserted. Multiple draws require the same order of draw as an evacuated system draw.
❑	10	After drawing, immediately mixes each tube that contains an additive. Gently inverts the tube five to ten times providing adequate mixing without causing hemolysis.
❑	5	Asks the patient to open hand and releases tourniquet.
❑	5	Lightly places a sterile gauze square or cotton ball above the venipuncture site.
❑	5	Removes the needle from the arm. Is certain to remove the last tube drawn before removing the needle.
❑	5	*Rationale:* This prevents blood from dripping off the tip of the needle.
❑	5	Applies pressure to the site for three to five minutes. Asks patient to assist by elevating the arm above heart level to reduce blood flow.
❑	15	Immediately discards the needle and disposable butterfly assembly in the appropriate waste containers.
❑	5	*Rationale:* All sharps must be discarded in a sharps container.
❑	15	Labels all tubes at the patient's side before leaving the examination room.
❑	5	Applies an adhesive bandage.
❑	5	Removes and discards gloves, goggles, and mask in a biohazard container.
❑	5	Washes hands.
❑	5	Documents procedure.
❑	5	Completed the tasks within 15 minutes.
❑	15	Results obtained were accurate.

______	Earned	ADD POINTS OF TASKS CHECKED
260	Points	TOTAL POINTS POSSIBLE
______	SCORE	DETERMINE SCORE (divide points earned by total points possible, multiply results by 100)

By Syringe

Task Performed	Possible Points	TASKS
❑	10	Positions and identifies the patient, asking the patient's name and verifying it with the computer label or identification number. Verifies compliance with fasting instructions, if appropriate.
❑	5	Washes hands and puts on gloves. Puts on goggles and mask if potential for blood spatter is present.
❑	5	Assembles equipment.
❑	5	Opens the butterfly needle system package. Attaches syringe.
❑	5	Before using, taps all tubes that contain additives to ensure that all additive is dislodged from the stopper and wall of the tube.
❑	10	Inserts the tube into the holder until the needle slightly enters the stopper. Avoids pushing the needle beyond the recessed guideline.
❑	5	*Rationale:* Understands that pushing beyond the recessed guideline may result in a loss of vacuum.
❑	5	If tube retracts slightly, leaves in the retracted position.
❑	5	Applies the tourniquet.
❑	5	Asks patient to close the hand and places the patient's arm in a downward position.

SKILLS COMPETENCY ASSESSMENT — continued

Procedure 33-4: Venipuncture by Butterfly Needle System

Task Performed	Possible Points	TASKS
❑	5	*Rationale:* Does not allow patient to pump hand, as pumping the hand will change the values of laboratory tests.
❑	10	Selects a vein, noting its location and direction.
❑	10	Cleans the venipuncture site with a 70 percent isopropyl alcohol swab.
❑	15	Does not touch the venipuncture site.
❑	10	Draws the patient's skin taut with the thumb; places the thumb one to two inches below the puncture site.
❑	10	Holds the wings of the butterfly with the bevel up. Lines up with needle with the vein and performs the venipuncture. Removes hand from drawing the skin taut.
❑	5	Draws blood with a butterfly system
❑	15	Aliquots blood into appropriate tube(s). Punctures the stopper of the evacuated tube with the syringe needle and allows the blood to enter the tube freely until the flow stops. Does not push on plunger. Mixes if any anticoagulant is present.
❑	5	Immediately discards the syringe and needle in the appropriate waste containers.
❑	5	*Rationale:* All sharps must be discarded in a sharps container.
❑	15	Labels all tubes before leaving the examination room.
❑	5	Applies an adhesive bandage.
❑	5	Removes and discards gloves, goggles, and mask in a biohazard container.
❑	5	Washes hands.
❑	5	Documents procedure.
❑	5	Completed the tasks within 15 minutes.
❑	15	Results obtained were accurate.

______	Earned	ADD POINTS OF TASKS CHECKED
210	Points	TOTAL POINTS POSSIBLE
______	SCORE	DETERMINE SCORE (divide points earned by total points possible, multiply results by 100)

Actual Student Time Needed to Complete Procedure: ____________

Student's Initials: ____________ Instructor's Initials: ____________ Grade: ____________

Suggestions for Improvement: ____________________________________

Evaluator's Name (print) ____________________________________

Evaluator's Signature____________________________________

Comments ____________________________________

DOCUMENTATION

Chart the procedure in the patient's medical record.

Date:____________________

Charting: ____________________________________

____

____

Student's Initials:____________

EVALUATION OF CHAPTER KNOWLEDGE

How has your instructor evaluated the knowledge you have achieved?

	Instructor Evaluation		
Knowledge	*Good*	*Average*	*Poor*
Understands the principles and usage of venipuncture procedures	_____	_____	_____
Identifies and describes venipuncture equipment and techniques	_____	_____	_____
Demonstrates understanding of the physiology of the circulatory system	_____	_____	_____
Differentiates between serum and plasma	_____	_____	_____
Describes purpose of additives and anticoagulants	_____	_____	_____
Demonstrates ability to respond correctly to adverse patient reactions to venipuncture	_____	_____	_____
Recalls vein stimulation techniques	_____	_____	_____
Identifies correct color-coded tubes used with specific anticoagulants	_____	_____	_____
Identifies correct order of draw for blood collection	_____	_____	_____
Facilitates therapeutic communication with patients, putting them at ease during venipuncture	_____	_____	_____
Observes aseptic technique and standard precautions for infection control, including proper disposal of sharps	_____	_____	_____
Understands effects of factors on accurate laboratory test results	_____	_____	_____
Possesses the ability to handle and process acceptable specimens for accurate analysis in the laboratory	_____	_____	_____

Student's Initials: ______ Instructor's Initials: ______

Grade: ________

CHAPTER 34

Hematology

PERFORMANCE OBJECTIVES

Hematology is the study of the blood in both normal and diseased states. As a diagnostic tool hematological tests are invaluable to the physician in determining illness, evaluating a patient's progress, and deciding upon treatment modalities. The most common hematological tests include: hemoglobin, hematocrit, white blood cell count, red blood cell count, platelet count, differential white blood cell count, erythrocyte sedimentation rate, and prothrombin time. Included in the study of hematology is the study of hemopoiesis, the formation of blood cells. It is important for the clinical medical assistant to understand the process of hemopoiesis, normal blood values, and how to perform various blood collection and testing procedures. Following safety and quality control guidelines will protect medical assistants and others and contribute to the accuracy of test results.

EXERCISES AND ACTIVITIES

Vocabulary Builder

A. To test your spelling skills, unscramble the key vocabulary terms below:

1. LETEMCOP ODBOL UNTOC ____________________
2. HEYOSRYTETCR ____________________
3. OCHYTREEMAMET ____________________
4. HOPINLOISE ____________________
5. LOBEHOMYPINHGOAT ____________________
6. RAYMOCPOHCITL ANSITS ____________________
7. MOTHEGLYAO ____________________
8. TIRCCMIOYC ____________________
9. YSNCAITSIOOS ____________________
10. DEEPINCAM LIPRINCEP ____________________
11. TYKULESOCE ____________________

SKILLS COMPETENCY ASSESSMENT

Procedure 34–1: Hemoglobin Determination (Manual Method Using a Spectrophotometer)

Student's Name: ______________________________ Date: ____________

Objective: To properly and safely perform a manual hemoglobin determination.

Conditions: The student demonstrates the ability to properly and safely perform a manual hemoglobin determination using a spectrophotometer to evaluate the oxygen-carrying capacity of the blood, using the following equipment and supplies: gloves, hand disinfectant, EDTA blood sample(s), spectrophotometer, hemoglobin standard solution, cuvettes, laboratory stretch film, 10 percent chlorine bleach solution, UNOHEME® hemoglobin system or supplies for manual hemoglobin, biohazard container. Consult operating manual for specific instructions for spectrophotometer.

Time Requirements and Accuracy Standards: 20 minutes. Points assigned reflect importance of step to meeting objective: Important = (5) Essential = (10) Critical = (15). Automatic failure results if any of the **critical** tasks are omitted or performed incorrectly.

STANDARD PRECAUTIONS:

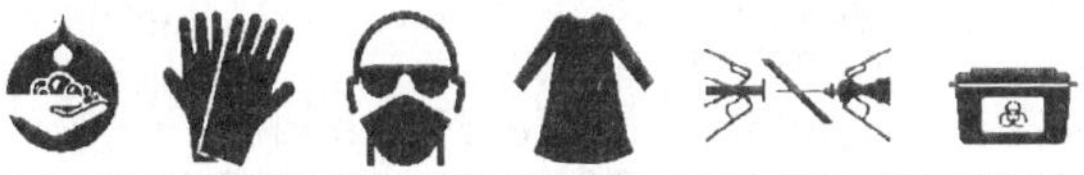

SKILLS ASSESSMENT CHECKLIST

Task Performed	Possible Points	TASKS
☐	5	Washes hands and puts on gloves.
☐	5	Assembles equipment and materials.
☐	10	Turns on spectrophotometer, sets wavelength at 540 nm.
		UNOHEME® Method
☐	5	Draws 20 μL of well-mixed blood into the UNOHEME capillary.
☐	15	Inserts capillary into UNOHEME reservoir and draws blood into reagent. Rinses capillary several times, taking care not to overflow pipette.
☐	5	Mixes contents by swirling; lets sit five minutes.
☐	10	Transfers contents of reservoir to a cuvette.
☐	15	Places diluting fluid from an unused UNOHEME reservoir into a cuvette labeled "blank."
☐	5	Pipettes 5 mL of a hemoglobin standard into cuvette labeled "Std."
	55	(Subtotal for UNOHEME® Method)
		or
		Manual Method
☐	5	Labels test tubes blank, standard, and unknown.

SKILLS COMPETENCY ASSESSMENT — continued

Procedure 34–1: Hemoglobin Determination (Manual Method Using a Spectrophotometer)

Task Performed	Possible Points	TASKS		
		❑	15	Dispenses 5.0 mL of Drabkins reagent into blank and unknown tubes and 5.0 mL of hemoglobin standard into standard tube.
		❑	10	Mixes blood samples for two minutes.
		❑	5	Draws up 0.02 mL of blood with micropipette, wiping off excess blood.
		❑	5	Dispenses blood sample into unknown tube.
		❑	15	Mixes contents thoroughly and lets stand for at least ten minutes.
			55	(Subtotal for Manual Method)
❑	10	Transfers contents of the tubes to cuvettes.		
❑	15	Places "blank" cuvette in spectrophotometer well; sets absorbance to zero following manufacturer's instructions.		
❑	10	Places "standard" cuvette into spectrophotometer well; reads and records absorbance.		
❑	10	Places "sample" cuvette into spectrophotometer well; reads and records absorbance.		
❑	15	Uses proper formula to calculate hemoglobin concentration; records results.		
❑	5	Properly discards specimens and disposes of waste in biohazard container.		
❑	5	Disinfects and cleans equipment and work area. Returns equipment to storage.		
❑	5	Removes gloves; properly disposes of gloves in biohazard container; washes hands with disinfectant soap.		
❑	10	Documents procedure.		
❑	5	Completed the tasks within 20 minutes.		
❑	15	Results obtained were accurate.		

________	Earned	ADD POINTS OF TASKS CHECKED
180	Points	TOTAL POINTS POSSIBLE
________	SCORE	DETERMINE SCORE (divide points earned by total points possible, multiply results by 100)

Actual Student Time Needed to Complete Procedure: ____________

Student's Initials: ____________ Instructor's Initials: ____________ Grade: ____________

Suggestions for Improvement: ____

Evaluator's Name (print) ____

Evaluator's Signature ____

Comments ____

DOCUMENTATION

Record test results in the patient's medical record.

Date: ____________________________

Charting: ____

____

____

Student's Initials: ________________

SKILLS COMPETENCY ASSESSMENT

Procedure 34–2: Hemoglobin Determination (Hemoglobin Analyzer)

Student's Name: ______________________________ Date: ____________

Objective: To properly and safely perform an automated hemoglobin determination.

Conditions: The student demonstrates the ability to properly and safely perform an automated hemoglobin determination to evaluate the oxygen capacity of the blood using the following equipment and supplies: gloves; hand disinfectant; 10 percent chlorine bleach solution; capillary puncture equipment or blood samples collected in EDTA; HbDirect™ System, HemoCue®, or other hemoglobin analyzer with appropriate supplies; biohazard container; sharps container.

Time Requirements and Accuracy Standards: 20 minutes. Points assigned reflect importance of step to meeting objective: Important = (5) Essential = (10) Critical = (15). Automatic failure results if any of the **critical** tasks are omitted or performed incorrectly.

STANDARD PRECAUTIONS: 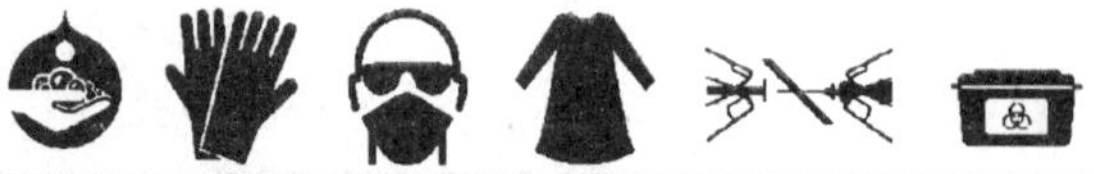

SKILLS ASSESSMENT CHECKLIST

Task Performed	Possible Points	TASKS
❑	5	Washes hands and puts on gloves.
❑	5	Assembles equipment and materials.
❑	5	Turns on, warms up, and calibrates or standardizes instruments following manufacturer's instructions.
❑	10	Performs a capillary puncture observing Bloodborne Pathogen Standards. Wipes away the first drop of blood with tissue or sterile cotton ball.
❑	15	Collects blood from puncture into capillary tube or cuvette appropriate for analyzer being used; avoids trapping air bubbles.
❑	5	Wipes off excess blood without touching open end of device.
		HbDirect™
❑	5	Inserts filled capillary tube into a cyanmethemoglobin vial and caps tightly.
❑	15	Inverts five to ten times to empty vial of blood; lets stand for five minutes at room temperature.
❑	10	Inverts vial slowly, holds horizontally for three seconds, slowly returns to upright position.
❑	5	Positions vial so capillary tube is at the back of the vial.
❑	5	Wipes fingerprints from sides of vial.
❑	5	Checks that the reagent vial is tightly capped.
❑	10	Properly inserts into Hemoglobin Analyzer.
❑	5	*Rationale:* Understands that following proper steps for insertion ensures that the analyzer light path is not obstructed.

Task Performed	Possible Points	TASKS		
		❑	5	Waits five seconds, reads the analyzer display; checks that capillary tube remains in upper half of vial.
			65	(Subtotal for Hb Direct™ Method)
		or		
		HemoCue®		
		❑	15	Inserts filled cuvette into HemoCue® photometer within ten minutes of filling.
		❑	10	Reads and records hemoglobin value.
			25	(Subtotal for HemoCue® Method)
❑	5	Properly disposes of contaminated waste in biohazard container.		
❑	5	Returns all equipment to proper storage.		
❑	5	Cleans and disinfects counters.		
❑	5	Removes gloves; properly disposes of gloves in biohazard container; washes hands with disinfectant soap. Documents procedure.		
❑	5	Completed the tasks within 20 minutes.		
❑	15	Results obtained were accurate.		

_______	Earned	ADD POINTS OF TASKS CHECKED
150	Points	TOTAL POINTS POSSIBLE FOR HbDIRECT™
110	Points	TOTAL POINTS POSSIBLE FOR HEMOCUE® METHOD
_______	SCORE	DETERMINE SCORE (divide points earned by total points possible, multiply results by 100)

Actual Student Time Needed to Complete Procedure: ____________

Student's Initials: ____________ Instructor's Initials: ____________ Grade: ____________

Suggestions for Improvement: ______________________________

Evaluator's Name (print) ______________________________

Evaluator's Signature ______________________________

Comments ______________________________

DOCUMENTATION

Record test results in the patient's medical record.

Date: ______________________

Charting: ______________________________

____

____

Student's Initials: ______________

SKILLS COMPETENCY ASSESSMENT

Procedure 34–3: Microhematocrit

Student's Name: ______________________________ Date: __________

Objective: To properly and safely perform the microhematocrit procedure.

Conditions: The student demonstrates the ability to properly and safely perform the microhematocrit procedure using a few microliters of blood in a capillary tube to separate the cellular elements of the blood from the plasma by centrifugation, using the following equipment and supplies: gloves; hand disinfectant; capillary tubes, plain and with heparin; acrylic safety shield; precalibrated capillary tubes (optional); sealing clay or disposable plastic sealing caps; microhematocrit centrifuge and reader; tube of anticoagulated venous blood; paper towels or soft laboratory tissue; 70 percent alcohol or alcohol swabs; sterile, disposable blood lancets; surface disinfectant; biohazard and sharps containers.

Time Requirements and Accuracy Standards: 20 minutes. Points assigned reflect importance of step to meeting objective: Important = (5) Essential = (10) Critical = (15). Automatic failure results if any of the **critical** tasks are omitted or performed incorrectly.

STANDARD PRECAUTIONS:

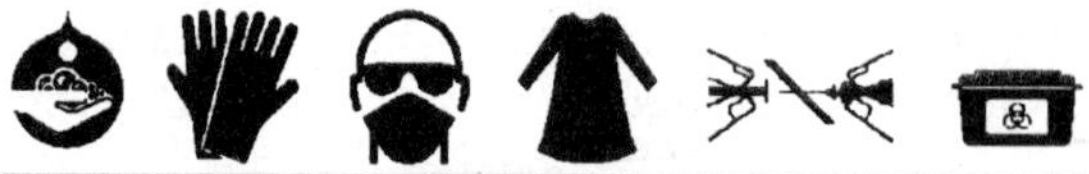

SKILLS ASSESSMENT CHECKLIST

Task Performed	Possible Points	TASKS		
☐	5	Washes hands and puts on gloves.		
☐	5	Assembles equipment and materials for capillary puncture and microhematocrit.		
☐	5	Fills two capillary tubes from a capillary puncture.		
		☐	5	Performs capillary puncture.
		☐	5	Wipes away first drop of blood.
		☐	10	Touches one end of heparinized capillary tube to the second drop of blood, fills tube ¾ full. For precalibrated tubes, fills to the line.
		☐	5	Fills second tube in same manner.
		☐	5	Wipes excess blood from sides of tubes.
		☐	10	Seals the capillary tubes by placing clean end into tray of sealing clay.
☐	5	Fills two capillary tubes using EDTA anticoagulated blood.		
		☐	10	Mixes blood for two minutes by gently rocking tube from end to end by mechanical mixer or fifty to sixty times by hand.
		☐	5	Uses acrylic safety shield to remove cap from tube.
		☐	5	Tilts tube, inserts tip of plain capillary tube, and fills ¾ full by capillary action. For precalibrated tubes, fills to the line.
		☐	15	Seals the tube. If using self-sealing tubes, checks that plug has expanded.

Task Performed	Possible Points	TASKS
	❑ 5	Fills second tube in same manner.
❑	10	Makes sure interior sealing clay edge appears level in tubes.
❑	10	Places tubes in the microhematocrit centrifuge with sealed ends securely against gasket; fastens both lids securely.
❑	15	Sets timer, centrifuges for prescribed time (varies from two to five minutes, depending upon the equipment used).
❑	5	Unlocks lids after centrifuge comes to complete stop.
❑	15	Determines microhematocrit values using the appropriate method.
❑	10	Averages the values from the two tubes and records results.
❑	5	Discards capillary tubes and used lancets into sharps container.
❑	5	Cleans and returns equipment to proper storage; cleans and disinfects work area.
❑	5	Removes and discards gloves into biohazard container; washes hands with disinfectant soap.
❑	5	Completed the tasks within 20 minutes.
❑	15	Results obtained were accurate.

______	Earned	ADD POINTS OF TASKS CHECKED
200	Points	TOTAL POINTS POSSIBLE
______	SCORE	DETERMINE SCORE (divide points earned by total points possible, multiply results by 100)

Actual Student Time Needed to Complete Procedure: __________

Student's Initials: __________ Instructor's Initials: __________ Grade: __________

Suggestions for Improvement: ______________________________

Evaluator's Name (print) ______________________________

Evaluator's Signature ______________________________

Comments ______________________________

DOCUMENTATION

Record test results in the patient's medical record.

Date:____________________

Charting: ______________________________

____

____

Student's Initials:______________

SKILLS COMPETENCY ASSESSMENT

Procedure 34–4: White Blood Cell Count (Unopette Method)

Student's Name: ______________________________ Date: ____________

Objective: To determine white blood cell count using a self-contained system.

Conditions: The student demonstrates the ability to properly and safely perform the white blood cell count using a self-contained system to determine the total number of white blood cells per cubic millimeter of blood using the following supplies and equipment: gloves, surface disinfectant, tube of EDTA blood or supplies for capillary puncture, hand disinfectant, unopette WBC or WBC/Platelet system, hemacytometer with coverglass, hand tally counter, 70 percent alcohol, microscope, lens paper, acrylic safety shield, biohazard and sharps waste containers. This procedure demonstrates use of the Unopette system; consult manufacturer's package insert for specific instructions.

Time Requirements and Accuracy Standards: 30 minutes. Points assigned reflect importance of step to meeting objective: Important = (5) Essential = (10) Critical = (15). Automatic failure results if any of the **critical** tasks are omitted or performed incorrectly.

STANDARD PRECAUTIONS:

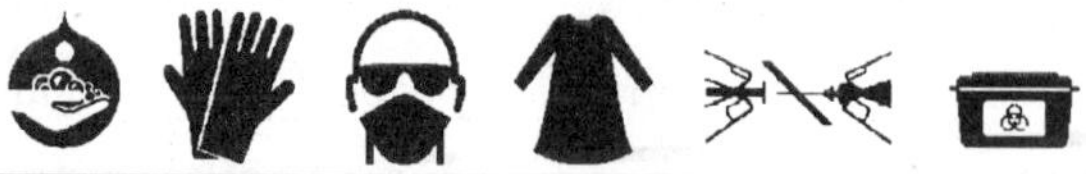

SKILLS ASSESSMENT CHECKLIST

Task Performed	Possible Points	TASKS
☐	5	Assembles equipment and materials.
☐	5	Places clean hemacytometer coverglass on a clean hemacytometer.
☐	5	Pierces the diaphragm of the Unopette reservoir with pipette shield.
☐	5	Sets up acrylic safety shield, washes hands, puts on gloves.
☐	5	Removes shield from pipette assembly. Uses safety shield as barrier from blood or blood solution.
☐	15	Fills capillary tube from capillary puncture or tube of well-mixed EDTA blood.
☐	10	Allows blood to rise in capillary until it automatically stops.
☐	5	Wipes off excess blood from exterior of pipette without touching the tip with the tissue.
☐	15	Squeezes the reservoir slightly, careful not to expel any liquid. Maintains pressure on reservoir and inserts capillary pipette, seating pipette firmly into the neck of the reservoir without expelling any liquid.
☐	5	Releases the pressure on the reservoir, drawing blood out of the capillary into the diluent.
☐	10	Squeezes reservoir gently three to four times to rinse remaining blood from the pipette without allowing blood-diluent mixture to flow out of the top.

Task Performed	Possible Points	TASKS
❑	10	Swirls to gently mix contents of reservoir; lets system sit for ten minutes (but not longer than one hour) to destroy red blood cells.
❑	10	Removes pipette from reservoir and inserts into neck of reservoir so pipette tip extends upward from the reservoir.
❑	5	Thoroughly mixes contents of reservoir, inverts reservoir, and gently squeezes to discard four or five drops onto paper towel.
❑	5	Touches tip of pipette to edge of coverglass and counting chamber. Fills both counting chambers.
❑	15	Places filled hemacytometer into a Petri dish beside a damp cotton ball; lets stand for ten minutes.
❑	5	Carefully places hemacytometer on the microscope stage to secure it; uses low-power objective (10×) to bring ruled area into focus.
❑	15	Counts white blood cells within all nine counting squares using the boundary rule; records results.
❑	10	Repeats count using other side of hemacytometer; records results.
❑	10	Averages results of the two sides.
❑	10	Calculates 10 percent of the average and adds that figure to the average; multiplies total by 100. Documents results.
❑	5	Places hemacytometer and coverglass in bleach solution for ten minutes; rinses with water, dries carefully with lens paper.
❑	5	Discards sharps and Unopette assemble in sharps container. Returns tube of blood to storage or discards appropriately.
❑	5	Returns equipment to storage.
❑	5	Cleans and disinfects work area.
❑	5	Removes and discards gloves in biohazard container.
❑	5	Washes hands with hand disinfectant.
❑	5	Completed the tasks within 30 minutes.
❑	15	Results obtained were accurate.

______	Earned	ADD POINTS OF TASKS CHECKED
230	Points	TOTAL POINTS POSSIBLE
______	SCORE	DETERMINE SCORE (divide points earned by total points possible, multiply results by 100)

SKILLS COMPETENCY ASSESSMENT — continued

Procedure 34–4: White Blood Cell Count (Unopette Method)

Actual Student Time Needed to Complete Procedure: ____________

Student's Initials: ____________ Instructor's Initials: ____________ Grade: ____________

Suggestions for Improvement: ____

Evaluator's Name (print) ____

Evaluator's Signature ____

Comments ____

DOCUMENTATION

Records results in the patient's medical record.

Date: ____________________

Charting: ____

____

____

Student's Initials: ________________

SKILLS COMPETENCY ASSESSMENT

Procedure 34–5: Red Blood Cell Count (Unopette Method)

Student's Name: ______________________________________ Date: ____________

Objective: To count red blood cells.

Conditions: The student demonstrates the ability to accurately count red blood cells using the Unopette method and the following equipment and supplies: gloves, hand disinfectant, materials for capillary puncture or blood sample anticoagulated with EDTA, hemacytometer with coverglass, test tube rack or beaker, Unopette for RBC count, microscope, lens paper, 70 percent alcohol, hand tally counter, surface disinfectant, sharps and biohazard containers, acrylic safety shield. Procedure follows use of Unopette system; consult package insert for specific instructions.

Time Requirements and Accuracy Standards: 30 minutes. Points assigned reflect importance of step to meeting objective: Important = (5) Essential = (10) Critical = (15). Automatic failure results if any of the **critical** tasks are omitted or performed incorrectly.

STANDARD PRECAUTIONS:

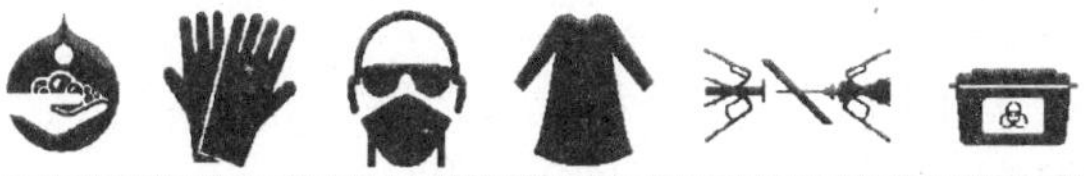

SKILLS ASSESSMENT CHECKLIST

Task Performed	Possible Points	TASKS
☐	5	Assembles equipment; sets up acrylic safety shield.
☐	5	Places clean hemacytometer coverglass over a clean hemacytometer.
☐	5	Washes hands and puts on gloves.
☐	10	Punctures diaphragm of the Unopette by holding reservoir firmly on flat surface with one hand and using the pipette shields tip to make a puncture large enough to easily accommodate the pipette.
☐	5	Removes shield from pipette assembly.
☐	15	Fills capillary pipette from capillary puncture or a well-mixed tube of EDTA anticoagulated blood. Pipette fills by capillary action and stops automatically.
☐	5	*Rationale:* Understands that pipette must be kept horizontal or at a slight (5°) upward angle to avoid overfilling.
☐	5	Wipes excess blood from exterior without allowing tissue to touch pipette tip.
☐	10	Squeezes reservoir slightly, careful not to expel liquid.
☐	15	Maintains pressure on reservoir and inserts capillary pipette into reservoir, seating pipette firmly into the reservoir neck without expelling any liquid.
☐	15	Releases pressure on reservoir, drawing blood out of capillary pipette into diluent.

SKILLS COMPETENCY ASSESSMENT — continued

Procedure 34–5: Red Blood Cell Count (Unopette Method)

Task Performed	Possible Points	TASKS
❑	10	Squeezes reservoir gently, three to four times, to rinse remaining blood from pipette without allowing blood-diluent mixture to flow out of the top.
❑	5	Gently swirls reservoir to mix contents.
❑	10	Withdraws pipette from the reservoir and inserts it into neck of reservoir in reverse position (pipette tip projects upward from reservoir).
❑	10	Thoroughly mixes reservoir contents. Inverts and gently squeezes to discard four to five drops onto a paper towel.
❑	15	Fills both sides of hemacytometer, places on microscope stage, and secures. Uses low-power (10×) objective to bring the ruled area into focus; locates large central square.
❑	10	Rotates high-power objective (45×) into position; uses fine adjustment knob to focus image.
❑	5	Adjusts light and/or condenser so red blood cells are visible.
❑	15	Counts cells in four corner squares and one center square within the large center square using left-to-right, right-to-left counting pattern; records results for each of the five squares.
❑	15	Repeats count using other side of hemacytometer; calculates RBC count using worksheet; records.
❑	5	Disinfects hemacytometer and coverglass. Discards specimens and disposable materials appropriately.
❑	5	Returns equipment to proper storage; cleans and disinfects work area.
❑	5	Removes gloves and discards in a biohazard waste container; washes hands with hand disinfectant.
❑	5	Completed the tasks within 30 minutes.
❑	15	Results obtained were accurate.

_______	Earned	ADD POINTS OF TASKS CHECKED
225	Points	TOTAL POINTS POSSIBLE
_______	SCORE	DETERMINE SCORE (divide points earned by total points possible, multiply results by 100)

Actual Student Time Needed to Complete Procedure: ____________

Student's Initials: ____________ Instructor's Initials: ____________ Grade: ____________

Suggestions for Improvement: ____________

Evaluator's Name (print) ____________

Evaluator's Signature ____________

Comments ____________

DOCUMENTATION

Record results in the patient's medical record.

Date: ____________

Charting: ____________

____

____

____

____

____

Student's Initials: ____________

SKILLS COMPETENCY ASSESSMENT

Procedure 34–6: Preparation of a Differential Blood Smear Slide

Student's Name: ______________________________ Date: __________

Objective: To properly and safely prepare an anticoagulated blood smear to microscopically view the cellular components.

Conditions: The student demonstrates the ability to properly prepare an anticoagulated blood smear and a capillary blood smear by spreading blood on a microscopic slide, altering the form, structure, and distribution of cells (morphology) as little as possible to microscopically view the cellular components. The student uses the following equipment and supplies: gloves, hand disinfectant, pencil, microscope slides (1″ × 3″), 95 percent ethyl alcohol, laboratory tissue, capillary tubes (plain and heparinized) slide drying rack, hot water, detergent, distilled water, methanol in coplin jar, fresh EDTA anticoagulated blood specimen, materials for capillary puncture, surface disinfectant, sharps and biohazard waste containers.

Time Requirements and Accuracy Standards: 30 minutes. Points assigned reflect importance of step to meeting objective: Important = (5) Essential = (10) Critical = (15). Automatic failure results if any of the **critical** tasks are omitted or performed incorrectly.

STANDARD PRECAUTIONS:

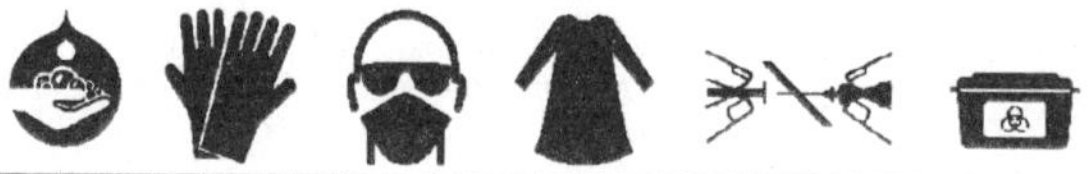

SKILLS ASSESSMENT CHECKLIST

Task Performed	Possible Points	TASKS
☐	5	Assembles equipment and materials.
☐	5	Places clean slide on flat surface, touching only edges with fingers; writes patient's ID on frosted area.
☐	5	Washes hands and puts on gloves.
☐	10	Uses anticoagulated blood sample supplied by instructor; mixes blood well and fills a plain capillary tube.
☐	10	Dispenses a small drop of blood from the capillary tube onto the slide ½″ to ¾″ from right end (if left-handed, reverse instructions).
☐	10	Places end of clean, polished unchipped spreader slide at 30–35° angle in front of the drop of blood, balancing spreader lightly with fingertips.
☐	10	Slides spreader back into the drop of blood until the blood spreads along three-fourths of the width of the spreader.
☐	5	*Rationale:* Spreader slide is held at a 30–35° angle to ensure proper thickness of the smear.
☐	10	Pushes the spreader forward with a quick, steady motion, using the other hand to keep the slide steady. Examines to see if smear is satisfactory.

Task Performed	Possible Points	TASKS
❑	15	Repeats procedure until two satisfactory smears are obtained.
❑	10	Places slide on end in slide drying rack and allows to air dry quickly.
❑	5	Places dried smear in absolute menthol for 30 to 60 seconds to preserve smear; removes and allows to air dry.
❑	5	Stores slide for staining.
❑	15	Performs a capillary puncture, wipes away the first blood drop, fills one or two heparinized capillary tubes, prepares two blood smears from capillary blood. Stores slides for staining.
❑	5	Discards blood specimens appropriately or stores for later use. Places contaminated materials in proper biohazard or sharps containers.
❑	5	Cleans equipment and returns it to proper storage, cleans and disinfects work area.
❑	5	Removes and discards gloves in biohazard waste container, washes hands with hand disinfectant.
❑	5	Completed the tasks within 30 minutes.
❑	15	Results obtained were accurate.

________	Earned	ADD POINTS OF TASKS CHECKED
155	Points	TOTAL POINTS POSSIBLE
________	SCORE	DETERMINE SCORE (divide points earned by total points possible, multiply results by 100)

Actual Student Time Needed to Complete Procedure: ____________

Student's Initials: ____________ Instructor's Initials: ____________ Grade: ____________

Suggestions for Improvement: ______________________________

Evaluator's Name (print) ______________________________

Evaluator's Signature ______________________________

Comments ______________________________

SKILLS COMPETENCY ASSESSMENT

Procedure 34–7: Staining a Differential Blood Smear Slide

Student's Name: ______________________________ Date: __________

Objective: To properly and safely apply a stain to a blood smear.

Conditions: The student demonstrates the ability to properly and safely apply a stain to a blood smear so the cells and structures may be more easily viewed through microscopic examination. The student uses the following equipment and supplies: gloves, hand disinfectant, freshly prepared or preserved blood smears, blood stain reagents, tube of EDTA anticoagulated blood (optional), staining rack, immersion oil, microscope, lens paper, forceps, laboratory tissue, lap apron or coat, staining jars for quick stains, surface disinfectant, sharps and biohazard waste containers, slide storage box. Stain characteristics may vary with stain lot; follow the manufacturer's instructions for best results.

Time Requirements and Accuracy Standards: 30 minutes. Points assigned reflect importance of step to meeting objective: Important = (5) Essential = (10) Critical = (15). Automatic failure results if any of the **critical** tasks are omitted or performed incorrectly.

STANDARD PRECAUTIONS:

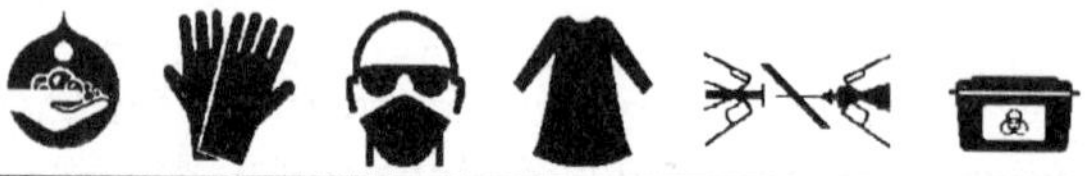

SKILLS ASSESSMENT CHECKLIST

Task Performed	Possible Points	TASKS
Two-Step Method		
❑	5	Washes hands, puts on gloves.
❑	5	Assembles equipment and materials.
❑	5	Prepares blood smear (see Procedure 34–6), or obtains a previously prepared, fixed smear.
❑	5	Stains a blood smear by one of the following methods:
❑	5	Places dried smear on staining rack or flat surface, blood side up.
❑	15	Floods smear with Wright's stain without allowing stain to flow over sides of slide; leaves stain on slide for exact time supplied by instructor (one to three minutes; time varies according to manufacturer's instructions).
❑	15	Adds buffer, dropwise, to stain until buffer volume is equal to the stain.
❑	5	Blows gently on fluid surface to mix the solutions. Observes for metallic green sheen.
❑	15	Leaves buffer on slide for exact time supplied by instructor (two to four minutes; time varies according to manufacturer's instructions); does not allow mixture to run off slide.
❑	5	Rinses thoroughly and continuously with gentle stream of tap or distilled water, drains water off.
❑	5	Wipes backs of slides with wet gauze to remove excess stain, stands smears on end to air dry.
❑	5	Completed the tasks within 30 minutes.

Task Performed	Possible Points	TASKS
❑	15	Results obtained were accurate.

________	Earned	ADD POINTS OF TASKS CHECKED
105	Points	TOTAL POINTS POSSIBLE
________	SCORE	DETERMINE SCORE (divide points earned by total points possible, multiply results by 100)

Three-Step Method

❑	20	Performs the first four steps of the Two-Step Method.
❑	15	Dips dry smear into solutions following manufacturer's instructions without allowing slide to dry between solutions; rinses slide if necessary.
❑	5	Removes excess stain from back of slide with wet gauze; stands slide on end to air dry.
❑	5	Places dry slide on microscope stage, stain side up; focuses on low power (10×) objective.
❑	10	Scans slide to find area where cells are barely touching each other.
❑	15	Places drop of immersion oil on slide, rotates oil immersion lens carefully into position, focuses with fine adjustment knob only.
❑	15	Observes erythrocytes, leukocytes, nuclei, neutrophil granules, and platelets for proper stain color.
❑	5	Rotates low power (10×) objective into position; removes slide from microscope stage.
❑	5	Cleans oil objective thoroughly with lens paper; gently wipes oil from slide with soft tissue.
❑	5	Cleans equipment and returns to proper storage; cleans work area with disinfectant.
❑	5	Removes and discards gloves in a biohazard waste container; washes hands with hand disinfectant.
❑	5	Completed the tasks within 30 minutes.
❑	15	Results obtained were accurate.

________	Earned	ADD POINTS OF TASKS CHECKED
125	Points	TOTAL POINTS POSSIBLE
________	SCORE	DETERMINE SCORE (divide points earned by total points possible, multiply results by 100)

Actual Student Time Needed to Complete Procedure: ____________

Student's Initials: ____________ Instructor's Initials: ____________ Grade: ____________

Suggestions for Improvement: ____

Evaluator's Name (print) ____

Evaluator's Signature ____

Comments ____

SKILLS COMPETENCY ASSESSMENT

Procedure 34–8: Differential Leukocyte Count

Student's Name: ______________________________ Date: __________

Objective: To properly and safely examine a stained blood smear for differential leukocyte count.

Conditions: The student demonstrates the ability to properly and safely examine a stained blood smear to observe, identify, and record 100 leukocytes and differentiate the five types of leukocytes by size, nuclear characteristics, and cytoplasmic characteristics. The student uses the following supplies and equipment: gloves, hand disinfectant, stained normal blood smears, microscope with oil immersion objective, immersion oil, lens paper, soft tissue or soft paper towels, blood cell atlas, tally counter or differential counter, worksheet, sharps and biohazard waste containers, surface disinfectant.

Time Requirements and Accuracy Standards: 30 minutes. Points assigned reflect importance of step to meeting objective: Important = (5) Essential = (10) Critical = (15). Automatic failure results if any of the **critical** tasks are omitted or performed incorrectly.

SKILLS ASSESSMENT CHECKLIST

Task Performed	Possible Points	TASKS
❑	5	Washes hands, puts on gloves.
❑	5	Assembles equipment and materials.
❑	5	Places stained smear on microscope stage and secures; uses low power (10×) objective to locate feathered edge of smear.
❑	5	Focuses cells using coarse adjustment.
❑	10	Scans smear to find area where red blood cells are barely touching.
❑	10	Places one drop of immersion oil on smear; rotates oil immersion objective carefully into position; focuses cells using fine adjustment.
❑	15	Allows maximum light into the objective by raising condenser and opening diaphragm; scans the smear to observe leukocytes.
❑	15	Studies smear to identify all five types of leukocytes, platelets, and red cells. Repeats procedural steps until cells can be readily identified.
❑	5	Using the same slide or a different one, restarts procedure, performing each procedural step through identification of cells.
❑	15	Counts 100 consecutive leukocytes using appropriate counting pattern. Moves the slide or movable stage so consecutive microscopic fields are viewed.
❑	10	Observes the red blood cells in at least ten fields, noting hemoglobin content and recording as normochromic or hypochromic.
❑	15	Observes red blood cell size, recording as normocytic, microcytic, or macrocytic. Uses appropriate method to record an approximation of the number of cells affected.

Task Performed	Possible Points	TASKS
❑	15	Observes platelets in at least ten fields, noting morphology and estimating number of platelets per oil immersion field and recording appropriately.
❑	5	Rotates low power (10×) objective into place; removes slide from stage.
❑	5	Cleans the oil immersion objective with lens paper and checks microscope stage and condenser for oil; cleans with soft tissue if necessary.
❑	5	Places slide properly in slide box or disposes of slide as instructed; cleans equipment and returns it to proper storage.
❑	5	Disposes of waste in appropriate sharps or biohazard waste container.
❑	5	Cleans and disinfects work area.
❑	5	Removes gloves and discards in biohazard container; washes hands with hand disinfectant.
❑	5	Completed the tasks within 30 minutes.
❑	15	Results are within acceptable range.

______	Earned	ADD POINTS OF TASKS CHECKED
190	Points	TOTAL POINTS POSSIBLE
______	SCORE	DETERMINE SCORE (divide points earned by total points possible, multiply results by 100)

Actual Student Time Needed to Complete Procedure: ____________

Student's Initials: ____________ Instructor's Initials: ____________ Grade: ____________

Suggestions for Improvement: ______________________________

Evaluator's Name (print) ______________________________

Evaluator's Signature ______________________________

Comments ______________________________

DOCUMENTATION

Record results in the patient's medical record.

Date: ____________________

Charting: ______________________________

____

____

Student's Initials: ____________

SKILLS COMPETENCY ASSESSMENT

Procedure 34–9: Erythrocyte Sedimentation Rate

Student's Name: ______________________________ Date: ____________

Objective: To properly and safely examine a blood sample to determine erythrocyte sedimentation rate.

Conditions: The student demonstrates the ability to properly and safely examine a blood sample by using either the Sediplast (Westergren) or Wintrobe method to record the erythrocyte sedimentation rate. The student uses the following equipment and supplies: gloves, hand disinfectant, sample of venous blood collected in EDTA, equipment for Sediplast kit or Wintrobe method, timer, 10 percent chlorine bleach solution, sharps and biohazard waste containers, acrylic safety shield. Consult the manufacturer's package insert for specific instructions for ESR kit use.

Time Requirements and Accuracy Standards: 75 minutes. Points assigned reflect importance of step to meeting objective: Important = (5) Essential = (10) Critical = (15). Automatic failure results if any of the **critical** tasks are omitted or performed incorrectly.

STANDARD PRECAUTIONS:

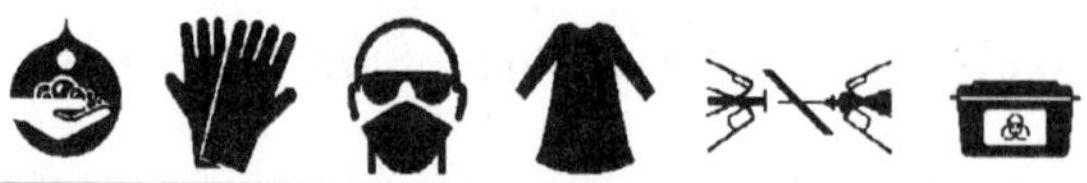

SKILLS ASSESSMENT CHECKLIST

Task Performed	Possible Points	TASKS
☐	5	Washes hands and puts on gloves.
☐	5	Assembles equipment and materials. Gently mixes blood sample for two minutes.
		Sediplast ESR (modified Westergren)
☐	15	Removes stopper from Sedivial and fills with 0.8 mL blood to indicated mark. Replaces stopper and inverts vial several times to mix.
☐	15	Places vial in Sediplast rack on level surface. Gently inserts disposable Sediblast pipette through pierceable stopper with twisting motion; pushes down until the pipette rests on the bottom of the vial. Pipette autozeros blood and excess flows into sealed reservoir compartment.
☐	10	Sets timer for one hour; returns blood sample to proper storage.
☐	15	Lets pipette stand undisturbed for exactly one hour; records results. Uses scale on the tube to measure the distance from the top of plasma to the top of red blood cells. Records sedimentation rate.
☐	10	Disposes of tube and vial in appropriate biohazard waste container.
☐	5	Completed the tasks within 75 minutes.
☐	15	Results obtained were accurate.

______	Earned	ADD POINTS OF TASKS CHECKED
95	Points	TOTAL POINTS POSSIBLE
______	SCORE	DETERMINE SCORE (divide points earned by total points possible, multiply results by 100)

Task Performed	Possible Points	TASKS
		Wintrobe Method
☐	10	Places tube in Wintrobe sedimentation rack; checks leveling bubble to ensure rack is level.
☐	15	Fills Wintrobe tube to the zero mark with well-mixed blood using Pasteur pipette and being careful not to overfill. Fills tube from bottom to avoid air bubbles.
☐	5	Sets timer for one hour, being certain tube is vertical.
☐	10	Returns blood sample to proper storage.
☐	15	After exactly one hour, correctly measures the distance the erythrocytes have fallen, in mm, and records the sedimentation rate.
☐	5	Disinfects and clean equipment, returning it to proper storage.
☐	5	Disposes of waste in appropriate biohazard or sharps container.
☐	5	Cleans and disinfects work area.
☐	5	Removes gloves and discards in a biohazard waste container; washes hands with hand disinfectant.
☐	5	Completed the tasks within 75 minutes.
☐	15	Results obtained were accurate.

_______	Earned	ADD POINTS OF TASKS CHECKED
95	Points	TOTAL POINTS POSSIBLE
_______	SCORE	DETERMINE SCORE (divide points earned by total points possible, multiply results by 100)

Actual Student Time Needed to Complete Procedure: ____________

Student's Initials: ____________ Instructor's Initials: ____________ Grade: ____________

Suggestions for Improvement: ________________________________

Evaluator's Name (print) ________________________________

Evaluator's Signature ________________________________

Comments ________________________________

DOCUMENTATION

Record results in the patient's medical record.

Charting: ________________________________

____

____

Student's Initials: ____________

EVALUATION OF CHAPTER KNOWLEDGE

How has your instructor evaluated the knowledge you have achieved?

	Instructor Evaluation		
Knowledge	*Good*	*Average*	*Poor*
Can discuss the role and importance of hematological studies as a diagnostic tool for physicians	_____	_____	_____
Can discuss clinical science of hematology	_____	_____	_____
Compares normal and abnormal values of CBC parameters and understands how CBC is used in diagnosis and treatment of disease	_____	_____	_____
Maintains aseptic technique and follows standard precautions throughout all procedures	_____	_____	_____
Understands the importance of following all quality control guidelines	_____	_____	_____
Displays the appropriate techniques in collecting and processing specimens	_____	_____	_____
Performs tests with competent skill necessary for entry-level employment	_____	_____	_____
Performs calculations accurately	_____	_____	_____
Documents all procedures according to laboratory policy	_____	_____	_____
Describes physiological reasons for different variations of test results in different states of health and disease	_____	_____	_____
Operates and maintains facility and equipment safely	_____	_____	_____
Exhibits empathy for patient and attends to patient's emotional needs during the collection of patient blood samples for analysis	_____	_____	_____

Student's Initials: ______ Instructor's Initials: ______

Grade: ________

CHAPTER 35

Urinalysis

PERFORMANCE OBJECTIVES

Urinalysis refers to the examination of urine as an aid in patient diagnosis or to follow the course of a disease. Urinalysis is a routine procedure in most physical examinations. Physicians often order a variety of tests on urine to help determine or rule out certain aberrations in order to make accurate patient diagnoses. It is essential that medical assistants understand both the importance of urinalysis and their own role in assisting in patient diagnosis and treatment. In this chapter, medical assisting students learn the basics of urinalysis, examination of urine specimens, including proper collection techniques for urine specimens, safety guidelines involved in collecting and handling specimens, and measures to ensure a consistent quality control program. Students learn to properly perform urinalysis testing and become cognizant of factors that may intervene with urinalysis accuracy. Observing standard precautions is mandatory in urinalysis procedures.

EXERCISES AND ACTIVITIES

Vocabulary Builder

A. *Match the following terms listed in Column A with corresponding definitions listed in Column B.*

Column A	Column B
1. Clinitest	22. A. Urine testing that includes physical, chemical, and microscopic testing of a urine sample.
2. Ketone	15. B. Crystalline material found in urine sediment; shapeless; possessing no definite form.
3. pH	____ C. Tiny structures usually formed by deposits of protein (or other substances) on the walls of renal tubes.
4. Urochrome	____ D. Reagent table test that confirms the presence of reducing sugars in the urine.

5. Sediment	E. Found in normal urine sediment, these structures generally have no particular significance; a few should be noted as they may indicate disease states.
6. Amorphous	F. Microorganisms cultivated in a nutrient medium.
7. Ictotest	G. Transparent, clear casts that are often hard to see in urine; these casts should be examined under subdued lighting.
8. Cultures	H. Confirmatory test for bilirubin.
9. Casts	I. Chemical compound produced during increased metabolism of fat; tested on a reagent strip.
10. Urinalysis	J. Curvature appearing in a liquid's upper surface when the liquid is placed in a container.
11. Acetest	K. Urine sample collected in the middle of the flow of urine.
12. Quality control	L. Test results that indicate a potentially life-threatening or greatly debilitating situation that must be reported to a physician immediately.
13. Specific gravity	M. Scale that indicates the relative alkalinity or acidity of a solution; measurement of hydrogen ion concentration.
14. Hyaline	N. Program that ensures accurate and dependable test results.
15. Crystals	O. Narrow strip of plastic on which pads containing reagents are attached; used in urinalysis to detect a variety of substances and values.
16. Midstream collection	P. Insoluble matter that settles to the bottom of a liquid; material examined in the urinalysis microscopic examination.
17. Panic values	Q. Ratio of weight of a given volume of a substance to the weight of the same volume of distilled water at the same temperature; test often performed during the urinalysis physical examination (can also appear on the reagent strip).
18. Reagent test strip	R. Opaque; lack of clarity.
19. Urea	S. Product used to test for the presence of abnormal amounts of acetone in the urine.
20. Meniscus	T. Principal end product of protein metabolism.
21. Turbid	U. Yellow pigment that provides color to urine.
22. Screening	V. Condition that occurs when the net rate at which the body produces acids or bases is equal to the net rate at which acids or bases are excreted.
23. Acid/base balance	W. Preliminary examination used to detect the most characteristic signs of a disorder that may entail further investigation.

B. Unscramble the following items to create the proper terms relating to urinalysis.

1. INUBBIRIL ____________________

   Orange-yellow pigment that forms from the breakdown of hemoglobin in broken-down red blood cells. It usually travels in the bloodstream to the liver, where it is converted to a water-soluble form and excreted into the bile.

2. ARUTAHEMI ______________________

   Abnormal presence of blood in urine, symptomatic of many disorders of the genitourinary system and renal diseases.

3. SLOGCUE ______________________

   Simple sugar that is a major source of energy in the human body; monitoring of its levels in the urine and blood is a vital diagnostic test in diabetes and other disorders; a test on a reagent strip.

4. TEKYLCOUE SEESATER ______________________

   Test on a reagent strip that indicates the presence of white blood cells in the urinary tract.

5. GENNUROBILIO ______________________

   Colorless compound produced in the intestine after the breakdown by bacteria of bilirubin.

6. GEARSTEN ______________________

   Chemical substances that detect or synthesize other substances in a chemical reaction and are used in laboratory analyses because they are known to react in a specific way.

7. CASISETOOKID ______________________

   Accumulation of ketones in the body, occurring primarily as a compilation of diabetes mellitus; if left untreated, it could cause coma.

8. NICCARDIA MHYRTH ______________________

   Pattern based on 24-hour cycle that emphasizes the repetition of certain physiologic phenomena such as eating and sleeping.

9. ERCTIENINA ______________________

   Waste product formed in muscle that is excreted by the kidneys; elevated in blood and urine when kidney function is abnormal.

10. FAREOTCRETEM ______________________

    Instrument that measures the refractive index of a substance or solution; used in the urinalysis chemical examination to measure the urine specimen's specific gravity.

11. RETINOMERU ______________________

    Device used to measure specific gravity; consists of a float with a calibrated stem.

12. STRAPTUNANE ______________________

    Urine that appears to be above the sediment when centrifuged; poured off before sediment is examined in the urinalysis microscopic examination.

13. MATM-LAFSHORL ______________________

    Mucoprotein excreted by the epithelial cells of the renal tubules.

Learning Review

Fill in the blanks in the following paragraphs with the appropriate terms.

1.

Urea	Soluble	Excess fluid
Filtration	Glomerulus	Urine
Tubule	Salts	Waste products
Homeostasis	Electrolytes	Metabolism
Nephron	Milliliters	

The formation and excretion of ________________ is the principal method by which the body excretes water and the ________________ waste products of ________________. The kidneys control this process and also regulate the fluid outside the cells of the body, carefully maintaining the body's balance of fluids eliminated or retained, or ________________ of body fluids. The kidneys are responsible for the ________________ of __________, __________ and ________________ from the blood. Substances filtered out of the body can include water, ammonia, ______________, glucose, amino acids, creatinine, and __________. These wastes leave the body through the eliminated urine. The filtering unit of the kidney is called the ________________. The ________________ is the part of the kidney that concentrates the filtered material. Together, these elements of the kidney form the ________________. Each minute, more than 1,000 ________________ of blood flows through the kidney to be cleansed.

2.

Creatinine	Amino acids	Concentration
Threshold	Glucose	Kidney
Protein	Blood	

While passing through the __________, some substances, such as __________ and __________, need to be reabsorbed into the __________. These substances are reabsorbed in relation to their __________ in the blood and are known as __________substances. Some of these substances need only be partially reabsorbed, such as __________ and __________.

3.

Urine	Kidney	Sodium
Drugs	Hydrogen	Ammonium
Secreted	Blood	

Toward the end of the ________________'s sojourn through the ________________, other substances that have not already been filtered are secreted into the ________________. For instance, substances such as ________________ and ________________ ions may be __________ in the urine in exchange for ________________. In addition, certain ________________ in the blood at this point may also be secreted into the urine.

4. A. After passing through a healthy kidney, urine composition is approximately ____ percent water and _____ percent dissolved substances, which generally come from dietary intake or metabolic waste products.

B. Identify each substance below as a normal (N) or an abnormal (AB) substance found in urine.

____ (1) Urobilinogen	____ (4) Multiple Leukocytes	____ (7) Erythrocytes
____ (2) Potassium	____ (5) Lipids	____ (8) Creatinine
____ (3) Uric acid	____ (6) 1+ Protein	____ (9) Chloride

C. When certain disease processes occur in the human body, changes in urine production can occur. List six possible changes.

(1) ______________________ (4) ______________________
(2) ______________________ (5) ______________________
(3) ______________________ (6) ______________________

5. When handling urine specimens, standard precautions must be followed to ensure that proper infection control standards are observed. In the space provided below, list five precautions used when handling urine specimens.
   (1) ______________________
   (2) ______________________
   (3) ______________________
   (4) ______________________
   (5) ______________________

Circle the correct response for each multiple choice question below.

6. Quality control (QC) programs
   A. provide a random spot-check of accuracy.
   B. ensure accurate and reliable results for the patient.
   C. provide comparisons with patient specimens necessary to interpret urinalysis test results.
7. Equipment and instruments used for urine testing
   A. must be disposed of properly in biohazard containers after each procedure.
   B. are self-calibrating and require no adjustment.
   C. should be checked daily for proper calibration.
8. Quality control procedures should be performed
   A. exactly as procedures are performed on patient specimens.
   B. on every other urine specimen tested.
   C. only by a licensed health care professional trained to interpret the results.
9. Urine control samples
   A. have no special storage requirements.
   B. are purchased commercially from manufacturers.
   C. are used to obtain baseline urinalysis results from healthy patients.
10. Documentation of quality control testing
    A. must be recorded in a daily urinalysis QC log and kept for at least three years.
    B. is not necessary unless the equipment is malfunctioning.
    C. should be recorded in the patient's medical record.
11. List six Clinical Laboratory Improvement Amendments (CLIA) regulations that apply to the clinical medical assistant performing urine testing:
    (1) ______________________
    (2) ______________________
    (3) ______________________
    (4) ______________________
    (5) ______________________
    (6) ______________________

12. A. One of the most important steps in the collection of urine specimens is to correctly identify the specimen through proper labeling. Using your own Social Security number as your ID number and Dr. Mark Woo as your physician, write out complete labeling information for a specimen of your own urine below.

Correct urine specimen label: ______________________________

____

B. What is the proper procedure for testing an unlabeled or incorrectly labeled specimen?

____

C. Name the four types of urine specimens frequently ordered by physicians.

(1) ______________ (3) ______________

(2) ______________ (4) ______________

D. Name the four methods of urine collected ordered by physicians.

(1) ______________ (3) ______________

(2) ______________ (4) ______________

13. A. What are the four steps in a physical examination of a urine specimen?

(1) ______________________________

(2) ______________________________

(3) ______________________________

(4) ______________________________

B. What does the specific gravity of urine indicate? ______________

____

C. Name three methods of measuring the specific gravity of a urine specimen and state the advantages or disadvantages of each. Which method is available in conjunction with chemical testing?

(1) ______________________________

(2) ______________________________

(3) ______________________________

14. Reagent test strips, or dipsticks, are used to test urine for many metabolic processes, including kidney and liver functions, urinary tract infection, and pH balance.

A. Match each test below to the information that best describes it.

______ 1. Glucose	______ 5. Nitrites	______ 8. Ketones
______ 2. pH	______ 6. Leukocyte	______ 9. Protein
______ 3. Urobilinogen	______ 7. Specific gravity	______ 10. Bilirubin
______ 4. Blood		

A. These occur during prolonged fasting. They appear when excessive amounts of fatty acids are broken down into simpler compounds and when glucose availability is limited.

B. Increased levels of this substance suggest liver disease or bleeding disorders. It is a degradation product of bilirubin formed by intestinal bacteria.

C. This substance in a urine sample indicates infection, urinary tract trauma, kidney bleeding, and menses.

D. This substance can increase during a high fever and also indicates injury to the kidney, specifically to the glomerular membrane.

E. This test indicates white blood cells in the urinary tract, presumably attracted by invading bacteria.

F. This test detects unsuspected diabetes or is used to check the efficiency of insulin therapy in diabetics.

G. This test changes color, depending on the ion concentration in urine. The highest reading available on the test is 1.030.

H. This test has a range of 4.6 to 8.0 and measures the acidity or alkalinity of the urine. A reading under 7.0 indicates increased acidity; above 7.0 indicates increased alkalinity.

I. The presence of this substance indicates a urinary tract infection, as it is normally absent from urine. It is formed from the conversion of nitrates by certain species of bacteria.

J. This substance, a product of the breakdown of hemoglobin, breaks down in the light; a urine sample should be protected from light during testing.

B. How should reagent test strips be handled and stored?

____

____

____

15. The results of reagent strips are screening results; some positive results must be confirmed by further testing. For each substance below, identify the confirming test used. Then match each entry to the information that best fits each test.

______________________ (1) Reducing sugars

______________________ (2) Protein

______________________ (3) Ketones

______________________ (4) Bilirubin

___ A. This test includes a tablet and an absorbent mat. A purple color will develop when a urine drop is placed on a moist mat if the substance is present.

___ B. This test is used to detect lactose and galactose and is performed when the glucose test is positive on the reagent test strip.

___ C. In this test, a 2+ result is cloudy and granular.

___ D. A drop of urine added to a tablet will produce a purple color when this substance, produced during an increased metabolism of fat, is present.

16. Microscopic examination of urine sediment is also a valuable diagnostic tool for physicians.

A. Match each type of sediment listed to the statement that best describes it.

A. White blood cells	D. Renal epithelial cells	G. Red blood cells
B. Yeast	E. Bacteria	H. Protozoa
C. Squamous epithelial cells	F. Artifacts	I. Sperm

____ 1. Hair, fiber, air bubbles, and oil are common examples.

____ 2. These skin cells are not medically significant and are sloughed off continuously in urine.

____ 3. *Trichomonas vaginalis* is the most common example.

____ 4. Cocci, bacilli, and spirilla.

____ 5. These cells appear as pale, light-refractive disks. They are counted in a microscopic field and reported as cells per high-power field (HPF).

____ 6. These cells are larger than erythrocytes, have a visible nucleus, and may appear granular. They are reported as cells per high-power field (HPF).

____ 7. These are reported only when seen in male urine, unless specifically requested by the physician.

____ 8. *Candida albicans* is the most common example.

____ 9. These cells can indicate kidney disease if present in large numbers and are easily confused with leukocytes and other skin cells. If suspected, the slide should be reviewed by the physician. They are reported as cells per high-power field (HPF).

B. In the circles below, draw an example of the sediment as seen under a microscope.

1. Fiber, hair, air bubble artifact 2. Yeast 3. Squamous epithelial cells 4. Bacteria

17. Crystals are the most insignificant part of urinary sediment and are not usually an important element of microscopic analysis, though many labs do report them. However, a few crystals may indicate disease states; name three.

(1) ____________________ (2) ____________________ (3) ____________________

18. Identification of casts in urine requires an experienced eye; medical assistants who encounter them should ask for assistance in confirming identification. Casts are formed when protein accumulates and precipitates in the kidney tubules and are then washed into the urine. Identify each cast below and draw an example in the circle provided.

A. **B.** **C.**

_______________ A. These casts contain remnants of disintegrated cells that have a fine or coarse appearance.

_______________ B. These casts contain leukocytes, erythrocytes, or skin cells.

_______________ C. These casts are difficult to see under the microscope without some light adjustment because of their near transparency.

Investigation Activity

Standard precautions are essential when performing urinalysis on patient urine specimens. As responsible health care professionals, medical assistants must be aware of the possible hazards of procedures performed in the ambulatory care setting and the proper techniques for preventing or reducing any potential risk to patients, employees, or visitors. Consider the urine Clinitest, which detects the presence of reducing sugars in specimens (Procedure 35–6). Complete the Office Procedures Safety Form below, which will become part of the medical practice's Office Procedures Manual for employees.

OFFICE PROCEDURES SAFETY FORM

Procedure: _______________ Type of hazard: _______________

Person performing procedure: _______________ PPE required: _______________

Proper techniques for safety: _______________

____

____

What is done with used materials and soiled instruments? _______________

____

____

____

What chemical products are involved? _______________

____

____

____

What are the specific risks of the procedure? _______________

____

____

____

Additional comments: _______________

____

____

Prepared by: _______________ Date: _______________

CASE STUDIES

Case 1

At Inner City Health Care, Wanda Slawson, CMA, gives patient Wendy Janus written directions for a 24-hour urine collection to be performed at home, but Wendy misplaces them. Wanda must give directions to Wendy over the telephone.

1. What directions should be given to the patient to correctly perform the urine collection?
2. What communication techniques should Wendy use to make sure the patient understands the collection procedures? What other potential alternatives for communicating the information, besides the telephone, are available?

Case 2

Wanda Slawson, CMA, is asked to give a male adolescent patient the proper procedure for a clean-catch specimen. The fifteen-year-old boy is visibly embarrassed and will not hold eye contact with Wanda as she relates the instructions for collection to him.

1. What instructions are relevant for a clean-catch specimen for this patient?
2. What communication techniques should Wanda use in working with this patient?

SUPPLEMENTARY RESOURCES

Study Guide Disk: Additional practice exercises for this chapter are available on the study guide disk found in the back of the textbook.

Medical Assisting Videos: Appropriate content is available on Delmar's Medical Assisting Videos, 2nd ed., Tape 14, for the following topics:

Quality Control in Collecting and Processing Specimens
Collect and Label Random Urine Specimens
Perform a Routine Urinalysis and Record Results
Perform Microscopic Examination of Urine

SKILLS COMPETENCY ASSESSMENT

Procedure 35-1: Assessing Urine Volume

Student's Name: ______________________________ Date: ____________

Objective: To accurately determine and document the volume of a urine sample.

Conditions: The student demonstrates the ability to determine and document the volume of a urine specimen using the following supplies: gloves, graduated urine container, graduated cylinder, biohazard container, and laboratory report form.

Time Requirements and Accuracy Standards: 5 minutes. Points assigned reflect importance of step to meeting objective: Important = (5) Essential = (10) Critical = (15). Automatic failure results if any of the **critical** tasks are omitted or performed incorrectly.

STANDARD PRECAUTIONS:

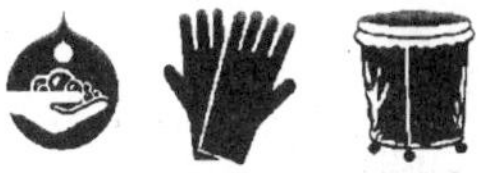

SKILLS ASSESSMENT CHECKLIST

Task Performed	Possible Points	TASKS
☐	5	Washes hands.
☐	5	Puts on gloves.
☐	5	Assembles equipment and materials.
☐	5	Follows all safety guidelines.
☐	5	Is careful not to splash urine. Wipes up any and all spills with antiseptic cleaner.
☐	5	Observes sample for proper labeling.
☐	5	*Rationale:* Understands that unlabeled urine is not tested and can state correct procedure for obtaining a new, properly labeled sample.
☐	15	Checks to see that urine container lid is tightly closed, then mixes the urine by inversion in the sealed container.
☐	5	Pours the urine into a suitable measuring device if the container is not graduated.
☐	15	Records the volume of the urine in milliliters. If urine volume is between 4 and 10 mL (or less), makes the proper documentation.
☐	10	Marks samples of less than 4 mL (except for newborns) with appropriate documentation. Insufficient samples are not tested.
☐	10	After volume is recorded, places an aliquot in a standard urinalysis centrifuge tube for continuation of urinalysis.
☐	5	Completed the tasks within 5 minutes.

SKILLS COMPETENCY ASSESSMENT — continued

Procedure 35-1: Assessing Urine Volume

Task Performed	Possible Points	TASKS
☐	15	Results obtained were accurate.

________	Earned	ADD POINTS OF TASKS CHECKED
110	Points	TOTAL POINTS POSSIBLE
________	SCORE	DETERMINE SCORE (divide points earned by total points possible, multiply results by 100)

Actual Student Time Needed to Complete Procedure: ____________

Student's Initials: ____________ Instructor's Initials: ____________ Grade: ____________

Suggestions for Improvement: ______________________________

Evaluator's Name (print) ______________________________

Evaluator's Signature ______________________________

Comments ______________________________

DOCUMENTATION

Record the volume of the urine sample in milliliters (mL): ____________

Record the proper documentation for a specimen of 4 to 10 mL ____________

____

If the urine volume is below 4 mL, the specimen is marked: ____________

Student's Initials: ________

SKILLS COMPETENCY ASSESSMENT

Procedure 35-2 Observing Urine Color

Student's Name: ______________________________ Date: ____________

Objective: To observe and record the color of a urine specimen.

Conditions: The student demonstrates the ability to observe and document the color of a urine specimen using the following supplies: gloves, urine specimen, centrifuge tube, white card, biohazard container, and laboratory report form.

Time Requirements and Accuracy Standards: 5 minutes. Points assigned reflect importance of step to meeting objective: Important = (5) Essential = (10) Critical = (15). Automatic failure results if any of the **critical** tasks are omitted or performed incorrectly.

STANDARD PRECAUTIONS:

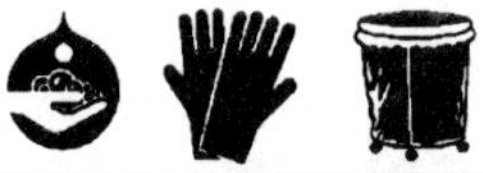

SKILLS ASSESSMENT CHECKLIST

Task Performed	Possible Points	TASKS
☐	5	Washes hands.
☐	5	Puts on gloves.
☐	5	Assembles equipment and materials.
☐	5	Follows all safety guidelines.
☐	5	Is careful not to splash urine. Wipes up any and all spills with antiseptic cleaner.
☐	10	Mixes the urine specimen thoroughly.
☐	15	Observes the color of the urine in a clear centrifuge tube using good light against a white background (white card).
☐	5	Records results on laboratory report form.
☐	5	Completed the tasks within 5 minutes.
☐	15	Results obtained were accurate.
______	Earned	ADD POINTS OF TASKS CHECKED
75	Points	TOTAL POINTS POSSIBLE
______	SCORE	DETERMINE SCORE (divide points earned by total points possible, multiply results by 100)

SKILLS COMPETENCY ASSESSMENT — continued

Procedure 35-2 Observing Urine Color

Actual Student Time Needed to Complete Procedure: ____________

Student's Initials: ____________ Instructor's Initials: ____________ Grade: ____________

Suggestions for Improvement: ____________

Evaluator's Name (print) ____________

Evaluator's Signature ____________

Comments ____________

DOCUMENTATION

Record the labeling of the urine specimen. ____________

____

Record the color of the urine sample. ____________

What is the proper documentation for each abnormally colored urine sample due to the causes listed?

(1) Hematuria: ____________

(2) Bladder infection treated with Pyridium: ____________

(3) Liver disease: ____________

(4) Vitamin intake: ____________

(5) Dehydration: ____________

Student's Initials: ____________

SKILLS COMPETENCY ASSESSMENT

Procedure 35-3: Observing Urine Clarity

Student's Name: ______________________________ Date: __________

Objective: To observe and record the clarity of a urine sample.

Conditions: The student demonstrates the ability to observe and document the clarity of a urine specimen using the following supplies: gloves, urine specimen, centrifuge tube, white sheet of paper with print, biohazard container, and laboratory report form.

Time Requirements and Accuracy Standards: 5 minutes. Points assigned reflect importance of step to meeting objective: Important = (5) Essential = (10) Critical = (15). Automatic failure results if any of the **critical** tasks are omitted or performed incorrectly.

STANDARD PRECAUTIONS:

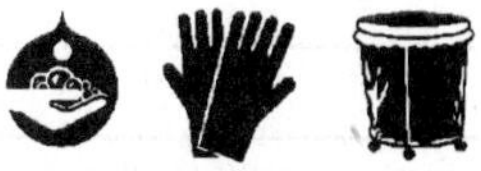

SKILLS ASSESSMENT CHECKLIST

Task Performed	Possible Points	TASKS
☐	5	Washes hands.
☐	5	Puts on gloves.
☐	5	Assembles equipment and materials.
☐	5	Follows all safety guidelines.
☐	5	Is careful not to splash urine. Wipes up any and all spills with antiseptic cleaner.
☐	15	Holds the centrifuge tube close to a printed piece of white paper.
☐	10	Observes the clarity and records results on laboratory report form.
☐	5	Dispose of all biohazardous wastes in the biohazard container.
☐	5	Completed the tasks within 5 minutes.
☐	15	Results obtained were accurate.

________	Earned	ADD POINTS OF TASKS CHECKED
75	Points	TOTAL POINTS POSSIBLE
________	SCORE	DETERMINE SCORE (divide points earned by total points possible, multiply results by 100)

SKILLS COMPETENCY ASSESSMENT — continued

Procedure 35-3: Observing Urine Clarity

Actual Student Time Needed to Complete Procedure: ____________

Student's Initials: ____________ Instructor's Initials: ____________ Grade: ____________

Suggestions for Improvement: ____

Evaluator's Name (print) ____

Evaluator's Signature ____

Comments ____

DOCUMENTATION

Record the labeling of the urine specimen. ____

____

Record observations regarding the color and clarity of the urine specimen.

____

____

Student's Initials: _________

SKILLS COMPETENCY ASSESSMENT

Procedure 35-4: Using the Refractometer to Measure Specific Gravity

Student's Name: ______________________________ Date: ____________

Objective: To measure and record the specific gravity of a urine specimen.

Conditions: The student demonstrates the ability to observe and document the specific gravity of a urine specimen using the following supplies: gloves, urine specimen, refractometer, pipettes, distilled water, 5 percent saline solution lint-free tissues, quality control urine sample, biohazard container, and laboratory report form.

Time Requirements and Accuracy Standards: 10 minutes. Points assigned reflect importance of step to meeting objective: Important = (5) Essential = (10) Critical = (15). Automatic failure results if any of the **critical** tasks are omitted or performed incorrectly.

STANDARD PRECAUTIONS:

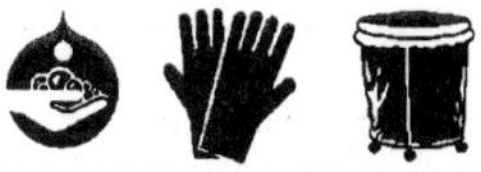

SKILLS ASSESSMENT CHECKLIST

Task Performed	Possible Points	TASKS
☐	5	Washes hands.
☐	5	Puts on gloves.
☐	5	Assembles equipment and materials.
☐	5	Follows all safety guidelines.
☐	5	Is careful not to splash urine. Wipes up any and all spills with antiseptic cleaner.
☐	10	Checks the value of the distilled water at 1.000 as a quality control check for the refractometer.
☐	5	Cleans surface of cover and prism with a lint-free cloth moistened with distilled water. Wipes dry.
☐	10	Closes the cover. Applies a drop of distilled water to the notched portion of the cover so it flows over the prism.
☐	10	Tilts the instrument to allow light to enter and reads specific gravity scale.
☐	5	Wipes the cover and prism.
☐	15	Tests sample of 5 percent saline solution, which should read 1.023 ± 0.001, thereby standardizing the equipment.
☐	15	Tests quality control urine sample and records results on quality control sheet.
☐	5	Wipes cover and prism.

SKILLS COMPETENCY ASSESSMENT — continued

Procedure 35-4: Using the Refractometer to Measure Specific Gravity

Task Performed	Possible Points	TASKS
❑	10	Tests patient urine specimen and records results on patient requisition form.
❑	5	Cleans area after finishing procedure, including wiping up any spills with antiseptic solution, wiping refractometer clean with a lint-free tissue and distilled water, and disposing of all biohazardous waste in the biohazard container.
❑	5	Completed the tasks within 10 minutes.
❑	15	Results obtained were accurate.

______	Earned	ADD POINTS OF TASKS CHECKED
135	Points	TOTAL POINTS POSSIBLE
______	SCORE	DETERMINE SCORE (divide points earned by total points possible, multiply results by 100)

Actual Student Time Needed to Complete Procedure: ____________

Student's Initials: ____________ Instructor's Initials: ____________ Grade: ____________

Suggestions for Improvement: ____

Evaluator's Name (print) ____

Evaluator's Signature ____

Comments ____

DOCUMENTATION

Record the labeling of the urine specimen: ____

____

Record the specific gravity of the quality control urine specimen in the quality control sheet:

____

Record the specific gravity of the patient urine specimen on the patient requisition form:

____

Student's Initials: __________

SKILLS COMPETENCY ASSESSMENT

Procedure 35-5: Performing a Urinalysis Chemical Examination

Student's Name: ______________________________ Date: __________

Objective: To detect any abnormal chemical constituents of a urine specimen.

Conditions: The student demonstrates the ability to perform a urinalysis chemical examination using the following supplies: gloves, dipsticks, urine specimen, biohazard container, and laboratory report form.

Time Requirements and Accuracy Standards: 10 minutes. Points assigned reflect importance of step to meeting objective: Important = (5) Essential = (10) Critical = (15). Automatic failure results if any of the **critical** tasks are omitted or performed incorrectly.

STANDARD PRECAUTIONS:

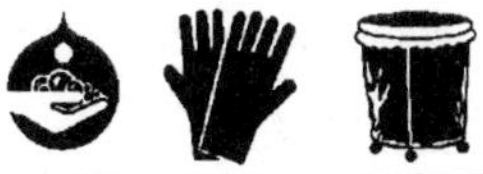

SKILLS ASSESSMENT CHECKLIST

Task Performed	Possible Points	TASKS
☐	5	Washes hands.
☐	5	Puts on gloves.
☐	5	Assembles equipment and materials.
☐	5	Follows all safety guidelines.
☐	5	Is careful not to splash urine. Wipes up any and all spills with antiseptic cleaner.
☐	10	Mixes the urine specimen well by inverting it several times, making sure the cover is on tightly before inverting.
☐	10	Removes test strip from a container, making sure the desiccant packet, which ensures dryness, remains in the container; replaces the cap tightly.
☐	10	Immerses strip completely in the uncentrifuged urine and removes it immediately.
☐	10	While removing the strip from urine, runs its edge against the rim of the container, tapping it lightly on the container to remove any excess urine. Does not allow urine drops to run down the strip from one reagent pad to another after tapping.
☐	5	*Rationale:* Understands that excess urine can bridge the gap between reagent pads, causing inaccurate results.
☐	15	Follows the proper timing listed on the dipstick container.
☐	5	*Rationale:* Understands that precise timing is critical to obtaining accurate results.
☐	15	Holds dipstick close to container. Compares the test areas to the proper area on the container and records results on the laboratory report form. Uses correct manufacturer's chart to determine test results.

SKILLS COMPETENCY ASSESSMENT— continued

Procedure 35-5: Performing a Urinalysis Chemical Examination

Task Performed	Possible Points	TASKS
☐	5	Properly disposes of the used reagent strips and other disposable items in the proper waste receptacles. Properly stores reagent strip container according to manufacturer's instructions. (Reagent strips should never be refrigerated or frozen.)
☐	5	Completed the tasks within 10 minutes.
☐	15	Results obtained were accurate.

_______	Earned	ADD POINTS OF TASKS CHECKED
130	Points	TOTAL POINTS POSSIBLE
_______	SCORE	DETERMINE SCORE (divide points earned by total points possible, multiply results by 100)

Actual Student Time Needed to Complete Procedure: ____________

Student's Initials: ____________ Instructor's Initials: ____________ Grade: ____________

Suggestions for Improvement: ____

Evaluator's Name (print) ____

Evaluator's Signature ____

Comments ____

DOCUMENTATION

Record the labeling of the urine specimen. ____

____

Record the results of the urinalysis chemical examination. ____

____

____

____

Student's Initials: ____________

SKILLS COMPETENCY ASSESSMENT

Procedure 35-6: Testing for Reducing Sugars

Student's Name: ______________________________ Date: ____________

Objective: To perform a Clinitest on a urine specimen to detect reducing sugars.

Conditions: The student demonstrates the ability to perform a Clinitest on a urine specimen using the following supplies: gloves, Clinitest tablets, urine specimen, clean glass test tube, distilled water, disposable pipettes, biohazard container, and laboratory report form.

Time Requirements and Accuracy Standards: 10 minutes. Points assigned reflect importance of step to meeting objective: Important = (5) Essential = (10) Critical = (15). Automatic failure results if any of the **critical** tasks are omitted or performed incorrectly.

STANDARD PRECAUTIONS:

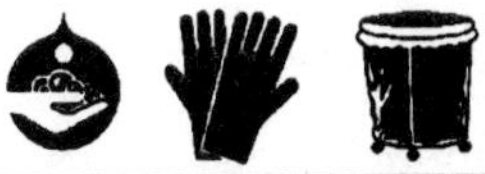

SKILLS ASSESSMENT CHECKLIST

Task Performed	Possible Points	TASKS
☐	5	Washes hands.
☐	5	Puts on gloves.
☐	5	Assembles equipment and materials.
☐	5	Follows all safety guidelines.
☐	5	Is careful not to splash urine. Wipes up any and all spills with antiseptic cleaner.
☐	10	Transfers five drops of urine (0.3 mL) into a clean glass test tube.
☐	10	Adds ten drops of water (0.6 mL) and mixes well. Is careful not to splash contents of tube.
☐	10	Drops one tablet into tube and watches mixture while the complete boiling takes place.
☐	5	*Rationale:* Understands that the bottom of the test tube becomes hot enough to cause severe burns.
☐	10	Does not shake the tube after adding the tablet until at least 15 seconds after the boiling stops.
☐	10	Gently shakes tube after appropriate waiting period to mix, without touching bottom of tube.
☐	15	Compares color of liquid to the proper color chart and documents it in laboratory report. Uses the percentage and/or trace through 4+ reporting methods. Ignores any changes in color that occur after the waiting period.
☐	15	Disposes of all biohazardous waste in the biohazard waste container.

SKILLS COMPETENCY ASSESSMENT — continued

Procedure 35-6: Testing for Reducing Sugars

Task Performed	Possible Points	TASKS
☐	5	Completed the tasks within 15 minutes.
☐	15	Results obtained were accurate.

________	Earned	ADD POINTS OF TASKS CHECKED
130	Points	TOTAL POINTS POSSIBLE
________	SCORE	DETERMINE SCORE (divide points earned by total points possible, multiply results by 100)

Actual Student Time Needed to Complete Procedure: ____________

Student's Initials: ____________ Instructor's Initials: ____________ Grade: ____________

Suggestions for Improvement: ____

Evaluator's Name (print) ____

Evaluator's Signature ____

Comments ____

DOCUMENTATION

Record labeling for the urine specimen: ____

____

Record the Clinitest results for the urine specimen: ____

____

____

____

____

Student's Initials: ________

SKILLS COMPETENCY ASSESSMENT

Procedure 35-7: Microscopic Examination of Urine Sediment

Student's Name: ______________________________ Date: ____________

Objective: To perform a microscopic examination of urine sediment.

Conditions: The student demonstrates the ability to perform a microscopic examination of urine sediment using the following supplies: gloves, microscope, centrifuge, microscope slides, cover slips, disposable pipettes, centrifuge tube, urine sediment, containing casts, urine atlas, biohazard container, and laboratory report form.

Time Requirements and Accuracy Standards: 20 minutes. Points assigned reflect importance of step to meeting objective: Important = (5) Essential = (10) Critical = (15). Automatic failure results if any of the **critical** tasks are omitted or performed incorrectly.

SKILLS ASSESSMENT CHECKLIST

Task Performed	Possible Points	TASKS
❑	5	Washes hands.
❑	5	Puts on gloves.
❑	5	Assembles equipment and materials.
❑	5	Follows all safety guidelines.
❑	5	Is careful not to splash urine. Wipes up any and all spills with antiseptic cleaner.
❑	5	Obtains a urine specimen and examines as quickly as possible thereafter.
❑	10	Mixes specimen well, then centrifuges a 10- to 15-mL aliquot at 1,500 revolutions per minute for five minutes.
❑	15	Pours off supernatant after centrifugation, leaving approximately 1 mL in the bottom of the centrifuge tube.
❑	10	Taps or flicks bottom of tube to resuspend the sediment in the remaining fluid.
❑	10	Places a drop of sediment on a microscope slide; places coverglass over drop of sediment.
❑	10	Places slide on microscope stage and immediately examines.
❑	5	*Rationale:* Understands optimum light and focus adjustments for best examination of specimen.
❑	5	Scans sediment using a 100× (low) magnification.
❑	5	*Rationale:* Understands procedure for achieving a 100× magnification.
❑	5	Views ten to fifteen fields and around the edges of the drop for casts.
❑	10	Records the average number of each type of cast viewed per LPF. Uses 45× objective, if necessary, to identify some of the casts.

SKILLS COMPETENCY ASSESSMENT — continued

Procedure 35-7: Microscopic Examination of Urine Sediment

Task Performed	Possible Points	TASKS
☐	10	Scans drop using a 400× (high) magnification. Counts and averages numbers of other formed elements in ten to fifteen fields.
☐	5	Records results on laboratory report form.
☐	5	Disposes of all biohazardous waste in the biohazard container. Cleans microscopic lenses with lens paper and wipes up all spills with antiseptic cleaner.
☐	5	Completed the tasks within 20 minutes.
☐	15	Results obtained were accurate.

______	Earned	ADD POINTS OF TASKS CHECKED
155	Points	TOTAL POINTS POSSIBLE
______	SCORE	DETERMINE SCORE (divide points earned by total points possible, multiply results by 100)

Actual Student Time Needed to Complete Procedure: ____________

Student's Initials: ____________ Instructor's Initials: ____________ Grade: ____________

Suggestions for Improvement: ____

Evaluator's Name (print) ____

Evaluator's Signature ____

Comments ____

DOCUMENTATION

Record labeling of urine specimen. ____

____

Record results of microscopic examination of the urine sediment specimen: ____________

____

____

____

Student's Initials: ________

SKILLS COMPETENCY ASSESSMENT

Procedure 35-8: Performing a Urinalysis

Student's Name: ______________________________ Date: ____________

Objective: To perform a complete urinalysis.

Conditions: The student demonstrates the ability to perform a complete urinalysis, including physical, chemical, and microscopic examinations using the following supplies: gloves, urine specimen, measuring cylinder, test tubes, pipettes, centrifuge tube, centrifuge, microscope, microscope slides, coverglasses, reagent strips, control urine sample, urine atlas, refractometer (or urinometer), distilled water, lint-free tissues, biohazard container, and laboratory report form.

Time Requirements and Accuracy Standards: 45 minutes. Points assigned reflect importance of step to meeting objective: Important = (5) Essential = (10) Critical = (15). Automatic failure results if any of the **critical** tasks are omitted or performed incorrectly.

STANDARD PRECAUTIONS: 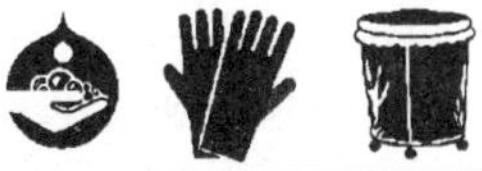

SKILLS ASSESSMENT CHECKLIST

Task Performed	Possible Points	TASKS
☐	5	Washes hands.
☐	5	Puts on gloves.
☐	5	Assembles equipment and materials.
☐	5	Follows all safety guidelines.
☐	5	Is careful not to splash urine. Wipes up any and all spills with antiseptic cleaner.
		PHYSICAL EXAMINATION
☐	10	Obtains a urine specimen.
☐	10	Measures amount of specimen in measuring cylinder and makes sure there is more than 12 mL of urine in specimen.
☐	5	Gently mixes and pours approximately 5 mL of urine into a test tube.
☐	15	Observes and records the color of the urine (see "Documentation").
☐	15	Observes and records the transparency of the urine (see "Documentation").
☐	10	Notes unusual odors of the urine.
☐	15	Measures specific gravity of urine using a refractometer or urinometer and records the results (see "Documentation").

SKILLS COMPETENCY ASSESSMENT — continued

Procedure 35-8: Performing a Urinalysis

Task Performed	Possible Points	TASKS
		Refractometer
❑	10	Places one drop of distilled water on the glass plate and closes.
❑	10	Looks through the ocular and reads specific gravity from the scale: 1.000.
❑	5	Wipes the water from the glass plate with lint-free tissues.
❑	5	Places one drop of urine on the plate and closes.
❑	10	Looks through the ocular, reads and records the specific gravity.
❑	5	Cleans the glass plate with water and dries with a tissue.
		Urinometer
❑	10	Pours 40 to 50 mL distilled water into the glass cylinder.
❑	5	Inserts urinometer with a spinning motion.
❑	15	Reads the specific gravity from the scale on the stem of the urinometer as it stops spinning: 1.000.
❑	5	Rinses the equipment with distilled water.
❑	5	Repeats the procedure using a urine specimen. Reads and records specific gravity.
❑	5	Cleans the equipment carefully using detergent, rinsing thoroughly with distilled water and drying carefully.
		CHEMICAL EXAMINATION
❑	5	Continues wearing gloves and uses the same specimen used in the physical examination.
❑	10	Tests the urine control sample with a reagent strip. Dips the strip into the sample, moistening all pads.
❑	5	Immediately removes strip, taps to remove excess urine.
❑	10	Observes reagent pads and compares colors to color chart at appropriate intervals.
❑	5	Properly disposes of reagent strip and records results on laboratory report form (see "Documentation").
❑	10	Performs appropriate tests on any positive results that need confirmation, following manufacturer's directions and all necessary safety precautions.
❑	5	Documents results of confirmatory tests on laboratory report form (see "Documentation").

Task Performed	Possible Points	TASKS
❑	5	Disposes of all biohazardous materials in a biohazard container.
		MICROSCOPIC EXAMINATION
❑	5	Continues to wear gloves and uses the same urine sample used in the physical and chemical examinations. Follows all necessary safety precautions.
❑	10	Pours 12 mL urine into a specimen tube and centrifuges the specimen at 1,500 to 2,500 rpm for five minutes.
❑	15	Decants the supernatant and resuspends the sediment.
❑	15	Pipettes one drop of resuspended urine on a clean glass slide.
❑	5	Places coverglass over drop of urine.
❑	5	Carefully places slide under microscope.
❑	10	Scans slide under low power (100×) and reduced light for casts. Refers to urine atlas as necessary.
❑	10	Rotates to high power (40× and 45× objective).
❑	10	Scans slide and identifies any blood cells, bacteria, yeast, protozoa, and epithelial cells.
❑	10	Identifies any crystals or amorphous deposits seen.
❑	5	Records all results on laboratory report form (see "Documentation").
❑	5	Discards all biohazardous materials in biohazard container.
❑	5	Cleans and returns equipment to proper storage.
❑	5	Cleans work area with disinfectant.
❑	5	Discards gloves in biohazard container.
❑	5	Thoroughly washes hands with disinfectant soap.
❑	5	Completed the tasks within 45 minutes.
❑	15	Results obtained were accurate.

______	Earned	ADD POINTS OF TASKS CHECKED
395	Points	TOTAL POINTS POSSIBLE
______	SCORE	DETERMINE SCORE (divide points earned by total points possible, multiply results by 100)

SKILLS COMPETENCY ASSESSMENT — continued

Procedure 35-8: Performing a Urinalysis

Actual Student Time Needed to Complete Procedure: ____________

Student's Initials: ____________ Instructor's Initials: ____________ Grade: ____________

Suggestions for Improvement: ____

Evaluator's Name (print) ____

Evaluator's Signature ____

Comments ____

DOCUMENTATION

Record labeling of urine specimen. ____

____

Record all observations pertaining to the physical examination.

Color, Transparency, and Specific Gravity ____

____

Record all observations pertaining to the chemical examination.

____

____

____

Record all observations pertaining to the microscopic examination.

____

____

____

____

Student's Initials: __________

EVALUATION OF CHAPTER KNOWLEDGE

Evaluate your comprehension of urinalysis, including proper collection and handling techniques; safety guidelines involved; and how to properly perform a complete urinalysis, including physical, chemical, and microscopic examinations. Compare this evaluation with the one provided by your instructor:

	Student Self-Evaluation			**Instructor Evaluation**		
Knowledge	*Good*	*Average*	*Poor*	*Good*	*Average*	*Poor*
Understands the importance of urinalysis as a diagnostic tool	____	____	____	____	____	____
Understands how urine is formed and excreted in the human body	____	____	____	____	____	____
Can define key terms related to urinalysis found in glossary	____	____	____	____	____	____
Understands the crucial role safety procedures and quality control play in performing urinalysis	____	____	____	____	____	____
Can accurately perform a physical examination of urine and explain causes of abnormal physical characteristics in urine specimens	____	____	____	____	____	____
Can accurately perform a chemical examination of urine and explain causes of abnormal chemical characteristics in urine specimens	____	____	____	____	____	____
Can accurately perform a microscopic examination of urine and explain causes of abnormal microscopic characteristics in urine specimens	____	____	____	____	____	____
Able to describe confirmatory tests for ketones, glucose, protein, and bilirubin	____	____	____	____	____	____
Can identify the proper method of preparing urine sediment for microscopic examination	____	____	____	____	____	____
Able to identify both normal and abnormal structures discovered during the microscopic examination of urine sediment	____	____	____	____	____	____
Is aware of and can describe factors that may interfere with urinalysis accuracy	____	____	____	____	____	____
Performs proper documentation of procedures	____	____	____	____	____	____
Follows standard precautions	____	____	____	____	____	____

Student's Initials: ______ Instructor's Initials: ______

Grade: ______

CHAPTER 36

Basic Microbiology

PERFORMANCE OBJECTIVES

Microbiology is an area of enormous importance in health care and one in which medical assistants play a role. Specimens are processed in either the physician's office laboratory (POL) or reference laboratory. The emergence of pathogens increasing in resistance to antibiotics makes this area even more significant to the health professions. Rapid and precise culturing and identification of pathogens allows for appropriate treatment of the patient. The quality of the diagnosis and treatment of an infection is rooted in the quality of the specimen obtained and processed. Although laboratories will vary in size and extent of work, one thing will remain constant—safety precautions and quality control procedures must be carefully followed for the protection of health care professionals and for the integrity of test results.

EXERCISES AND ACTIVITIES

Vocabulary Builder

Find the key vocabulary terms in the word search puzzle.

Aerobic
Aerosols
Anaerobic
Biochemical tests
Broth tubes
Check cell slides
Concentration method
counterstain
culture
decolorizer
dermatophyte
DNA
Enterobacteriaceae
Expectorate
Fastidious bacteria
Genus
Gram stain
Holding media
Immunosuppressed
Inoculate
Kirby Bauer
Lumbar puncture
Microbiology
Mordant
Morphology
Mycobacteria
Mycology
Nematode
Normal flora
Nosocomial
Ova
Parasitology
Pathogen
Petri dish
Protozoa
Quality control

Reagents
Sensitivity
Species
Stab culture
Taxonomy
Tetrads
Virology
Wood's lamp

N	Y	R	S	D	A	R	T	E	T	G	K	A	D	S	E	M	L	B	R	I	X	D	S	K	K	H	Q	C	Q	Z
P	E	Z	E	U	T	P	V	F	Y	R	F	N	C	E	D	Y	B	Z	X	N	A	A	T	Q	B	J	U	I	C	A
E	R	G	W	A	N	V	H	V	T	A	N	A	E	I	O	C	B	Y	O	O	Z	R	C	H	X	K	A	X	W	T
H	T	O	O	N	G	E	M	X	C	M	C	E	S	C	T	O	B	V	F	C	C	O	Y	F	L	D	L	L	P	Q
S	S	A	T	H	L	E	G	R	A	S	F	R	W	E	A	L	J	U	L	U	V	L	U	S	E	I	I	W	E	I
I	D	L	R	O	T	A	N	J	K	T	D	O	Q	P	M	O	M	L	U	L	L	F	H	R	U	B	T	R	Q	B
D	Q	A	O	O	Z	A	I	T	N	A	V	B	P	S	E	G	E	Z	M	A	Q	L	M	O	L	U	Y	X	B	D
I	A	H	E	L	T	O	P	M	S	I	G	I	K	D	N	Y	Y	E	B	T	Q	A	X	K	M	C	C	Q	F	D
R	G	M	X	K	D	C	A	M	O	N	V	C	I	R	F	R	N	A	A	E	T	M	Y	D	C	X	O	L	V	Q
T	P	B	I	O	C	H	E	M	I	C	A	L	T	E	S	T	S	A	R	O	G	R	O	D	Z	F	N	J	O	R
E	Z	R	W	Q	N	E	X	P	C	S	O	A	N	J	E	K	C	P	P	C	A	O	P	M	V	C	T	Y	J	W
P	O	V	Y	Z	T	C	A	P	X	C	E	S	V	R	A	P	M	H	U	T	X	N	Z	I	H	M	R	M	Y	L
E	D	S	Q	O	C	K	Y	I	A	E	L	B	O	E	S	V	Y	Y	N	J	C	R	Y	N	I	J	O	Y	S	P
E	R	U	T	L	U	C	D	A	D	R	P	B	U	N	B	T	O	W	C	D	I	V	W	C	C	Y	L	E	R	T
G	U	H	T	U	C	E	S	A	X	E	A	L	O	T	E	V	Q	T	T	O	R	S	R	N	M	Y	N	W	D	Q
B	I	M	N	W	S	L	R	J	U	C	M	S	V	S	H	J	W	W	U	W	B	O	J	O	P	S	V	V	N	L
Y	X	L	K	A	O	L	Y	W	T	I	U	G	I	A	R	T	B	V	R	A	B	A	N	V	I	Z	I	U	X	L
K	Q	K	O	S	Q	S	Z	E	X	D	Z	R	N	T	E	Y	O	A	E	I	P	O	C	T	V	R	Y	G	E	L
R	Q	D	O	X	N	L	R	D	N	S	P	E	T	I	O	R	C	R	O	B	X	P	I	T	O	J	E	U	Q	J
Z	P	R	R	E	Z	I	R	O	L	O	C	E	D	D	D	L	O	L	B	A	Z	V	V	L	E	W	D	K	B	Q
F	E	D	U	X	A	D	Y	U	M	O	B	T	B	V	R	L	O	B	T	O	I	M	O	Y	W	R	A	K	T	Q
A	N	N	K	C	K	E	W	L	Z	V	K	P	U	O	X	G	O	G	I	T	Q	G	J	T	S	Y	I	J	J	V
A	R	M	E	V	B	S	R	C	N	K	P	J	B	B	Y	Z	I	H	Y	C	Y	A	X	G	D	F	F	A	I	X
J	U	A	B	T	W	G	D	E	D	O	H	T	E	M	N	O	I	T	A	R	T	N	E	C	N	O	C	I	U	W
N	E	O	C	O	U	N	T	E	R	S	T	A	I	N	W	O	O	D	S	L	A	M	P	C	A	C	D	X	W	L
A	I	R	E	T	C	A	B	S	U	O	I	D	I	T	S	A	F	R	E	U	A	B	Y	B	R	I	K	A	K	W
I	M	M	U	N	O	S	U	P	P	R	E	S	S	E	D	U	E	M	F	Z	T	N	A	D	R	O	M	W	Z	E
Y	G	O	L	O	H	P	R	O	M	E	R	U	T	L	U	C	B	A	T	S	N	U	X	T	Z	X	M	K	E	E

Learning Review

1. Infections from parasites have increased as more people travel and public awareness of the symptoms grow.

   A. The most common parasite infections seen in the laboratory are ________________ ________________, a nematode that causes pinworm infections and ________________ ________________, a flagellate causing a sexually transmitted disease in both men and women.

   B. Specimens collected for parasites need to be checked for ________________, ________________, and ________________.

C. Labeling specimens sent for testing with ________________, ________________, and ________________ collected is important, as well as noting if the patient has been ________________ to a specific place, and what the physician suspects.

D. To diagnose the presence of a parasite, either the ____________ ____________ or ________________ must be located in the specimen.

E. Obtaining the specimen to test for pinworms is performed by using a ____________ ____________ ____________ that is placed sticky side down to the skin around the anal area.

F. ________________ ________________ ________________ should be worn when working with specimens. Assuming that all specimens are ________________ is an important element of following standard precautions for infection control.

G. The practice of proper aseptic ________________ ________________ several times a day, including after glove removal, is essential and should become a ________________.

2. Specimen containers will arrive at the laboratory inside plastic bags to avoid danger to laboratory personnel. What precautions are taken before opening the bags?

____

____

3. A laboratory's success in finding and identifying the pathogenic organism depends on multiple factors. Name nine:

(1) ________________ (6) ________________

(2) ________________ (7) ________________

(3) ________________ (8) ________________

(4) ________________ (9) ________________

(5) ________________

4. Describe how you feel about working with patients who have an infection, which is possibly communicable. What, if anything, concerns you? What resources do you have in addressing your concerns?

____

____

____

5. The medical assistant in a physician's office will most likely frequently assist in the care and treatment of patients with sore throats.

Why is it necessary to rapidly identify the cause? ________________

What test would be used? ________________________________

What five rules should be followed?

(1) ____________________

(2) ____________________

(3) ____________________

(4) ____________________

(5) ____________________

6. *Label the parts of the cell and check off "some" for the parts that are sometimes present and "all" for the parts that are always present.*

Basic Bacterial Cell

		Some	All
A.	____________	❑	❑
B.	____________	❑	❑
C.	____________	❑	❑
D.	____________	❑	❑
E.	____________	❑	❑
F.	____________	❑	❑

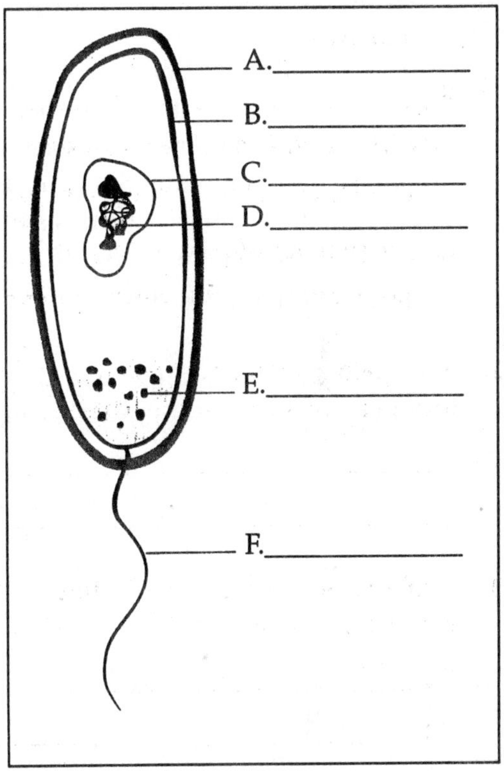

Investigation Activity

Laboratories have many responsibilities in the safety arena. These exist internally, as in the area of employee safety, and externally, as in reporting of the isolation and identification of organisms that are of public health concern. For each example below, research both of these areas at the library, a laboratory, the Public Health Department, or through a regulatory agency.

A. Identify what your course of action might be if you are asked to work without appropriate Personal Protective Equipment (PPE) or to place hazardous waste in the regular waste container.

B. The physician has ordered throat cultures for several patients who are from the same-area school. They are quite ill, with a high fever and sore throat; the physician states that one patient appears to be developing scarlet fever. To whom is this occurrence reported? Is this obligatory for public health? What agency makes the recommendations for public health? Where can you find a list of communicable diseases that laboratories must report? What international agency classifies infectious diseases?

CASE STUDY

Case 1

Winston Lewis, M. D., has ordered a series of three sputum cultures for Herb Fowler, who has been suffering with a productive cough for several months and extreme fatigue. Audrey Jones, CMA, is assigned to obtain the cultures. When each culture is obtained from Mr. Fowler, Audrey brings it to the physician's office laboratory (POL) for culturing.

Discuss the following:

1. What is the procedure for obtaining a sputum specimen? Why are detailed patient instructions critical?
2. Mr. Fowler wishes to give all three specimens in one day to save on the transportation to and from the physician's office. Audrey explains that the specimens must be obtained one each day, upon awakening, for three days. What is the reason for this?
3. What microorganisms might the physician suspect and how should the specimen be treated in the physician's office laboratory (POL)? Under what circumstances should the specimen be sent to an outside reference laboratory for further testing?

Case 2

Mary O'Keefe calls for an emergency appointment for her 3-year-old son Chris because he awakened during the night with a high fever and severe pain in his right ear, which is draining. Dr. King performs the examination, assisted by Ellen Armstrong, CMA. During the examination Dr. King takes a specimen of the fluid ear discharge for laboratory analysis, which the physician suspects will confirm a clinical diagnosis of otitis media. Dr. King asks Ellen to perform a Gram stain on a portion of the patient specimen and to send the remainder of the specimen to an outside reference laboratory for culturing.

Discuss the following:

1. What equipment will Ellen require to perform the Gram staining of the specimen?
2. What standard precautions must Ellen observe while performing the Gram stain procedure?
3. If a strain of *Streptococcus* or *Staphylococcus* bacteria is responsible for the infection producing the patient's condition of otitis media, what Gram staining result will Ellen receive? What will the Gram stained specimen look like under the microscope? *Consult a medical reference or encyclopedia, if necessary.*

SUPPLEMENTARY RESOURCES

Study Guide Disk: Additional practice exercises for this chapter are available on the study guide disk found in the textbook.

Medical Assisting Videos: Appropriate content is available on Delmar's Medical Assisting Videos, 2nd ed., for the following topics:

Tape 5: Perform Medical Aseptic Technique of Hand Washing
Infections in the Office

Tape 14: Quality Control in Collecting and Processing Specimens
Collect a Stool Specimen
Perform a Hemoccult Test
Collect a Sputum Specimen
Collect a Throat Culture
Perform a Strep Screen
Collect Vaginal Samples
Streak a Culture Plate
Make a Gram Stain

SKILLS COMPETENCY ASSESSMENT

Procedure 36-1: Preparing a Bacteriological Smear

Student's Name: ______________________________ Date: __________

Objective: To prepare a bacteriological smear.

Conditions: The student demonstrates the ability to prepare a bacterial suspension for staining to examine bacteria microscopically using the following equipment: PPE, clean glass slide, distilled water, loop or swab, organism, heat, staining rack, tray, and stains.

Time Requirements and Accuracy Standards: 30 minutes. Points assigned reflect importance of step to meeting objective: Important = (5) Essential = (10) Critical = (15). Automatic failure results if any of the **critical** tasks are omitted or performed incorrectly.

STANDARD PRECAUTIONS:

SKILLS ASSESSMENT CHECKLIST

Task Performed	Possible Points	TASKS
❑	5	Washes hands and puts on PPE.
❑	5	Assembles equipment.
❑	15	Applies thin film of bacteria to slide using a sterile or flamed loop or rolling a swab onto the surface of the slide, making a smear about the size of a nickel.
❑	15	If bacteria is in a liquid suspension, applies directly to the slide; if not, adds a drop of sterile water to the slide first.
❑	10	Allows the bacteria time to air dry.
❑	5	*Rationale:* Can state what will happen if heat is applied before bacteria is completely air dried.
❑	10	Heat fixes slide by passing it through the flame two or three times.
❑	5	*Rationale:* Can state the consequences if heat fixing is omitted or overdone.
❑	10	Allows slide to cool before staining.
❑	5	Follows all safety precautions.
❑	5	Completed the tasks within 30 minutes.
❑	15	Results obtained were accurate.

________	Earned	ADD POINTS OF TASKS CHECKED
105	Points	TOTAL POINTS POSSIBLE
________	SCORE	DETERMINE SCORE (divide points earned by total points possible, multiply results by 100)

Actual Student Time Needed to Complete Procedure: __________

Student's Initials: __________ Instructor's Initials: __________ Grade: __________

Suggestions for Improvement: ______________________________

Evaluator's Name (print) ______________________________

Evaluator's Signature ______________________________

Comments ______________________________

SKILLS COMPETENCY ASSESSMENT

Procedure 36-2: Gram Stain

Student's Name: ______________________________ Date: ____________

Objective: To Gram stain and read a bacteriological slide.

Conditions: The student demonstrates the ability to identify Gram-negative and Gram-positive bacteria microscopically through the staining technique using the following equipment: PPE, distilled water in beaker or plastic squeeze bottle, prepared bacteriological smears, heat, Gram stain reagents or kit, bibulous paper, tray, and paper towels.

Time Requirements and Accuracy Standards: 20 minutes. Points assigned reflect importance of step to meeting objective: Important = (5) Essential = (10) Critical = (15). Automatic failure results if any of the **critical** tasks are omitted or performed incorrectly.

STANDARD PRECAUTIONS:

SKILLS ASSESSMENT CHECKLIST

Task Performed	Possible Points	TASKS
❑	5	Washes hands and applies PPE.
❑	5	Assembles equipment and supplies.
❑	15	Floods the prepared slide with crystal violet for accurate time, following manufacturer's instructions.
❑	10	Rinses stain off the slide with a gentle stream of distilled water; tilts slide to remove excess water.
❑	15	Floods the slide with Gram's iodine for the recommended time.
❑	5	Rinses slide as before, removing excess water.
❑	15	Holds slide by the short edge using forceps. Adds acetone-alcohol decolorizer by squeeze bottle or pasteur pipette until purple no longer runs off slide.
❑	5	Rinses immediately, as before, removing excess water.
❑	15	Counterstains the smears by flooding the slides with safranin for the recommended time.
❑	10	Rinses slide as before, removing excess water. Wipes back of slide to remove excess stain; stands slide on end or carefully blots between sheets of bibulous paper to dry.
❑	5	Reads and records results according to laboratory policy.
❑	5	Completed the tasks within 20 minutes.

Task Performed	Possible Points	TASKS
☐	15	Results obtained were accurate.

________	Earned	ADD POINTS OF TASKS CHECKED
125	Points	TOTAL POINTS POSSIBLE
________	SCORE	DETERMINE SCORE (divide points earned by total points possible, multiply results by 100)

Actual Student Time Needed to Complete Procedure: ____________

Student's Initials: ____________ Instructor's Initials: ____________ Grade: ____________

Suggestions for Improvement: ______________________________

Evaluator's Name (print) ______________________________

Evaluator's Signature ______________________________

Comments ______________________________

DOCUMENTATION

Record the results according to the laboratory policy.

Date: ________________

Charting: ______________________________

____

Student's Initials:__________

SKILLS COMPETENCY ASSESSMENT

Procedure 36-3: Ziehl-Neelsen Staining

Student's Name: ______________________________________ Date: ____________

Objective: To perform Ziehl-Neelsen staining.

Conditions: The student demonstrates the ability to use Ziehl-Neelsen staining to identify acid-fast and non-acid-fast organisms using the following equipment: PPE, organism, glass slide, distilled water, heat, Ziehl-Neelsen stain reagents, and staining rack and tray.

Time Requirements and Accuracy Standards: 20 minutes. Points assigned reflect importance of step to meeting objective: Important = (5) Essential = (10) Critical = (15). Automatic failure results if any of the **critical** tasks are omitted or performed incorrectly.

STANDARD PRECAUTIONS: 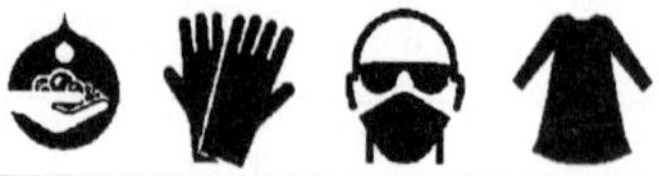

SKILLS ASSESSMENT CHECKLIST

Task Performed	Possible Points	TASKS
☐	5	Washes hands and puts on PPE.
☐	5	Assembles equipment and materials.
☐	15	Places prepared slide on rack, carefully applies heat, staining with carbolfuchsin. Applies heat under slide until steaming. Does not let stain dry on the slide; applies the carbolfuchsin liberally.
☐	10	Uses distilled water to wash off the stain.
☐	10	Decolorizes with acid alcohol for two minutes, then washes it off with distilled water.
☐	10	Applies counterstain of metheylene blue or malachite green for thirty seconds, then washes off slide with distilled water.
☐	5	Dries slide completely by air or heat block.
☐	5	Caution is shown in following laboratory safety precautions. This type of staining is done under a safety hood.
☐	5	*Rationale:* Knows why this type of slide is prepared under a safety hood.
☐	5	Disposes of hazardous mask appropriately, removes PPE, and washes hands.
☐	5	Documents results.
☐	5	Completed the tasks within 20 minutes.

Task Performed	Possible Points	TASKS
❑	15	Results obtained were accurate.

________	Earned	ADD POINTS OF TASKS CHECKED
100	Points	TOTAL POINTS POSSIBLE
________	SCORE	DETERMINE SCORE (divide points earned by total points possible, multiply results by 100)

Actual Student Time Needed to Complete Procedure: ____________

Student's Initials: ____________ Instructor's Initials: ____________ Grade: ____________

Suggestions for Improvement: ____

Evaluator's Name (print) ____

Evaluator's Signature ____

Comments ____

DOCUMENTATION

Charts the results according to the laboratory policy.

Date: ________________

Charting: ____

____

Student's Initials: ____________

SKILLS COMPETENCY ASSESSMENT

Procedure 36-4: Wet Slide and Hanging Drop Slide Preparation

Student's Name: ______________________________ Date: ____________

Objective: To prepare a wet slide and hanging drop slide.

Conditions: The student demonstrates the ability to prepare slides for viewing motility and characteristics of live organisms using the following equipment: Glass slides with concave well, PPE, clean glass slides with coverslips, petroleum jelly, dropper, and bacterial suspension.

Time Requirements and Accuracy Standards: 5 minutes. Points assigned reflect importance of step to meeting objective: Important = (5) Essential = (10) Critical = (15). Automatic failure results if any of the **critical** tasks are omitted or performed incorrectly.

STANDARD PRECAUTIONS: 

SKILLS ASSESSMENT CHECKLIST

Task Performed	Possible Points	TASKS
❑	5	Washes hands and puts on PPE.
❑	5	Assembles equipment and supplies.
		Wet Slide Preparation:
❑	10	Places bacterial suspension on clean glass slide.
❑	15	Places petroleum jelly on cover slip and places it appropriately on bacterial slide.
❑	5	*Rationale:* Knows the need to prepare this accurately to prevent drying out and to allow observation microscopically at any power.
		Hanging Drop Slide Preparation:
❑	10	Bacterial suspension placed appropriately on cover slip with petroleum jelly on the edge.
❑	15	Inverts slide with the concave well over the cover slip.
❑	10	Turns slide right side up and examines.
❑	5	Follows all laboratory safety precautions.
❑	5	*Rationale:* Can state why these precautions are so necessary in this procedure.
❑	5	Records results according to laboratory policy.
❑	5	Completed the tasks within 5 minutes each.

Task Performed	Possible Points	TASKS
❑	15	Results obtained were accurate.

______	Earned	ADD POINTS OF TASKS CHECKED
110	Points	TOTAL POINTS POSSIBLE
______	SCORE	DETERMINE SCORE (divide points earned by total points possible, multiply results by 100)

Actual Student Time Needed to Complete Procedure: ______________

Student's Initials: ______________ Instructor's Initials: ______________ Grade: ______________

Suggestions for Improvement: ______________________________

Evaluator's Name (print) ______________________________

Evaluator's Signature ______________________________

Comments ______________________________

DOCUMENTATION

Date: ______________

Chart this procedure as laboratory policy indicates. ______________________________

____

____

Student's Initials: ______________

SKILLS COMPETENCY ASSESSMENT

Procedure 36-5: Specimen Inoculation and Dilution Streaking

Student's Name: ______________________________ Date: __________

Objective: To perform specimen inoculation and dilution streaking.

Conditions: The student demonstrates the ability to inoculate solid media to study bacterial growth on agar using the following equipment: PPE, plates, heat, agar plates, inoculation loop, and bacterial specimens.

Time Requirements and Accuracy Standards: 10 minutes. Points assigned reflect importance of step to meeting objective: Important = (5) Essential = (10) Critical = (15). Automatic failure results if any of the **critical** tasks are omitted or performed incorrectly.

STANDARD PRECAUTIONS: 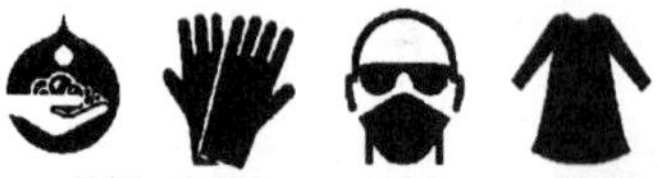

SKILLS ASSESSMENT CHECKLIST

Task Performed	Possible Points	TASKS
☐	5	Washes hands and puts on PPE.
☐	5	Assembles equipment and materials.
☐	10	Flames the loop (if metal loop is used) and allows to cool. Applies specimen to plate with sterile flamed loop or specimen's swab. Once applied, flames the loop again.
☐	15	Uses loop to streak specimen, being careful not to dig up the agar; remembers to turn plate after each of the three episodes and flames the loop appropriately.
☐	5	Implements all laboratory safety measures, including plating cultures under a safety hood.
☐	5	Records results according to laboratory policy.
☐	5	Completed the tasks within 10 minutes.
☐	15	Results obtained were accurate.

________	Earned	ADD POINTS OF TASKS CHECKED
65	Points	TOTAL POINTS POSSIBLE
________	SCORE	DETERMINE SCORE (divide points earned by total points possible, multiply results by 100)

Actual Student Time Needed to Complete Procedure: ____________

Student's Initials: ____________ Instructor's Initials: ____________ Grade: ____________

Suggestions for Improvement: ____________

Evaluator's Name (print) ____________

Evaluator's Signature ____________

Comments ____________

DOCUMENTATION

Chart the procedure as laboratory policy indicates. ____________

Student's Initials: ____________

SKILLS COMPETENCY ASSESSMENT

Procedure 36-6: Broth Tube Inoculation

Student's Name: ______________________________ Date: ____________

Objective: To inoculate a broth tube with bacteria.

Conditions: The student demonstrates the ability to inoculate liquid media to observe bacterial growth using the following equipment: PPE, broth, inoculating loop, liquid specimen, and heat.

Time Requirements and Accuracy Standards: 5 minutes. Points assigned reflect importance of step to meeting objective: Important = (5) Essential = (10) Critical = (15). Automatic failure results if any of the **critical** tasks are omitted or performed incorrectly.

STANDARD PRECAUTIONS:

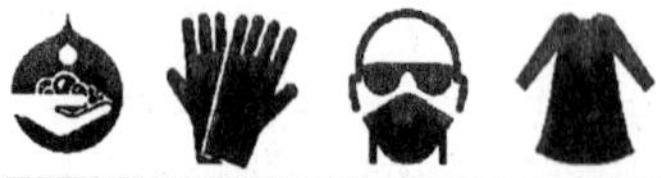

SKILLS ASSESSMENT CHECKLIST

Task Performed	Possible Points	TASKS
☐	5	Washes hands and puts on PPE.
☐	5	Assembles equipment and materials.
☐	5	Flames the loop, if it is metal.
☐	10	Picks up the specimen with the inoculating loop.
☐	15	Lifts the broth tube with care, slants the tube as required, touches the tube so the inoculation is submerged when upright.
☐	15	Gently mixes the tube to inoculate liquid media for bacterial growth.
☐	5	Follows all laboratory safety measures, particularly using the safety hood when appropriate.
☐	5	Records test results according to laboratory policy.
☐	5	Completed the tasks within 5 minutes.
☐	15	Results obtained were accurate.

______	Earned	ADD POINTS OF TASKS CHECKED
85	Points	TOTAL POINTS POSSIBLE
______	SCORE	DETERMINE SCORE (divide points earned by total points possible, multiply results by 100)

Actual Student Time Needed to Complete Procedure: ____________

Student's Initials: ____________ Instructor's Initials: ____________ Grade: ____________

Suggestions for Improvement: ________________________________

Evaluator's Name (print) ________________________________

Evaluator's Signature ________________________________

Comments ________________________________

DOCUMENTATION

Chart as required by laboratory policy.

Date: ______________

Charting: ________________________________

____

____

Student's Initials: ____________

SKILLS COMPETENCY ASSESSMENT

Procedure 36-7: Deep Inoculation/Slant

Student's Name: ______________________________ Date: ____________

Objective: To perform deep inoculation of slant media.

Conditions: The student demonstrates the ability to use deep inoculation of slant media to study motility or biochemical reactions using the following equipment: PPE, inoculating needle, deep agar or slant, heat, and isolated bacteria.

Time Requirements and Accuracy Standards: 5 minutes. Points assigned reflect importance of step to meeting objective: Important = (5) Essential = (10) Critical = (15). Automatic failure results if any of the **critical** tasks are omitted or performed incorrectly.

STANDARD PRECAUTIONS:

SKILLS ASSESSMENT CHECKLIST

Task Performed	Possible Points	TASKS
☐	5	Washes hands and puts on PPE.
☐	5	Assembles equipment and materials.
☐	15	Inoculates slant at 30 to 40 degree angle, stabbing to the bottom, making sure to flame needle before and after procedure.
☐	10	Using a needle, makes an "S" motion to streak up the slanted portion of the agar.
☐	5	Makes a straight deep stab into the upright agar.
☐	5	*Rationale:* Knows the reasoning behind inoculating the agar in these different ways.
☐	5	Follows all laboratory safety procedures.
☐	5	Uses safety hood as required for certain types of plating.
☐	5	Records procedure as laboratory requires.
☐	5	Completed the tasks within 5 minutes.
☐	15	Results obtained were accurate.

________	Earned	ADD POINTS OF TASKS CHECKED
80	Points	TOTAL POINTS POSSIBLE
________	SCORE	DETERMINE SCORE (divide points earned by total points possible, multiply results by 100)

Actual Student Time Needed to Complete Procedure: ____________

Student's Initials: ____________ Instructor's Initials: ____________ Grade: ____________

Suggestions for Improvement: ____

Evaluator's Name (print) ____

Evaluator's Signature ____

Comments ____

DOCUMENTATION

Chart the procedure as required by laboratory standards.

Date: ________________

Charting: ____

____

____

Student's Initials: ____________

EVALUATION OF CHAPTER KNOWLEDGE

How has your instructor evaluated the knowledge you have achieved?

Knowledge	Instructor Evaluation: Good	Average	Poor
Identifies the components of Personal Protective Equipment and important safety procedures	_____	_____	_____
Identifies quality control measures and describes uses	_____	_____	_____
Understands the importance and methods of collecting high-quality specimens	_____	_____	_____
Lists different types of specimens and stains	_____	_____	_____
Describes bacterial cell structure and can discuss identification systems for bacteria	_____	_____	_____
Identifies parasites and fungi	_____	_____	_____
Describes sensitivity testing	_____	_____	_____
Describes the difference between the presence of microorganisms as normal flora and as pathogens	_____	_____	_____
Understands the importance of patient education in obtaining specimens	_____	_____	_____
Can relate what happens when heat is used too long or too little in smear preparation for staining	_____	_____	_____
Understands the importance of the use of quality controls in the laboratory and with equipment	_____	_____	_____
Describes the need to discard media and reagents that have passed the expiration date	_____	_____	_____
Recognizes the role of the CMA in the laboratory	_____	_____	_____
Applies knowledge of microbiological classifications and nomenclature to appropriate use in the laboratory	_____	_____	_____
Follows precisely the procedures in performing tests in the laboratory	_____	_____	_____

Student's Initials: _____ Instructor's Initials: _____

Grade: _____

CHAPTER 37

Specialty Laboratory Tests

PERFORMANCE OBJECTIVES

More tests than ever before are performed in the ambulatory care setting. As a result, the medical assistant's role in laboratory testing is expanding. To meet the challenge, medical assistants must have a solid understanding of medical terminology, laboratory procedures, safety procedures, and standard precautions for infection control. Quality control programs and accuracy in the collection and handling of specimens, including blood specimens obtained by venipuncture, ensure accurate and reliable test results. Therapeutic communication, which helps gain the patient's cooperation in obtaining a good specimen for analysis, is an important skill for medical assistants to develop.

EXERCISES AND ACTIVITIES

Vocabulary Builder

A. *Insert the following key vocabulary terms into the sentences that follow.*

ABO blood group
agglutination
antibody
antigen
antiserum
bilirubin
blood urea nitrogen
cholesterol
choriocarcinoma
Cushing's syndrome
diabetes mellitus
ectopic
Epstein-Barr virus
Guthrie screening test
heterophile antibodies
high-density lipoprotein
human chorionic gonadotrophin (hCG)
hydatidiform
hemolytic anemia
hyperglycemia
hypoglycemia
infectious mononucleosis
immunoassay
insulin
latex beads
low-density lipoprotein
Mantoux test
phenylketonuria (PKU)
purified protein derivative (PPD)
Rh factor
semen
tine test
triglyceride
tuberculosis
wheal

1. Although the __________ is still used in some areas to test for ______________, most physicians, including Drs. Lewis and King, use the Mantoux test.

2. When a patient's glucose levels test high, Audrey Jones, CMA, knows it could be an indication of diabetes mellitus. She understands, however, that the high glucose levels could also be a sign of _______________ _______________, a hormonal disorder caused by an excess of corticosteriod hormones secreted by the adrenal glands, or a sign of acute stress response. A glucose tolerance test should be performed.

3. When Mary O'Keefe's enzyme _______________ test is positive, Ellen Armstrong, CMA, suspects that this positive reaction indicates a normal pregnancy. However, detection of hCG, _______________, can also indicate abnormal conditions such as an _______________ pregnancy; a developing _______________ mole of the uterus; _______________, a very rare malignant neoplasm, usually of the uterus.

4. When Ellen Armstrong, CMA, performs a test for pregnancy using a slide test, she makes sure that after she adds hCG _______________ (_______________ to hCG) to the urine on a microscope slide, she then adds an _______________ reagent containing _______________ coated with hCG to the mixture.

5. Bruce Goldman, CMA, commonly performs tests for blood glucose levels at Inner City Health Care. The results are used to screen for carbohydrate disorders such as _______________, in which a patient has a low blood glucose level.

6. Joe Guerrero, CMA, performs a slide test for pregnancy, remembering that negative _______________ indicates positive pregnancy.

7. When renal disease is suspected, a physician will order, as one of several tests, a BUN or _______________ _______________ _______________ test, which measures the concentration of urea in the blood.

8. Abigail Johnson has been diagnosed with _______________, which is a type of carbohydrate disorder usually characterized by a deficiency of _______________, a hormone secreted by the pancreas.

9. High levels of _______________, the "bad" cholesterol, are associated with an increased risk of coronary artery disease. Cholesterol bound to _______________, the "good" cholesterol, is transported to the liver where it is excreted in the form of bile.

10. To determine the severity of _______________, the quantity of _______________ in the amniotic fluid of pregnant women is evaluated.

11. Serum _______________ concentration will rise moderately after ingesting a meal containing fat, peaking four to five hours later.

12. When a _______________ sample is required of a male patient for analysis, Wanda Slawson, CMA, instructs patients to avoid ejaculation for three days prior to collection of the sample.

13. Liz Corbin performs a ______________ on Lenny Taylor's arm, raising a ______________ where 0.1mL of PPD was administered properly with an intradermal injection.

14. Bruce Goldman, CMA, explains to Corey Boyer that his case of IM, ______________ ______________, is a result of infection of the lymphocytes by the ______________ (EBV). Dr. Whitney confirmed the diagnosis from hematological and clinical findings combined with the detection of ______________ ______________.

15. Nora Fowler was born with ______________, an inherited condition in which the amino acid phenylalanine is not metabolized.

16. To evaluate a newborn for PKU, Audrey Jones, CMA, uses the ______________ to evaluate the baby's blood.

17. The symptoms of ______________ are similar to those of diabetes mellitus: excessive thirst; passing large amounts of urine; glycosuria, high levels of glucose in the urine; and ketosis, the high levels of ketones.

18. Patients exhibiting a positive or questionable ______________ reaction should have a chest Xray to examine for tubercules and a sputum sample should be stained to search for acid-fast rods. The presence of tubercules and acid-fast rods confirms active tuberculosis.

19. Two categories of blood typing are for the ______________ and the ______________.

Learning Review

1. A. Name three reasons for performing a semen analysis on a male patient.

(1) ______________

(2) ______________

(3) ______________

B. When a semen analysis is performed as part of a fertility workshop, seminal fluid is analyzed to determine what three factors?

(1) ______________ (2) ______________ (3) ______________

2. A. Name the four blood group categories.

(1) ________ (2) ________ (3) ________ (4) ________

B. Fill in the missing information in the chart below.

Blood Group/Type	Antigen on RBC	Serum Antibodies
1. AB	______________	______________
2. ______________	B	______________
3. ______________	______________	No anti-D

C. The Rh type of most North Americans is __________. How can most cases of hemolytic disease of the newborn (HDN) be prevented?

Circle the best answer or answers to the following questions.

3. Which of the following factors can alter the results of semen analysis?
   A. eating foods containing garlic
   B. smoking cigarettes
   C. riding a bicycle on the day of the analysis
   D. drinking milk

4. To ensure an accurate reading, the following precautions should be taken when performing a pregnancy test.
   A. The patient should abstain from having sex within two days of the test.
   B. Refrigerated urine samples and test reagents should be allowed to come to room temperature before testing.
   C. The patient should drink at least eight glasses of water in the six hours preceding the test.
   D. First morning urine or urine with a specific gravity of at least 1.010 should be used.

5. The wheal produced on a patient's arm in response to a Mantoux test is positive for a past or present infection of *Mycobacterium tuberculosis* if it is:
   A. almost invisible.
   B. 15 mm or more of induration.
   C. 10 mm or more of induration.
   D. exactly 2 mm of induration.

6. *Fill in the blanks with the correct term.*
   A. Glucose is the principal carbohydrate found circulating in the ________________.
   B. In glucose analyzers based on ________________, the glucose in the sample reacts with the reagents in the pad, causing a color to develop.
   C. Excess glucose is converted into ________________ for short-term storage in the liver and muscle cells.
   D. The blood glucose level of ________________ patients usually peaks thirty to sixty minutes after consumption of the glucose test solution leading to a level of 160–180 mg/dL and then returns to the fasting level after two to three hours.
   E. A patient should be instructed to eat a diet high in ________________ for three days prior to the glucose tolerance test.
   F. To determine whether diabetic patients are consistently adhering to their diets, physicians can administer the ________________ test.

7. A. Describe the cholesterol molecule.

   ____

   ____

   B. Explain the difference between saturated, monounsaturated, and polyunsaturated fats and give an example of each.

   ____

   ____

C. Look at table 37–6, reference values for total blood cholesterol. What are the levels found in the U. S. population for your age and sex?____________

D. Describe the function of cholesterol.

____

____

Investigation Activity

Learning as much as possible about the characteristics of particular diseases or conditions can help medical assistants provide assistance and support to patients who are undergoing testing.

A. Choose one disease or condition in this chapter and list the tests used to diagnose it.

Disease or Condition: ____________________________________

Test(s): ____

B. Contact a national or local health organization, such as the National Institutes of Health or the ODPHP National Health Information Center (Office of Disease Prevention and Health Promotion), to obtain information and resources about the disease or condition you have chosen. Ask for information on topics related to the disease or condition, such as statistics, treatments, diet/exercise programs, patient education, and so on. Use the Internet to conduct a search, or consult your local or school library for other health organizations of interest. National health organizations can be valuable resources for both health care professionals and patients. What organization will you contact?

Organization Name: ____________________________________

Address: ____

____

Telephone Number: ____________________________________

C. Imagine that you are a patient waiting to hear the test results for this disease or condition. How would you feel? What would you be thinking?

D. What confidentiality issues are involved with the reporting of laboratory test results? Why is patient privacy an important consideration in laboratory analysis?

CASE STUDY

Mary Alexander is an established patient of Dr. Eposito's at Inner City Health Care. Mary, 32 years old, is about 10 pounds overweight for her height. Mary has been diagnosed with Type I insulin-dependent diabetes mellitus since childhood. Dr. Esposito's treatment plan includes administration of 30 units of U-100 NPH insulin by injection every day. Dr. Esposito knows that Mary has trouble complying with the dietary restrictions included in her treatment plan and in observing regular mealtimes. Every now and then, the lifetime rigor of the diet wears Mary down and she begins to eat whatever she likes, whenever she feels like it. To guard against this, Mary must report her average glucose levels to Bruce Goldman, CMA, twice monthly as a safeguard.

At her next regular follow-up examination with Dr. Esposito, the physician orders a glycosated hemoglobin determination and discovers that Mary has been cheating on her diet again and has been reporting inaccurate glucose levels to the physician's office, hoping she would not get caught.

Discuss the following:

1. Why is Dr. Esposito able to tell from the glycosated hemoglobin determination that Mary is not adhering to her diet and health guidelines?
2. What is glycosated hemoglobin?
3. What is the role of the medical assistant in this situation?

SUPPLEMENTARY RESOURCES

Study Guide Disks: Additional practice exercises for this chapter are available on the study guide disks found in the back of the textbook.

Medical Assisting Videos: Appropriate content is available on Delmar's Medical Assisting Videos, 2nd edition, Tape 13, on the following topics:

Basic Information for Specimen Taking and Laboratory Work
When the Physician Orders a Specimen
Collect and Label a Blood Specimen
Perform Blood Chemistry Tests and Record the Results
Perform Immunologic Tests and Record the Results

SKILLS COMPETENCY ASSESSMENT

Procedure 37–1: Pregnancy Tests

Student's Name: ____ Date: ____________

Objective: To accurately perform pregnancy tests.

Conditions: The student demonstrates the ability to perform the enzyme immunoassay and agglutination inhibition tests to detect hCG in urine to determine positive or negative pregnancy results. The student uses the following equipment and supplies: gloves, hand disinfectant, urine specimen, stopwatch, surface disinfectant, biohazard container, hCG negative urine control, hCG positive urine control, pregnancy test kits for enzyme immunoassay and/or the agglutination inhibition pregnancy tests.

Time Requirements and Accuracy Standards: 15 minutes. Points assigned reflect importance of step to meeting objective: Important = (5) Essential = (10) Critical = (15). Automatic failure results if any of the **critical** tasks are omitted or performed incorrectly.

STANDARD PRECAUTIONS:

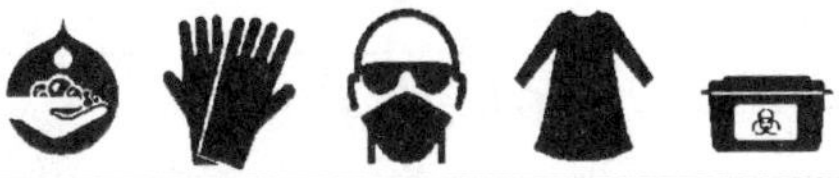

SKILLS ASSESSMENT CHECKLIST

Task Performed	Possible Points	TASKS
☐	5	Washes hands and puts on gloves.
☐	5	Assembles all equipment and supplies.
☐	15	*Enzyme Immunoassay Test (EIA)* Performs a modified enzyme immunoassay test for hCG following the manufacturer's instructions.
☐	10	Obtains test kit materials, reagents, and urine specimen.
☐	5	Applies urine to the test unit using dispenser provided.
☐	5	Waits appropriate time interval.
☐	5	Applies first reagent/antibody to test unit using dispenser provided.
☐	5	Rinses unreacted reagent from unit after appropriate time.
☐	10	Applies color reagent/substrate to test unit.
☐	10	Observes color development after appropriate time interval.
☐	5	Stops reaction.
☐	5	Records results; consults manufacturer's package insert to interpret test results.
☐	15	Repeats previous steps for modified enzyme immunoassay test for hCG, using both positive and negative urine controls.

SKILLS COMPETENCY ASSESSMENT — continued

Procedure 37–1: Pregnancy Tests

Task Performed	Possible Points	TASKS
❑	10	Proceeds with agglutination inhibition pregnancy test.
❑	5	Completed the tasks within 15 minutes.
❑	15	Results obtained were accurate.
______		Earned ADD POINTS OF TASKS CHECKED
	130	Points TOTAL POINTS POSSIBLE
______		SCORE DETERMINE SCORE (divide points earned by total points possible, multiply results by 100)
		Agglutination Inhibition Pregnancy Test
❑	15	Performs an agglutination inhibition test for hCG following the manufacturer's instructions.
❑	10	Obtains slide test kit, reagents, and urine specimen.
❑	10	Places one drop of antiserum in the center of the circled area of slide.
❑	5	Dispenses one drop of urine beside the drop of antiserum.
❑	5	Mixes urine and antiserum with stirrer provided.
❑	5	Rocks the slide in a figure-eight motion for the appropriate time.
❑	10	Applies one drop of well-mixed indicator particles to mixture on slide.
❑	15	Mixes indicator particles with antiserum-urine mixture and spreads the mixture over the entire circled area of the slide using a stirrer.
❑	5	Rocks slide slowly in a figure-eight motion for the appropriate time.
❑	10	Observes slide for agglutination at the end of the time interval and records the results.
❑	15	Repeats agglutination inhibition test for hCG following the manufacturer's instructions using positive and negative urine controls.
❑	5	Disinfects reusable equipment by soaking in 10 percent chlorine bleach solution a minimum of ten minutes; washes and rinses equipment thoroughly.
❑	5	Discards disposable supplies into biohazard container.
❑	5	Disposes of specimen as instructed.
❑	5	Cleans work area with surface disinfectant.
❑	5	Removes gloves and discards into biohazard container.

Task Performed	Possible Points	TASKS
☐	5	Washes hands with hand disinfectant.
☐	5	Documents procedure.
☐	5	Completed the tasks within 15 minutes.
☐	15	Results obtained were accurate.

________	Earned	ADD POINTS OF TASKS CHECKED
160	Points	TOTAL POINTS POSSIBLE
________	SCORE	DETERMINE SCORE (divide points earned by total points possible, multiply results by 100)

Actual Student Time Needed to Complete Procedure: ____________

Student's Initials: ____________ Instructor's Initials: ____________ Grade: ____________

Suggestions for Improvement: ____________________________________

Evaluator's Name (print) ____________________________________

Evaluator's Signature ____________________________________

Comments ____________________________________

DOCUMENTATION

Chart the procedure as laboratory policy indicates.

Date: ____________

Charting: ____________________________________

____

____

Student's Initials: ____________

SKILLS COMPETENCY ASSESSMENT

Procedure 37–2: Slide Test for Infectious Mononucleosis

Student's Name: ______________________________________ Date: ____________

Objective: To perform a slide test for infectious mononucleosis.

Conditions: The student demonstrates the ability to perform an accurate test of serum or plasma sample to detect the presence or absence of heterophile antibodies of infectious mononucleosis. The student uses the following equipment and supplies: gloves, hand disinfectant, sample serum or plasma, stopwatch, surface disinfectant, test kit for infectious mononucleosis, biohazard container.

Time Requirements and Accuracy Standards: 15 minutes. Points assigned reflect importance of step to meeting objective: Important = (5) Essential = (10) Critical = (15). Automatic failure results if any of the **critical** tasks are omitted or performed incorrectly.

STANDARD PRECAUTIONS:

SKILLS ASSESSMENT CHECKLIST

Task Performed	Possible Points	TASKS
☐	5	Washes hands and puts on gloves.
☐	5	Assembles all equipment and supplies.
☐	5	Places the Monospot slide on a flat work surface.
☐	10	Mixes the reagent vials several times by inversion.
☐	15	Fills the capillary pipette to the top mark: • Places the rubber bulb on the end of the capillary pipette with the heavy black line. • Inserts the pipette into the vial of indicator cells. • Allows the pipette to fill by capillary action to the top mark.
☐	10	Places the index finger over the hole in the bulb and squeezes gently to dispense one-half the cells on a corner of square I of the slide.
☐	10	Delivers the remaining cells to a corner of square II.
☐	15	Places one drop of thoroughly mixed reagent I in the center of square I.
☐	15	Places one drop of thoroughly mixed reagent II in the center of square II.
☐	15	Adds one drop of serum to the center of each square using the disposable plastic pipette provided.
☐	10	Uses a clean applicator stick to mix Reagent I with the serum; uses at least ten stirring motions and avoids touching the indicator cells.
☐	15	Blends in the indicator cells in square I with the applicator stick, using no more than ten stirring motions and spreading the mixture over the entire surface of the square.
☐	15	Repeats previous two steps using reagent II in square II, using a clean applicator stick.
☐	10	Starts the stopwatch upon completion of the mixing of both squares.

Task Performed	Possible Points	TASKS
☐	5	Does not pick up or move the slide.
☐	10	Observes for agglutination at the end of one minute without moving the slide or picking it up.
☐	15	Records the agglutination in each square and interprets the results.
☐	5	Records test results as positive or negative.
☐	10	Repeats the test procedure using positive and negative control sera.
☐	5	Discards contaminated materials into biohazard container.
☐	10	Disposes of specimen appropriately and disinfects reusable materials by soaking in 10 percent chlorine bleach solution for at least ten minutes; washes and rinses materials thoroughly.
☐	5	Cleans work area with surface disinfectant.
☐	5	Removes gloves and discards into biohazard container.
☐	5	Washes hands with hand disinfectant.
☐	5	Documents results.
☐	5	Completed the tasks within 15 minutes.
☐	15	Results obtained were accurate.
	______	Earned ADD POINTS OF TASKS CHECKED
	225	Points TOTAL POINTS POSSIBLE
	______	SCORE DETERMINE SCORE (divide points earned by total points possible, multiply results by 100)

Actual Student Time Needed to Complete Procedure: ____________

Student's Initials: ____________ Instructor's Initials: ____________ Grade: ____________

Suggestions for Improvement: ____________________

Evaluator's Name (print) ____________________

Evaluator's Signature ____________________

Comments ____________________

DOCUMENTATION

Chart the procedure as laboratory policy indicates.

Date:__________

Charting: ____________________

____

____

Student's Initials:________

SKILLS COMPETENCY ASSESSMENT

Procedure 37–3: Analyzing Semen

Student's Name: ______________________________ Date: ____________

Objective: To properly analyze semen.

Conditions: The student demonstrates the ability to analyze semen to determine the total sperm count, percent of motility, and percent of normally formed sperm cells using the following equipment and supplies: gloves, 10 mL graduated cylinder, pH test paper, automatic pipette, hemacytometer, diluting fluid, sodium bicarbonate, distilled water, slides and coverslips, Petri dishes, microscope, and coplin jar.

Time Requirements and Accuracy Standards: 10 minutes. Points assigned reflect importance of step to meeting objective: Important = (5) Essential = (10) Critical = (15). Automatic failure results if any of the **critical** tasks are omitted or performed incorrectly.

STANDARD PRECAUTIONS:

SKILLS ASSESSMENT CHECKLIST

Task Performed	Possible Points	TASKS
		Macroscopic Examination
❑	5	Washes hands and applies gloves.
❑	5	Assembles all equipment and supplies.
❑	15	Rates viscosity while pouring specimen into a graduated cylinder (rates viscosity within 30 minutes of the time the specimen is taken).
❑	15	Measures volume of specimen.
❑	15	Measures the pH using pH test paper.
❑	5	Removes gloves and washes hands.
❑	5	Documents results.
❑	5	Completed the tasks within 10 minutes.
❑	15	Results are within acceptable range.
	______	Earned ADD POINTS OF TASKS CHECKED
	85	Points TOTAL POINTS POSSIBLE
	______	SCORE DETERMINE SCORE (divide points earned by total points possible, multiply results by 100)
		Microscopic Examination
❑	5	Washes hands and applies gloves.
❑	5	Assembles all equipment and supplies.
❑	10	Mixes semen sample.

Task Performed	Possible Points	TASKS
☐	10	Places one drop of liquified sample and covers with a coverslip; examines for motility.
☐	15	Determines sperm count. • Uses automatic pipettes to make a 1:20 dilution of sample with sodium bicarbonate solution and mixes well. • Fills both sides of the hemocytometer and allows the sperm to settle for five to ten minutes. • Counts the sperm in two large WBC squares or 5 RBC squares and calculates sperm per milliliter.
☐	15	Prepares sperm sample for morphology evaluation by a pathologist or trained technologist. • Prepares two slides using the technique to make a blood smear; does not allow the slides to air dry; immediately immerses both slides into a coplin jar containing 95 percent alcohol. • Delivers the slides to the pathologist to view for morphology.
☐	5	Removes gloves and washes hands.
☐	5	Documents results.
☐	5	Completed the tasks within 10 minutes.
☐	15	Results obtained were accurate.

_______	Earned	ADD POINTS OF TASKS CHECKED
90	Points	TOTAL POINTS POSSIBLE
_______	SCORE	DETERMINE SCORE (divide points earned by total points possible, multiply results by 100)

Actual Student Time Needed to Complete Procedure: ____________

Student's Initials: ____________ Instructor's Initials: ____________ Grade: ____________

Suggestions for Improvement: ____

Evaluator's Name (print) ____

Evaluator's Signature ____

Comments ____

DOCUMENTATION

Chart the procedure as laboratory policy indicates.

Date: __________

Charting: ____

____

____

Student's Initials: ________

SKILLS COMPETENCY ASSESSMENT

Procedure 37–4: Obtaining Blood Sample for Phenylketonuria (PKU) Test

Student's Name: ______________________________ Date: ____________

Objective: To obtain a blood sample for a phenylketonuria (PKU) test.

Conditions: The student demonstrates the ability to obtain a blood sample using a PKU test card or "filter paper" to determine phenylalanine levels in newborns who are at least three to four days old. The student uses the following equipment and supplies: gloves, PKU filter paper test card and mailing envelope, alcohol swabs, cotton balls, sterile pediatric-sized lancet, biohazard waste container.

Time Requirements and Accuracy Standards: 15 minutes. Points assigned reflect importance of step to meeting objective: Important = (5) Essential = (10) Critical = (15). Automatic failure results if any of the **critical** tasks are omitted or performed incorrectly.

STANDARD PRECAUTIONS:

SKILLS ASSESSMENT CHECKLIST

Task Performed	Possible Points	TASKS
☐	5	Washes hands and puts on gloves.
☐	10	Identifies the infant; explains the purpose of the test and the procedure to the parents.
☐	5	Discusses the feeding pattern of the infant prior to beginning the procedure.
☐	5	*Rationale:* Understands that certain antibiotics, aspirin, or vomiting problems may cause false results.
☐	10	Selects and cleans an appropriate puncture site.
☐	15	Grasps the infant's foot, taking care not to touch the cleansed area; makes a puncture approximately 2-3 mm deep in the infant's heel, making sure the lateral portion of the infant's heel pad is used.
☐	5	Wipes away the first drop of blood with a cotton ball.
☐	5	*Rationale:* The first drop is diluted with alcohol and should not be collected for the test.
☐	15	Collects blood for the test by pressing the back side of the filter paper test card against the infant's heel while exerting gentle pressure on the heel.
☐	10	Makes sure the blood completely soaks through the paper and fills all of the circles on the test card completely.
☐	5	Holds a cotton ball over the puncture and applies gentle pressure until the bleeding stops.
☐	5	Properly disposes of all waste in biohazard container.

Task Performed	Possible Points	TASKS
❑	5	Removes gloves and washes hands.
❑	15	Allows the PKU test card to completely dry on a nonabsorbent surface at room temperature.
❑	5	After the test card is dry, puts on gloves and completes the PKU test card with all patient and physician information.
❑	10	Places the test card in the mailer envelope and sends it to the laboratory within two days.
❑	5	Removes gloves and washes hands.
❑	5	Documents the procedure in the patient's medical record.
❑	5	Documents test results when they are returned in the patient's medical record.
❑	5	Completed the tasks within 15 minutes.
❑	15	Results obtained were accurate.

________	Earned	ADD POINTS OF TASKS CHECKED
165	Points	TOTAL POINTS POSSIBLE
________	SCORE	DETERMINE SCORE (divide points earned by total points possible, multiply results by 100)

Actual Student Time Needed to Complete Procedure: ____________

Student's Initials: ____________ Instructor's Initials: ____________ Grade: ____________

Suggestions for Improvement: ____________________

Evaluator's Name (print) ____________________

Evaluator's Signature ____________________

Comments ____________________

DOCUMENTATION

Chart the procedure in the patient's medical record.

Date: __________

Charting: ____________________

____

____

Student's Initials: ________

SKILLS COMPETENCY ASSESSMENT

Procedure 37–5: Obtaining Urine Sample for Phenylketonuria (PKU) Test

Student's Name: ______________________________ Date: __________

Objective: To obtain a urine sample for a phenylketonuria (PKU) test.

Conditions: The student demonstrates the ability to obtain a urine sample using the diaper test or the Phenistik® test to determine phenylalanine levels in newborns who are at least six weeks old. The student uses the following equipment and supplies: gloves, 10 percent ferric acid for the diaper test or Phenistik for the Phenistik Method Test, biohazard waste container.

Time Requirements and Accuracy Standards: 10 minutes. Points assigned reflect importance of step to meeting objective: Important = (5) Essential = (10) Critical = (15). Automatic failure results if any of the **critical** tasks are omitted or performed incorrectly.

STANDARD PRECAUTIONS: 

SKILLS ASSESSMENT CHECKLIST

Task Performed	Possible Points	TASKS
❑	15	Identifies the infant; verifies that the infant is at least six weeks old; explains the purpose of the test and the procedure to the parents.
❑	5	Washes hands and applies gloves.
❑	15	Follows one of the two following procedures: • *Diaper Test:* Applies several drops of 10 percent ferric chloride to a diaper that contains fresh urine. • *Phenistik Test:* Dips the Phenistik test strip into fresh urine or presses it against a diaper containing fresh urine.
❑	15	Follows up a positive urine test with a blood test.
❑	5	Properly disposes of waste in a biohazard container.
❑	5	Removes gloves and washes hands.
❑	10	Documents the procedure and results in the patient's medical record.
❑	5	Completed the tasks within 10 minutes.
❑	15	Results obtained were accurate.

______	Earned	ADD POINTS OF TASKS CHECKED
90	Points	TOTAL POINTS POSSIBLE
______	SCORE	DETERMINE SCORE (divide points earned by total points possible, multiply results by 100)

Actual Student Time Needed to Complete Procedure: ____________

Student's Initials: ____________ Instructor's Initials: ____________ Grade: ____________

Suggestions for Improvement: ____

Evaluator's Name (print) ____

Evaluator's Signature ____

Comments ____

DOCUMENTATION

Chart the procedure in the patient's medical record.

Date:__________

Charting: ____

____

____

Student's Initials:________

SKILLS COMPETENCY ASSESSMENT

Procedure 37–6: Mantoux Test

Student's Name: ______________________________ Date: __________

Objective: To properly perform a Mantoux test.

Conditions: The student demonstrates the ability to safely and accurately inject 0.1 mL of intermediate strength (5 TU) purified protein derivative (PPD) intradermally to develop an indurated wheal to determine if an active or inactive tuberculous infection is present. The student uses the following equipment and supplies: gloves, goggles, tuberculin syringe, short (3/8–1/2 inches) 26- or 27-gauge needle, PPD (5 TU strength), alcohol, cotton balls or gauze, sharps container, biohazard waste container.

Time Requirements and Accuracy Standards: 15 minutes. Points assigned reflect importance of step to meeting objective: Important = (5) Essential = (10) Critical = (15). Automatic failure results if any of the **critical** tasks are omitted or performed incorrectly.

STANDARD PRECAUTIONS:

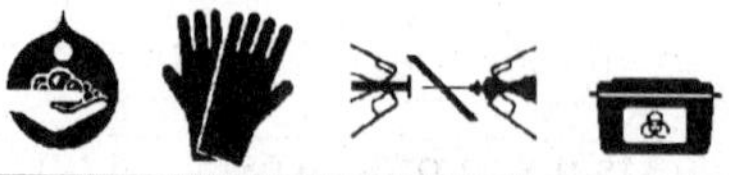

SKILLS ASSESSMENT CHECKLIST

Task Performed	Possible Points	TASKS
❑	5	Washes hands and puts on gloves and goggles.
❑	5	Identifies the patient and explains the procedure.
❑	10	Selects a site approximately three to four inches from the bend of the arm on the anterior side.
❑	10	Cleans the site with alcohol and allows the surface to dry; does not touch the site after cleaning.
❑	5	Uses a 1.0 mL tuberculin syringe fitted with a 3/8 – 1/2 inches, 26- or 27-gauge needle.
❑	10	Draws 0.1 mL of 5 TU strength PPD into the syringe, being careful to draw the exact amount of PPD into the syringe.
❑	5	*Rationale:* Too much or too little PPD will cause erroneous results.
❑	5	Holds the patient's forearm just under the chosen site to prevent movement during the injection.
❑	15	Slowly injects the PPD intradermally into the skin of the anterior portion of the arm to produce a wheal approximately 6–10 mm. Does not rub the injection site. (See Procedure 29–7: Administering an Intradermal Injection.)
❑	5	Disposes of the syringe and needle in a sharps container.
❑	15	Watches the patient carefully and notifies the physician immediately of any adverse reactions to the medication.
❑	10	Instructs the patient to return within 48–72 hours of the injection for test interpretation.

Task Performed	Possible Points	TASKS
❑	5	Removes gloves and washes hands.
❑	5	Documents procedure in the patient's medical record.
❑	5	Completed the tasks within 5 minutes.
❑	15	Results obtained were accurate.
	_______	Earned ADD POINTS OF TASKS CHECKED
	130	Points TOTAL POINTS POSSIBLE
	_______	SCORE DETERMINE SCORE (divide points earned by total points possible, multiply results by 100)
		When patient returns for test interpretation
❑	5	Washes hands.
❑	10	Bends the patient's arm at the elbow; inspects the injection site. Gently rubs a finger across the induration to evaluate its size, then measures in millimeters.
❑	15	Reads the test results; retests if site produces questionable results; documents the test results in the patient's medical record.
❑	5	Completed the tasks within 5 minutes.
❑	15	Results obtained were accurate.
	_______	Earned ADD POINTS OF TASKS CHECKED
	50	Points TOTAL POINTS POSSIBLE
	_______	SCORE DETERMINE SCORE (divide points earned by total points possible, multiply results by 100)

Actual Student Time Needed to Complete Procedure: _______________

Student's Initials: _______________ Instructor's Initials: _______________ Grade: _______________

Suggestions for Improvement: _______________________________________

Evaluator's Name (print) _______________________________________

Evaluator's Signature _______________________________________

Comments _______________________________________

DOCUMENTATION

Chart the procedure in the patient's medical record.

Date: ____________

Charting: _______________________________________

____

____

Student's Initials: __________

SKILLS COMPETENCY ASSESSMENT

Procedure 37–7: Measurement of Blood Glucose Using an Automated Analyzer

Student's Name: ______________________________ Date: __________

Objective: To measure a patient's blood glucose using an automated analyzer.

Conditions: The student demonstrates the ability to analyze blood glucose at timed intervals following the patient's ingestion of a standard glucose dose to aid in the diagnosis and management of diabetes or in the management of hypoglycemia. The student uses the following equipment and supplies: gloves, goggles, sterile lancet, alcohol swabs or 70 percent alcohol and cotton swabs, glucose analyzer, control solutions for glucose analyzer, test strips for glucose analyzer, laboratory tissue.

Time Requirements and Accuracy Standards: 15 minutes. Points assigned reflect importance of step to meeting objective: Important = (5) Essential = (10) Critical = (15). Automatic failure results if any of the **critical** tasks are omitted or performed incorrectly.

STANDARD PRECAUTIONS: 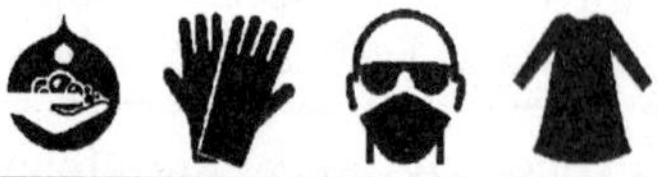

SKILLS ASSESSMENT CHECKLIST

Task Performed	Possible Points	TASKS
☐	5	Reviews the manufacturer's manual for the specific glucose analyzer being used; turns on the analyzer.
☐	5	Cleans the work area and assembles all materials and supplies.
☐	5	Washes hands.
☐	5	Puts on gloves and goggles.
☐	10	Records the control ranges, control lot number, and test strip lot number.
☐	10	Performs the check test and the control test according to the manufacturer's instructions; proceeds to the glucose test if both tests are within range; repeats both tests if either is out of acceptable range.
		To perform the glucose test
☐	5	Removes a test strip from the bottle and replaces the lid.
☐	15	Performs a capillary puncture.
☐	10	Applies a large drop of blood to the test strip.
☐	5	Blots the test strip with tissue after the time interval recommended by the manufacturer.
☐	5	Inserts the test strip into the test chamber.
☐	15	Reads the glucose concentration after the appropriate time interval has passed.

Task Performed	Possible Points	TASKS
❑	5	Documents the results.
❑	5	Removes gloves and washes hands.
❑	5	Disposes of all waste in a biohazard container.
❑	5	Completed the tasks within 15 minutes.
❑	15	Results obtained were accurate.

_______	Earned	ADD POINTS OF TASKS CHECKED
135	Points	TOTAL POINTS POSSIBLE
_______	SCORE	DETERMINE SCORE (divide points earned by total points possible, multiply results by 100)

Actual Student Time Needed to Complete Procedure: ____________

Student's Initials: ____________ Instructor's Initials: ____________ Grade: ____________

Suggestions for Improvement: ______________________________

Evaluator's Name (print) ______________________________

Evaluator's Signature ______________________________

Comments ______________________________

DOCUMENTATION

Chart the procedure in the patient's medical record.

Date: ______________________________

Charting: ______________________________

____

____

Student's Initials:________

SKILLS COMPETENCY ASSESSMENT

Procedure 37–8: Cholesterol Testing

Student's Name: ______________________________ Date: __________

Objective: To test a patient's total cholesterol level.

Conditions: The student demonstrates the ability to determine a patient's total cholesterol level to aid in the diagnosis of coronary artery disease using the following equipment and supplies: gloves, blood-collecting equipment, pipettes with disposable tips, chlorine bleach, commercial kit for manual determination of cholesterol, controls and standards, marking pen, biohazard container.

Time Requirements and Accuracy Standards: 15 minutes. Points assigned reflect importance of step to meeting objective: Important = (5) Essential = (10) Critical = (15). Automatic failure results if any of the **critical** tasks are omitted or performed incorrectly.

STANDARD PRECAUTIONS:

SKILLS ASSESSMENT CHECKLIST

Task Performed	Possible Points	TASKS
☐	5	Assembles all necessary equipment and materials.
☐	10	Washes hands, applies gloves and goggles.
☐	10	Obtains a blood sample from the patient, either by fingerstick or venipuncture (see Procedures 16–1 through 16–4), depending on the manufacturer's instructions.
☐	15	Follows the manufacturer's instructions to perform the cholesterol test.
☐	10	Properly disposes of all waste in a biohazard container.
☐	5	Documents results.
☐	5	Completed the tasks within 15 minutes.
☐	15	Results obtained were accurate.

________	Earned	ADD POINTS OF TASKS CHECKED
75	Points	TOTAL POINTS POSSIBLE
________	SCORE	DETERMINE SCORE (divide points earned by total points possible, multiply results by 100)

Actual Student Time Needed to Complete Procedure: ____________

Student's Initials: ____________ Instructor's Initials: ____________ Grade: ____________

Suggestions for Improvement: ____

Evaluator's Name (print) ____

Evaluator's Signature ____

Comments ____

DOCUMENTATION

Chart the procedure in the patient's medical record.

Date: ______________

Charting: ____

____

____

Student's Initials: ____________

EVALUATION OF CHAPTER KNOWLEDGE

How has your instructor evaluated the knowledge you have achieved?

Knowledge	Instructor Evaluation *Good*	*Average*	*Poor*
Identifies the three main precautions to be observed during all tests and the collection of samples	_____	_____	_____
Knows how to collect samples and perform and interpret test results	_____	_____	_____
Can discuss factors to be considered when evaluating test results	_____	_____	_____
Can discuss transmission, incubation period, and symptoms of EBV infectious mononucleosis	_____	_____	_____
Knows the blood group antigens and antibodies found in each of the four ABO groups and the Rh factor	_____	_____	_____
Identifies the cause of PKU and the symptoms caused by untreated PKU	_____	_____	_____
Recognizes normal and elevated levels of phenylalanine and the dietary restrictions to be observed by PKU patients	_____	_____	_____
Understands the cause of tuberculosis and some major characteristics of *Mycobacterium tuberculosis*	_____	_____	_____
Recognizes the role of insulin in the regulation of blood glucose levels	_____	_____	_____
Knows the differences between the normal values for fasting blood glucose, two-hour postprandial glucose, and the glucose tolerance test	_____	_____	_____
Can explain the importance of cholesterol and triglyceride testing to identify patients at high risk for coronary heart disease	_____	_____	_____
Knows the average values of cholesterol for adults, children, infants, and newborns	_____	_____	_____
Knows the acceptable level of LDL in persons with or without coronary heart disease and the role of HDL and LDL in coronary heart disease	_____	_____	_____
Identifies the normal values of urea nitrogen for adults, children, infants, and newborns and the significance of elevated blood urea levels	_____	_____	_____
Recognizes the importance of quality control programs, including instrument maintenance, reagent shelf life, and test controls	_____	_____	_____
Documents results accurately	_____	_____	_____
Is respectful of the patient's emotional needs	_____	_____	_____

Student's Initials: ______ Instructor's Initials: ______

Grade: _______

CHAPTER 38

The Medical Assistant As Office Manager

PERFORMANCE OBJECTIVES

In the ambulatory care setting, the office manager is an important and essential staff member involved in the daily operation of the practice. The office manager is responsible for a wide variety of duties, including supervision, time management, finances, purchasing, marketing, education, and personnel. In some cases, the same individual serves as both the office manager and the human resources manager. With more facilities turning to managed care as a way to ensure consumer use of the appropriate level of care and to facilitate cost containment, opportunities exist for medical assistants to advance to the office manager (OM) position. Use this workbook chapter to explore the role of the office manager in the ambulatory care setting.

EXERCISES AND ACTIVITIES

Vocabulary Builder

Insert the proper key vocabulary terms into the sentences that follow.

Agenda	"Going Bare"	Practicum
Ancillary services	Liability	Procedures manual
Benchmarking	Malpractice	Professional liability insurance
Benefits	Marketing	Risk management
Bond	Minutes	Teamwork
Embezzle	Negligence	Work statement
Externs		

1. ______________________________ refers to professional occupational companies hired to complete a specific job.
2. Legal responsibility is commonly referred to as ________________.
3. ______________________________ describes the situation of a physician who does not carry professional liability insurance.

4. Making a comparison between different organizations relative to how they accomplish tasks, remunerate employees, and so on, is called ______________________________.
5. ______________________________ is designed to protect assets in the event a liability claim is filed and awarded.
6. ______________________________ are a written record of topics discussed and actions taken during meeting sessions.
7. A ______________________________ provides a concise description of the work you plan to accomplish.
8. A ______________________________ is a binding agreement with an employee insuring recovery of financial loss should funds be stolen or embezzled.
9. A printed list of topics to be discussed during a meeting is called an ______________________________.
10. ______________________________ is the process by which the provider of services makes the consumer aware of the scope and quality of those services. Examples might include public relations, brochures, patient education seminars, and newsletters.
11. ______________________________ involves persons synergistically working together.
12. The failure to perform an act that a reasonable and prudent physician would or would not perform is ______________________________
13. The student ______________________________ is a transitional stage providing an opportunity to apply theory learned in the classroom to a health care setting through practical, hands-on experience.
14. Remuneration that is in addition to the salary is a ______________________________.
15. The office manager should schedule an informational interview with the ______________________________ student before the practicum begins.
16. To appropriate fraudulently for one's own use is to ______________________________.
17. ______________________________ involves the identification, analysis, and treatment of risks within the medical office or facility.
18. The ______________________________ provides detailed information relative to the performance of tasks within the job description.
19. ______________________________ is the term commonly used today to describe professional liability.

Learning Review

1. The office manager of a medical office or ambulatory care facility can have many varied responsibilities based on individual facility needs. What are five duties that are the responsibility of the office manager in a health care setting?

   (1) ____

   (2) ____

(3) ____________________
(4) ____________________
(5) ____________________

2. Most marketing tools used in a medical environment provide educational and office services information to patients, potential patients, and the local community. Match the following marketing tools with their potential use in the ambulatory care facility setting.

A. Seminars
B. Brochures
C. Newsletters
D. Press Releases
E. Special Events

1. _____ Used for announcing new equipment, new staff, expanded or remodeled office space, and so on.
2. _____ Typically come in two types—patient education and office services, and present a professional image of the ambulatory care setting.
3. _____ An effective way to join with other community organizations to promote wellness.
4. _____ Can educate patients and provide good will in the community. All facility staff can work as a team to organize these.
5. _____ Can include a wide range of information from health-related topics to staff introductions to insurance updates. May form the nucleus of a marketing program.

3. What are five attributes needed to perform as a quality manager in any office setting?

(1) ____________________
(2) ____________________
(3) ____________________
(4) ____________________
(5) ____________________

Investigation Activity

Office managers Marilyn Johnson and Shirley Brooks have received feedback from patients and medical assistants at the offices of Drs. Lewis & King requesting nutrition information and guidelines to help patients understand and comply with the nutritional requirements of their treatment plans. With the approval of the physician-employers, the office managers implement a plan to produce one-page nutritional newsletters to be mailed out to patients four times each year.

Using the agreed-upon format, assist the office managers by drafting a copy of the first newsletter sent to patients. This issue of the nutrition newsletter discusses the advantages of a low-fat, high-fiber diet and explains the food pyramid. Consult chapter 27, "Nutrition in Health and Disease," and other nutrition references for ideas and information. Be creative. You can even include a recipe.

LEWIS & KING, MD
2501 CENTER STREET
NORTHBOROUGH, OH 12345

NUTRITION NEWSLETTER

The Advantages of Low-Fat, High-Fiber Diets and the Food Pyramid Explained

Why is a low-fat diet so important to my health?

"An apple a day keeps the doctor away..." How to Get More Fiber into Your Diet

Everything You Wanted to Know About the Food Pyramid...and More!

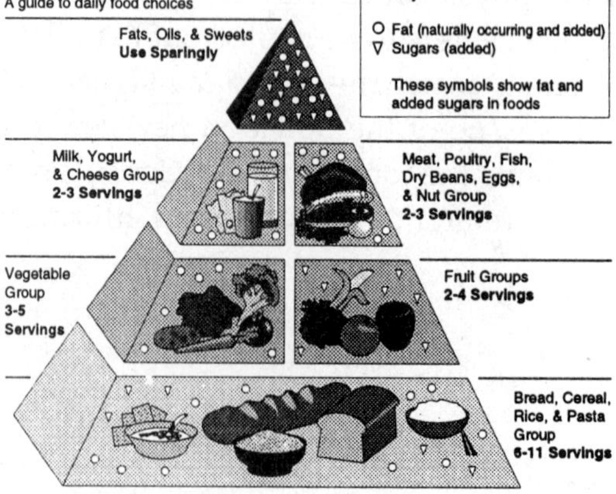

CASE STUDY

Office manager Shirley Brooks is responsible for the preparation and distribution of payroll checks at the offices of Drs. Lewis & King. As the group practice is in the process of upgrading the computer system to accommodate a recent influx of new patients, Shirley is temporarily preparing the payroll using the manual write-it-once bookkeeping system. She is careful to consult payroll records for each employee, which include the employee's name, address, and telephone number; social security number; number of exemptions claimed on the W-4 form; gross salary; deductions withheld for all taxes, including Social Security, federal, state, local, unemployment, and disability; and date of employment.

Discuss the following:

1. As Shirley writes out the payroll check for Audrey Jones, CMA, what information should be included on the paycheck stub?
2. What must the physician's office have to process payroll?
3. What responsibility does the office manager have with regard to the confidentiality of payroll records? How might employees' rights to privacy be maintained?

SUPPLEMENTARY RESOURCES

Study Guide Disks: Additional practice exercises for this chapter are available on the study guide disks found in the back of the textbook.

Medical Assisting Videos: Appropriate content is available on Delmar's Medical Assisting Videos, 2nd ed., for the following topics:

Tape 1: Work As a Team Member
Communication Skills
Tape 2: Apply Legal Concepts To Practice
Practice Risk Management Measures To Prevent Professional Liability
Tape 3: Perform Administrative Duties
Electronic Banking

SKILLS COMPETENCY ASSESSMENT

Procedure 38-1: Supervise Student Practicum

Student's Name: ______________________________ Date: ____________

Objective: To prepare a training path for a student extern being assigned to the office. To make the involved office personnel aware of their responsibilities. To preplan which jobs the student extern performs and in what sequence they will be assigned. To make the externship successful by providing as much supervision and assistance as necessary.

Conditions: The student demonstrates the ability to supervise student practicums in the medical facility setting using a scheduling log, calendar, and office policies manual.

Accuracy Standards: Points assigned reflect importance of step to meeting objective: Important = (5) Essential = (10) Critical = (15). Automatic failure results if any of the **critical** tasks are omitted or performed incorrectly.

SKILLS ASSESSMENT CHECKLIST

Task Performed	Possible Points	TASKS
❑	10	Determines the amount of supervision the extern will require.
❑	5	Identifies the supervisor who will be immediately responsible for the extern.
❑	15	Plans which tasks the extern will be allowed or encouraged to perform.
❑	15	Creates a schedule outlining the time the extern will be assigned to each unit.
❑	10	Begins orientation for the extern as soon as he or she arrives at the office. Includes a tour of the office and an introduction to the staff.
❑	10	Gives the extern a copy of the Office Policy Manual and the work schedule for the entire externship. Answers any questions the extern might have.
❑	10	Maintains an accurate record of the hours the extern works. Logs the date and reason for any missed days, late arrivals, or early dismissals.
❑	10	Checks with the extern frequently to be sure the extern is receiving meaningful training from the work experience.
❑	15	Consults physicians and staff members with whom the extern has worked for their opinion of the student's capabilities. Follows up on any problems that might be identified.
❑	10	Reports the extern's progress to the medical assisting supervisor from the educational institution. This person usually visits once or twice each rotation.

Task Performed	Possible Points	TASKS
❑	15	Prepares the student extern evaluation report from comments provided by the supervisor assigned and each employee who worked with the extern.

________	Earned	ADD POINTS OF TASKS CHECKED
125	Points	TOTAL POINTS POSSIBLE
________	SCORE	DETERMINE SCORE (divide points earned by total points possible, multiply results by 100)

Actual Student Time Needed to Complete Procedure: ____________

Student's Initials: ____________ Instructor's Initials: ____________ Grade: ____________

Suggestions for Improvement: ____

____

____

____

Evaluator's Name (print) ____

Evaluator's Signature ____

Comments ____

SKILLS COMPETENCY ASSESSMENT

Procedure 38-2: Developing and Maintaining a Procedures Manual

Student's Name: ______________________________ Date: __________

Objective: To develop and maintain a comprehensive, up-to-date procedures manual covering each medical, technical, and administrative procedure in the office, with step-by-step directions and rationales for performing each task.

Conditions: The student demonstrates the ability to develop and maintain a procedures manual using the following equipment and supplies: computer or electronic typewriter, binder (such as three-ring binder), paper, and standard procedures manual format.

Accuracy Standards: Points assigned reflect importance of step to meeting objective: Important = (5) Essential = (10) Critical = (15). Automatic failure results if any of the **critical** tasks are omitted or performed incorrectly.

SKILLS ASSESSMENT CHECKLIST

Task Performed	Possible Points	TASKS
☐	15	Writes detailed, step-by-step procedures and rationales for each medical, technical, and administrative function. Ensures that each procedure is written by experienced employees close to the function and then reviewed by a supervisor and/or office manager. Explains that rationales help employees understand why something is done.
☐	15	Collects the procedures into the Office Procedures Manual.
☐	10	Stores one complete manual in a common library area. Provides a completed copy to the physician/employer and the office manager. Distributes appropriate sections to the various departments.
☐	5	Reviews the procedures manual annually and adds any new procedures, deletes or modifies as necessary, and indicates the revision date.
☐	15	Results obtained were accurate.
________	Earned	ADD POINTS OF TASKS CHECKED
60	Points	TOTAL POINTS POSSIBLE
________	SCORE	DETERMINE SCORE (divide points earned by total points possible, multiply results by 100)

Actual Student Time Needed to Complete Procedure: __________

Student's Initials: __________ Instructor's Initials: __________ Grade: __________

Suggestions for Improvement: ______________________________

____

Evaluator's Name (print) ______________________________

Evaluator's Signature ______________________________

Comments ______________________________

EVALUATION OF CHAPTER KNOWLEDGE

How has your instructor evaluated the knowledge you have achieved?

	Instructor Evaluation		
Knowledge	*Good*	*Average*	*Poor*
Understands payroll processing and other employee-related financial duties, including taxes	_____	_____	_____
Exercises efficient time management techniques	_____	_____	_____
Understands risk management issues	_____	_____	_____
Understands the importance of developing and maintaining Policy and Procedures Manuals	_____	_____	_____
Understands methods of public relations for the ambulatory care setting	_____	_____	_____
Describes liability coverage and bonding	_____	_____	_____
Describes the qualities of an effective office manager	_____	_____	_____
Able to describe the process of supervising a student practicum	_____	_____	_____
Understands the importance of teamwork and its role in supervising personnel	_____	_____	_____

Student's Initials: ______ Instructor's Initials: ______

Grade: _______

CHAPTER 39

The Medical Assistant As the Human Resources Manager

PERFORMANCE OBJECTIVES

In some health care practices, particularly that of the solo practitioner, the office manager also functions as the human resources manager. In other cases, these management functions are assumed by two separate individuals. The human resources manager is concerned with both group and individual employee issues. The human resources manager performs such duties as formulating job descriptions, recruitment and hiring, payroll and salary review, training, retirement, health insurance, advancement, grievances, dismissals, and maintaining employee personnel records. Use this workbook chapter to explore the role of the human resources manager in the ambulatory care setting.

EXERCISES AND ACTIVITIES

Vocabulary Builder

Insert the proper key vocabulary terms into the following sentences.

Conflict resolution	Job description	Overtime
Educational history	Letter of reference	Probation
Evaluation	Letter of resignation	Resumes
Exit interview	Mentor	Salary review
Involuntary dismissal	Networking	Work history

1. Clinical medical assistant Anna Preciado, approaching one year of employment at the offices of Drs. Lewis & King, is due to have her ____________________to assess her job performance.
2. Due to an unexpected staffing shortfall, Audrey Jones, CMA, has volunteered to work ____________________ this week. She will receive one and one-half times the regular rate of pay for hours above her regular forty-hour week.
3. Office manager Marilyn Johnson, acting as the human resources manager, will conduct a __________________________ at the beginning of the new calendar year with each employee. If necessary, she will then inform the employee of their revised base pay rate.

4. An ______________________________ has been scheduled for administrative/clinical medical assistant Liz Corbin before she leaves the clinic to continue her education. This session will give Liz an opportunity to provide her positive and negative opinions of the position and the facility.
5. Jane O'Hara, co-office manager at Inner City Health Care, has been asked by her physician-employers to use ______________________________ to solve several problems occurring between two coworkers at the facility.
6. Office manager Marilyn Johnson has received a ______________________________from the former instructor of a current job applicant describing the applicant's performance, attitude, and qualifications.
7. In interviews for a new CMA position, office manager Walter Seals asks applicants to outline their ______________________________, including employers, positions, duties, and responsibilities.
8. Office manager Walter Seals reviews ________________________ received from applicants for the new medical assisting position to ensure that the applicants interviewed meet the physician-employer's minimum qualifications for education and work experience.
9. The ____________________________ listed on each resume reveals to the office manager the applicants' places of learning and degrees or certificates earned.
10. The violation of office policies at Inner City Health Care led to the ______________________ of one of the part-time employees.
11. Administrative medical assistant Ellen Armstrong, in her first job since leaving school, has had office manager Marilyn Johnson as her ________________________, to assist in the training, guidance, and coaching she will need in her first position.
12. Winston Lewis, M. D. is very active in his State Medical Society; the ____________________ has resulted in beneficial and long-lasting social, business, and professional relationships.
13. Liz Corbin, CMA, submitted a ______________________________ to her current employer when she decided to leave her present position to return to school to pursue an advanced degree.
14. Office manager Marilyn Johnson will inform all of the job applicants that they will be on ____________________ for their first six months on the job. During this time period, the employee and supervisory personnel can determine if the environment and the position are satisfactory for the employee.
15. Office manager Jane O'Hara, updating the employee manual, includes a ____________________ for every position in the office that details tasks, duties, and responsibilities.

Learning Review

1. The manual that identifies clear guidelines and directions required of all employees is known as the policy manual. What are four topics that would be included in a policy manual regardless of the size of the practice or specific problems that are to be addressed?

(1) ______________________________

(2) ______________________________

(3) ______________________________

(4) ______________________________

2. Office manager Marilyn Johnson has the responsibility of dismissing an employee for a serious violation of office policies. From the list below, select key points to keep in mind when dismissal is necessary by circling the letters of the statements that apply.

A. Have employee pack his or her belongings from desk.
B. The dismissal should be made in private.
C. Take no longer than twenty minutes for the dismissal.
D. Be direct, firm, and to the point in identifying reasons.
E. Explain terms of dismissal (keys, clearing out area, final paperwork).
F. Do not listen to the employee's opinion and emotions.
G. If he or she insists, allow the employee to finish the work of the day.
H. Do not engage in an in-depth discussion of performance.

3. The job description must have enough information to provide both the supervisor and the employee with a clear outline of what the job entails. Name four items that must be included in a job description.

(1) ______________ (3) ______________

(2) ______________ (4) ______________

4. The interview worksheet is an excellent tool to make certain that the interviews with each candidate are fair and equitable. Provide six items that should be included on any interview worksheet.

(1) ______________ (4) ______________

(2) ______________ (5) ______________

(3) ______________ (6) ______________

Investigation Activity

GENERAL SELF-PERFORMANCE RATING

Complete this self-performance review to evaluate your rate of performance as a medical assisting student.

Performance Definitions:

5 = Outstanding	Superior performance
4 = Above Standard	Commendable performance
3 = Standard	Competent and consistent performance
2 = Below Standard	Performance needs improvement
1 = Unsatisfactory	Performance is unacceptable

General Criteria	Rating	Comments Supporting Rating
1. *Patient Relations:* How well do you communicate a "we care" image to patients, visitors, health care professionals, fellow students, and the instructor?		
2. *Work Responsibilities:* What is the quality of your student work relative to quality, quantity, and timeliness?		
3. *Teamwork:* Do you have a team spirit? Do you interact well with other students and the instructor?		
4. *Adaptability:* Are you open to change and new ideas? Are you flexible to changes in routine, workload, or assignments?		
5. *Personal Appearance:* Do you maintain a professional and appropriate personal appearance, including attire and hygiene?		
6. *Communications:* Do you communicate well? Is information given and received clearly? Do you have good verbal skills? written skills?		
7. *Dependability:* Can you be relied upon for good attendance? Do you perform and follow through on work without supervisory intervention and assistance?		

TOTAL = ____________

24 points and higher = above standard performance
20 to 23 points = competent performance
19 points and below = below standard performance

CASE STUDY

Since the offices of Drs. Lewis & King have expanded to cover a rapidly growing patient load, including the hiring of a co-office manager and a new clinical medical assistant, the work pace has been hectic, but challenging. At the suggestion of Dr. Lewis, the office managers decide to hold a staff meeting to talk about ways to keep the lines of communication open and process the many changes occurring at the growing medical practice. Marilyn Johnson and Shirley Brooks encourage staff to be vocal with their feedback, suggestions, and concerns.

Discuss the following:

1. What other techniques can the office managers use to prevent or solve conflicts in the workplace during this period of growth and transition?
2. Why is effective communication one of the most important goals of the human resources manager?

SUPPLEMENTARY RESOURCES

Study Guide Disks: Additional practice exercises for this chapter are available on the study guide disks found in the back of the textbook.

Medical Assisting Videos: Appropriate content is available on Delmar's Medical Assisting Videos, 2nd ed., on the following topics:

Tape 1: Work As a Team Member
Career-seeking Skills
Communication Skills
Tape 3: Perform Administrative Duties
Triage Skills

SKILLS COMPETENCY ASSESSMENT

Procedure 39–1: Develop and Maintain a Policy Manual

Student's Name: ______________________ Date: __________

Objective: To develop and maintain a comprehensive, up-to-date policy manual of all office policies relating to employee practices, benefits, office conduct, and so on.

Conditions: The student demonstrates the ability to develop and maintain a comprehensive, up-to-date policy manual of all office policies using the following equipment and supplies: computer or electronic typewriter, binder, paper, standard policy manual format.

Accuracy Standards: Points assigned reflect importance of step to meeting objective: Important = (5) Essential = (10) Critical = (15). Automatic failure results if any of the **critical** tasks are omitted or performed incorrectly.

SKILLS ASSESSMENT CHECKLIST

Task Performed	Possible Points	TASKS
❑	15	Follows office format, develops precise, written office policies detailing all necessary information pertaining to the staff and their positions. Ensures that the information includes benefits, vacation, sick leave, hours, dress codes, evaluations, rules of conduct, and grounds for dismissal.
❑	15	Identifies procedures for reimbursing overtime, preventing discrimination and harassment, creating a safe working environment, and allowing for jury duty.
❑	10	Includes a policy statement related to smoking.
❑	15	Identifies steps to follow should an employee become disabled during employment.
❑	10	Determines what employee opportunities for continuing education, if any, will be reimbursed; includes requirements for recertification or licensure.
❑	10	Provides a copy of the policy manual for each employee.
❑	10	Reviews and updates the policy manual regularly. Adds or deletes items as necessary, dating each revised page.
❑	15	Results obtained were accurate.

______	Earned	ADD POINTS OF TASKS CHECKED
100	Points	TOTAL POINTS POSSIBLE
______	SCORE	DETERMINE SCORE (divide points earned by total points possible, multiply results by 100)

Actual Student Time Needed to Complete Procedure: __________

Student's Initials: __________ Instructor's Initials: __________ Grade: __________

Suggestions for Improvement: ______________________

Evaluator's Name (print) ______________________

Evaluator's Signature ______________________

Comments ______________________

SKILLS COMPETENCY ASSESSMENT

Procedure 39–2: Preparing a Job Description

Student's Name: ______________________________ Date: __________

Objective: To provide a precise definition of the tasks assigned to a job, to determine the expectations and level of competency required, and to specify the experience, training, and education needed to perform the job for purposes of recruiting and performance evaluation.

Conditions: The student demonstrates the ability to prepare a complete and precise job description using the following equipment and supplies: computer or electronic typewriter, paper, standard job description format.

Time Requirements and Accuracy Standards: 60 minutes. Points assigned reflect importance of step to meeting objective: Important = (5) Essential = (10) Critical = (15). Automatic failure results if any of the **critical** tasks are omitted or performed incorrectly.

SKILLS ASSESSMENT CHECKLIST

Task Performed	Possible Points	TASKS
❑	10	Details each task that creates a job.
❑	10	Lists special medical, technical, or clerical skills required.
❑	15	Determines the level of education, training, and experience required for the position.
❑	15	Determines where the job fits into the overall structure of the office.
❑	10	Specifies any unusual working conditions (hours, locations, etc.) that may apply.
❑	5	Describes career path opportunities.
❑	5	Completed the tasks within 60 minutes.
❑	15	Results obtained were accurate.

_______	Earned	ADD POINTS OF TASKS CHECKED
85	Points	TOTAL POINTS POSSIBLE
_______	SCORE	DETERMINE SCORE (divide points earned by total points possible, multiply results by 100)

Actual Student Time Needed to Complete Procedure: __________

Student's Initials: __________ Instructor's Initials: __________ Grade: __________

Suggestions for Improvement: ______________________________

____

Evaluator's Name (print) ______________________________

Evaluator's Signature ______________________________

Comments ______________________________

SKILLS COMPETENCY ASSESSMENT

Procedure 39–3: Interviewing

Student's Name: ______________________________ Date: ____________

Objective: To screen applicants for training, experience, and characteristics to select the best candidate to fill the vacant position.

Conditions: The student demonstrates the ability to interview candidates using the following equipment and supplies: resumes, interview worksheets, notepad.

Time Requirements and Accuracy Standards: 60 minutes. Points assigned reflect importance of step to meeting objective: Important = (5) Essential = (10) Critical = (15). Automatic failure results if any of the **critical** tasks are omitted or performed incorrectly.

SKILLS ASSESSMENT CHECKLIST

Task Performed	Possible Points	TASKS
❑	5	Reviews resumes and applications received.
❑	10	Selects candidates who most closely match the education and experience being sought.
❑	15	Creates an interview worksheet for each candidate, listing points to cover.
❑	5	Selects an interview team; makes sure this team includes the human resources or office manager and the immediate supervisor to whom the candidate will report.
❑	5	Calls personally to schedule interviews to judge the applicant's telephone manner and voice.
❑	15	Reminds the interviewers of various legal restrictions concerning questions to be asked.
❑	10	Conducts interviews in a private, quiet setting.
❑	5	Puts the applicant at ease by beginning with an overview about the practice and staff, briefly describing the job and answering preliminary questions.
❑	10	Asks questions about the applicant's work experience and educational background, using the resume and interview worksheet as a guide.
❑	10	Provides the most promising applicants with additional information on benefits and a tour of the office, if practical.
❑	5	Discusses the applicant's general salary requirements, but avoids discussion of a specific salary until a formal offer is tendered.
❑	10	Informs the applicant when a decision will be made and thanks the applicant for participating in the interview.
❑	5	Does not make a job offer until all the candidates have been interviewed.

SKILLS COMPETENCY ASSESSMENT — continued

Procedure 39–3: Interviewing

Task Performed	Possible Points	TASKS
❑	15	Checks references of all prospective employees.
❑	15	Establishes a second interview between the physician-employer(s) and the qualified candidate, if necessary.
❑	15	Confirms accepted job offers in writing, specifying details of the offer and acceptance.
❑	15	Notifies all unsuccessful applicants by letter when the position has been filled.
❑	5	Completed the tasks within 60 minutes.
❑	15	Results obtained were accurate.

______	Earned	ADD POINTS OF TASKS CHECKED
190	Points	TOTAL POINTS POSSIBLE
______	SCORE	DETERMINE SCORE (divide points earned by total points possible, multiply results by 100)

Actual Student Time Needed to Complete Procedure: __________

Student's Initials: __________ Instructor's Initials: __________ Grade: __________

Suggestions for Improvement: ______________________________

____

____

____

Evaluator's Name (print) ______________________________

Evaluator's Signature ______________________________

Comments ______________________________

SKILLS COMPETENCY ASSESSMENT

Procedure 39–4: Orient and Train Personnel

Student's Name: ______________________________ Date: ____________

Objective: To acquaint new employees with office policies, staff, what the job encompasses, procedures to be performed, and job performance expectations.

Conditions: The student demonstrates the ability to orient and train personnel using the following equipment and supplies: office policy and procedures manual, employee-related documents.

Time Requirements and Accuracy Standards: 60 minutes. Points assigned reflect importance of step to meeting objective: Important = (5) Essential = (10) Critical = (15). Automatic failure results if any of the **critical** tasks are omitted or performed incorrectly.

SKILLS ASSESSMENT CHECKLIST

Task Performed	Possible Points	TASKS
☐	5	Tours the facility and introduces the office staff.
☐	10	Completes employee-related documents and explains their purposes.
☐	5	Explains the benefits programs.
☐	5	Presents the office policy manual and discusses its key elements.
☐	5	Reviews federal and state regulatory precautions for medical facilities.
☐	5	Reviews the job description.
☐	15	Explains and demonstrates procedures to be performed and the use of procedure manuals supporting these procedures.
☐	10	Demonstrates the use of office equipment.
☐	15	Assigns a mentor from the staff to help with the orientation.
☐	5	Completed the tasks within 60 minutes.
☐	15	Results obtained were accurate.

______	Earned	ADD POINTS OF TASKS CHECKED
95	Points	TOTAL POINTS POSSIBLE
______	SCORE	DETERMINE SCORE (divide points earned by total points possible, multiply results by 100)

Actual Student Time Needed to Complete Procedure: ____________

Student's Initials: ____________ Instructor's Initials: ____________ Grade: ____________

Suggestions for Improvement: ______________________________

Evaluator's Name (print) ______________________________

Evaluator's Signature ______________________________

Comments ______________________________

EVALUATION OF CHAPTER KNOWLEDGE

How has your instructor evaluated the knowledge you have achieved?

	Instructor Evaluation		
Knowledge	*Good*	*Average*	*Poor*
Possesses the ability to describe the role of the human resources manager	_____	_____	_____
Explains the function of the office policy manual	_____	_____	_____
Identifies methods of recruiting employees for a medical practice	_____	_____	_____
Relates the interview process	_____	_____	_____
Describes appropriate evaluation tools for employees	_____	_____	_____
Recalls dismissal procedures	_____	_____	_____
Identifies items in employee personnel files	_____	_____	_____
Defines laws relating to personnel management	_____	_____	_____
Understands effective strategies for conflict resolution	_____	_____	_____

Student's Initials: ______ Instructor's Initials: ______

Grade: _______

CHAPTER 40

Preparing For Externship

PERFORMANCE OBJECTIVE

Medical assisting is a fast-growing profession, as all health-related occupations experience a surge in employment that is expected to continue for many years. The externship is an important part of the complete training program for medical assisting students, serving as a transition between the classroom and employment in an ambulatory care facility. In a professional health care setting, students see how classroom learning applies, while gaining additional knowledge from experience "on the job."

EXERCISES AND ACTIVITIES

Vocabulary Builder

Match the key vocabulary terms to the aspect of externship that applies.

_____ 1. Accreditation
_____ 2. Career orientation objective
_____ 3. Combination placement
_____ 4. Conditions
_____ 5. Council on Accreditation of Allied Health Education Programs (CAAHEP)
_____ 6. Criterion
_____ 7. Evaluation
_____ 8. Externship
_____ 9. Human relations objective
_____ 10. One-site placement
_____ 11. Performance objectives
_____ 12. Rotation
_____ 13. Skills acquisition objectives
_____ 14. Skills application/development objective

A. The level of acceptable performance.
B. Related to improving communication and interpersonal skills.
C. Related to one's personal career goal or career growth.
D. Concerned with development of new on-the-job skills or learning new tasks or concepts.
E. What is expected to be performed to demonstrate accomplishment.

F. Ensures quality education programs for allied health professions.
G. Assessment; significance or value of a situation.
H. Statements of the circumstances under which the objective will be achieved, and with what supplies and equipment.
I. Utilizes school's health services facility and/or advisory committee representatives.
J. Externship completed in only one facility.
K. A national, voluntary, specialized, not-for-profit corporation.
L. Improvement and development of skills already learned.
M. Transition stage between the classroom and actual employment; may also be referred to as internship or co-operative education.
N. Opportunity to spend two or three weeks in a variety of health care settings.

Learning Review

1. Although some variations will exist depending on the school, there are three main types of externship programs available to medical assisting students. In the space below, identify each type of program.

   (1) ______________ (2) ______________ (3) ______________

   Which type of externship do you find the most interesting and challenging? Why?

   ____

   ____

2. With proper planning and supervision, the externship experience should be mutually beneficial to both the externship site and the student/trainee. What are four benefits the student/trainee may receive from the externship experience?

   (1) ____
   (2) ____
   (3) ____
   (4) ____

   What are four benefits that the externship site/facility may receive from the student externship experience?

   (1) ____
   (2) ____
   (3) ____
   (4) ____

3. The ______________________________(CAAHEP) is a national, non-profit corporation providing accreditation and other related coordination services to ensure that allied health professionals receive quality education programs. The sites selected for externship should include ______________, ______________, and ______________ areas to provide a full range of experience. The site of first choice is the office or clinic of a

____. The site of second choice is the office of a ____. The site of third choice is ____________________.

4. The student/trainee must always realize that the externship experience is akin to employment. The externship should be treated as an employment situation, not a classroom experience. Name four ways the student/trainee can show responsibility within the externship environment.

(1)______________________________ (3) ______________________________

(2)______________________________ (4) ______________________________

5. Which of the following statements would correctly describe the externship experience? Circle the correct response(s).

A. The medical assisting student will not receive pay for the externship experience.
B. The student should be placed in an office in lieu of regular office personnel.
C. The physician in the externship office must be willing to devote his or her time to ensuring that the extern receives a broad exposure to all facets of the practice.
D. A minimum of three visits and one telephone call will be made to the facility by the coordinator of the externship program during the student's/trainee's training.

Investigation Activity

To begin the process of choosing the right externship for you, complete the form below to consider the factors that will affect your decision—including the location of the practice, a comparison of your schedule and the practice's business hours, and the type of practice you would find most challenging and exciting for the externship experience. All of these factors impact upon the success of the externship experience for both the student and the externship facility. Consider your responses carefully.

Medical Assistant Externship — Preliminary Participant Information

NAME:__________ PROGRAM:__________
STREET ADDRESS: __________ PHONE: __________
CITY, STATE, ZIP: ____________________
DO YOU HAVE RELIABLE TRANSPORTATION? __________
DO YOU RELY ON THE METRO BUS SYSTEM? __________
ARE YOU EMPLOYED OUTSIDE OF SCHOOL? ______ WHERE? __________
WILL THIS EMPLOYMENT CONTINUE WHEN WORK EXPERIENCE BEGINS? __________
WHAT ARE YOUR WORK HOURS? __________
Days Per Week Hours
ARE THESE HOURS FLEXIBLE? __________
CAN YOU WORK SHIFT HOURS? __________
CAN YOU WORK WEEKENDS? __________

WHAT TYPE OF FACILITY AND WHAT CITY DO YOU PREFER FOR WORK EXPERIENCE?
____
____
____

Keep in mind that externship hours are considered educational service rather than paid service. The accrediting agencies state that students be placed in facilities where they can receive the best all-around training in clinical, administrative, and general responsibilities.

____

OFFICE USE ONLY

PLACEMENT: __________
ADDRESS: __________ PHONE: __________
____
HOURS AVAILABLE FOR STUDENT: __________
SUPERVISOR: __________

CASE STUDY

Michelle Lucas is preparing for externship. Michelle is an excellent student, detail-oriented, responsible, and professional in her dress and attitude. Michelle is eager to do her externship with a large general practice or clinic with open hours built into the schedule for emergency patients, such as Inner City Health Care. Michelle is intrigued by the idea of working with a group of physicians and a diverse patient population where she can really work on improving her triage skills. Michelle, however, is shy and quiet; she has difficulty meeting new people and relies on a core group of friends.

Discuss the following:

1. Is Michelle really suited to externship at Inner City Health Care? What are the potential advantages or disadvantages of this externship placement?
2. Consider your own short- and long-range goals. How important is it to challenge yourself, personally and professionally, with experiences that contribute to your growth and knowledge? How can you use your externship placement to work toward fulfilling your goals?

SUPPLEMENTARY RESOURCES

Study Guide Disks: Additional practice exercises for this chapter are available on the student practice disks found in the textbook.

Medical Assisting Videos: Appropriate content is available on Delmar's Medical Assisting Videos, 2nd ed., Tape 1, on the following topics:

Career-seeking Skills
Examinations and Certification through AAMA
Explanation of DACUM
Communication Skills

EVALUATION OF CHAPTER KNOWLEDGE

How has your instructor evaluated the knowledge you have achieved?

	Instructor Evaluation		
Knowledge	*Good*	*Average*	*Poor*
Understands externship opportunities available to students	____	____	____
Understands requirements of the externship as a component of the requirements needed for graduation from a CAAHEP-accredited education program	____	____	____
Recognizes and applies concept of performance objectives in setting and achieving goals	____	____	____
Describes CAAHEP's role in externship	____	____	____
Explores the benefits of externship as a learning and growth experience that will help prepare the student for a professional medical assisting career	____	____	____
Displays professionalism	____	____	____

Student's Initials: ______ Instructor's Initials: ______

Grade: ________

CHAPTER 41

Preparing For Medical Assisting Credentials

PERFORMANCE OBJECTIVES

Certification provides established, consistent criteria for evaluating the professional competence of a medical assistant. The certification examination is offered by the American Association of Medical Assistants (AAMA). An individual who successfully passes the exam is awarded the Certified Medical Assistant (CMA) credential. In addition, the American Medical Technologists (AMT) organization conducts the examination that leads to the Registered Medical Assistant (RMA) credential. Certification is an important part of professional development and is highly valued by employers in the health care workplace. Use this workbook chapter to determine the specifics of the certification process.

EXERCISES AND ACTIVITIES

Vocabulary Builder

Match each key vocabulary term to the aspect of the certification process that best describes it.

______ **1.** Certification Examination

______ **2.** Certified Medical Assistant (CMA)

______ **3.** Continuing Education Units (CEUs)

______ **4.** National Board of Medical Examiners (NBME)

______ **5.** Recertification

______ **6.** Registered Medical Assistant (RMA)

______ **7.** Revalidation

______ **8.** Task Force for Test Construction

A. Maintaining current RMA status.
B. Method for earning points toward recertification.
C. A standardized means of evaluating medical assistant competency.
D. Maintaining current CMA status.
E. Credential awarded for successfully passing the Certification Examination.
F. Committee of professionals whose responsibility is to update the CMA exam annually to reflect changes in medical assistants' responsibilities, and to include new developments in medical knowledge and technology.
G. Credential awarded for successfully passing the AMT Examination.
H. Consultants for the Certification Examination.

Learning Review

1. The AAMA Certification Examination is a comprehensive test of the knowledge actually utilized in today's medical office. The test is updated annually to include the latest changes in medical assistants' daily responsibilities. In addition, the updates include the latest developments in medical knowledge and technology. Name the three major areas tested in the Certification Examination and describe what each includes.

   (1) ______________________________

   (2) ______________________________

   (3) ______________________________

2. A. Health care professionals today should maintain a lifelong commitment to

   ____

   B. To keep their ____________________ current, CMAs are required to recertify every

   ____________________.

   C. A total of ________ points is necessary to recertify the basic CMA credential.

   D. Continuing education courses are offered by ______________________________ groups.

3. A. What is the address and telephone number for obtaining an application for the Certification Examination?

   ____

   ____

   B. What guide for the Certification Examination is available from the AAMA?

   ____

   C. What program and what bimonthly publication does the AAMA make available to members who are interested in pursuing continuing education credits?

   Program ______________________________

   Publication ______________________________

Investigation Activity

The *Candidate's Guide to the AAMA Certification Examination* contains a sample 120-question examination that can help students prepare for the actual certification examination. Write to the AAMA to request this booklet and take the sample test at least three months before you are scheduled to take the Certification Examination. Use your score on the practice examination to determine areas for extra study and focus. Form a study group with students who are also preparing for the examination and who share your special study needs.

CASE STUDY

Michele Lucas is performing an externship at Inner City Health Care under the direction of office manager Jane O'Hara. Michele has purchased a certification review study guide and has taken the sample 120-question Certification Examination available from the AAMA. From her studies, she has determined that she needs more work in the area of collections and insurance processing. Part-time administrative medical assistant Karen Ritter is responsible for these duties at Inner City Health Care, under Jane's supervision.

Discuss the following:

1. How can Michele use her externship experience to help her concentrate on improving her skills in the area of collections and insurance processing?
2. What are your own personal strengths and weaknesses in preparing for the CMA Certification Examination? What can you do to improve your areas of weakness?

SUPPLEMENTARY RESOURCES

Study Guide Disks: Additional practice exercises for this chapter are available on the student practice disks found in the textbook.

Medical Assisting Videos: Appropriate content is available on Delmar's Medical Assisting Videos, 2nd ed., Tape 1,on the following topics:

Examinations and Certification through AAMA
RMA/AMT

EVALUATION OF CHAPTER KNOWLEDGE

How has your instructor evaluated the knowledge you have achieved?

	Instructor Evaluation		
Knowledge	*Good*	*Average*	*Poor*
Describes approved methods of training	_____	_____	_____
Differentiates between being certified and being registered	_____	_____	_____
Identifies the benefits of certification	_____	_____	_____
Understands the qualifications to sit for the AAMA Certification Examination	_____	_____	_____
Knows when the AAMA Certification Examination is offered and the registration deadlines	_____	_____	_____
Describes methods for obtaining CEUs	_____	_____	_____
Understands the recertification process and its importance	_____	_____	_____
Understands the importance of enhancing skills through continuing education and the importance of maintaining professional growth throughout the career as a medical assistant	_____	_____	_____

Student's Initials: ______ Instructor's Initials: ______

Grade: _______

CHAPTER 42

Employment Strategies

PERFORMANCE OBJECTIVES

Once medical assisting students have completed their studies, it is time for them to start a career in their chosen field. There are various employment strategies that will greatly aid in obtaining a quality position in an ambulatory care setting. It is important that the job applicant adopt a strategy for job finding that includes self-assessment, job analysis and research, and budgetary needs analysis. In addition, there are several techniques that can make a difference in the success of the job-finding mission. Resume preparation is one of the essential ingredients of the job hunt. A well-constructed resume summarizing your work, education, and volunteer experience will make a vital connection in the interviewer's mind between what you can do and how these skills can benefit the organization. The construction of the cover letter or completion of the application form is also an important step in the success of the job-search process. The cover letter introduces the applicant to the potential employer with the goal of obtaining an interview. Once you have obtained an interview, you can prepare for it by learning what to expect in an interview and how to increase your chances for success.

EXERCISES AND ACTIVITIES

Vocabulary Builder

Match each key vocabulary term to the aspect of the job-seeking process that best describes it.

_____ 1. Accomplishment statements

_____ 2. Application form

_____ 3. Application/cover letter

_____ 4. Bullet point

_____ 5. Career objective

_____ 6. Chronological resume

_____ 7. Contact tracker

_____ 8. Functional resume

_____ 9. Interview

_____ 10. Power verbs

_____ 11. References

_____ 12. Resume

_____ 13. Targeted resume

A. Expresses your career goal and the position for which you are applying.
B. Resume format used to highlight specialty areas of accomplishments and strengths.
C. A form devised by a prospective employer to collect information relative to qualifications, education, and experience in employment.
D. Individuals who have known or worked with you long enough to make an honest assessment and recommendation regarding your background history.
E. Resume format utilized when focusing on a clear, specific job.
F. A statement that begins with a power verb and gives a brief description of what you did, and the demonstrable results that were produced.
G. Asterisk or dot followed by a descriptive phrase.
H. A written summary data sheet or brief account of your qualifications and progress in your chosen career.
I. Action words used to describe your attributes and strengths.
J. A letter used to introduce yourself and your resume to a prospective employer with the goal of obtaining an interview.
K. Resume format used when you have employment experience.
L. A meeting in which you discuss employment opportunities and strengths that you can bring to the organization.
M. Form used to keep track of employment contact information, such as name of employer, name of contact person, address and telephone number, date of first contact, resume sent, interview date, and follow-up information and dates.

Learning Review

1. A variety of references should be included on your resume or listed on a separate sheet of paper that closely matches your resume. Give the appropriate response to the following questions:
   A. Choose references who are well-respected and are ______________________.
   B. List three types of professional references that would make excellent reference choices.
   (1) ______________ (2) ______________ (3) ______________
   Identify someone you know or have contact with who fits each professional reference type listed above.
   (1) ______________ (2) ______________ (3) ______________

2. There are various styles of resumes that can be used depending on your employment strengths and abilities. Each particular style has advantages and disadvantages; and can be used singly or in combination. In some cases, a medical facility may prefer a certain resume style.
   A. Identify situations when using a targeted resume is advantageous by circling the number next to the statements that apply.
   (1) You are just starting your career and have little experience, but you know what you want and you are clear about your capabilities.
   (2) You want to use one resume for several different applications.
   (3) You are not clear about your abilities and accomplishments.
   (4) You can go in several directions, and you want a different resume for each.
   (5) You are able to keep your resume on a computer disk.

B. Identify the situations in which using a chronological resume is advantageous by circling the number next to the statements that apply.
   (1) You have been in the same job for many years.
   (2) Your job history shows real growth and development.
   (3) You are trained and employed in highly traditional fields (health care, government).
   (4) You are looking for your first job.
   (5) You are staying in the same field as prior jobs.

C. Identify the situations in which using a functional resume is advantageous by circling the number next to the statements that apply.
   (1) You have extensive specialized experience.
   (2) Your most recent employers have been highly prestigious.
   (3) You have had a variety of different, apparently unconnected, work experiences.
   (4) You want to emphasize a management growth pattern.
   (5) Much of your work has been volunteer, freelance, or temporary.

3. If you are sending your resume to a potential employer, you will need to mail a cover letter with it. A well-written cover letter introduces you, tells the reader why you are writing and what you are sending, highlights your qualifications and experience, and enhances the information on your resume. There are numerous guidelines to follow when writing a cover letter for submission to a potential employer. List four guidelines that are essential when preparing an effective cover letter.
   (1) ______________________________
   (2) ______________________________
   (3) ______________________________
   (4) ______________________________

4. When Ellen Armstrong, CMA, began her job search she encountered several employers that required her to complete an application form. Ellen could recall six points that were particularly important when filling out a job application. List four items that are important when completing a job application.
   (1) ______________________________
   (2) ______________________________
   (3) ______________________________
   (4) ______________________________

5. A. Bob Thompson has an interview at Inner City Health Care for a new clinical medical assisting position. He is confident he has prepared well for the interview. On the way to the interview, Bob reminds himself of three principles he has learned about interviewing.
   (1) ____________________ before answering questions, trying to provide the information requested in a ____________________ manner.
   (2) ____________________ carefully so that you understand what information the interviewer is requesting.
   (3) ____________________ for ____________________ if you are uncertain.

B. Bob Thompson also recalls that it is not appropriate to ask questions about certain subjects during a first interview, but instead to concentrate on the value and skills one can contribute to the organization. Name four items you should not ask questions about in a first interview:

(1) ______________________ (3) ______________________

(2) ______________________ (4) ______________________

Investigation Activity

Power words are essential tools when preparing your resume for prospective employers. Using verbs that engage the reader brings confidence and focus to your achievements, knowledge, and skills. In the spaces provided below, use power words to describe ten different aspects of your personality, experience, or accomplishments that may be relevant in formulating your professional resume. Choose a new power word for each accomplishment statement that you compose.

1. ______________________
2. ______________________
3. ______________________
4. ______________________
5. ______________________
6. ______________________
7. ______________________
8. ______________________
9. ______________________
10. ______________________

CASE STUDY

You are the subject of this case study. Complete the Self-Evaluation Worksheet that follows. Use your answers to help you determine the working environment you are most interested in and suited for. The worksheet can become a useful tool when researching prospective employers to target for your exciting first job in the medical assisting profession.

SUPPLEMENTARY RESOURCES

Study Guide Disks: Additional practice exercises for this chapter are available on the study guide disks found in the back of the textbook.

Medical Assisting Videos: Appropriate content is available on Delmar's Medical Assisting Videos, 2nd ed., Tape 1, on the following topics:

Your Career As a Medical Assistant
Display Professionalism
Career-seeking Skills
Communication Skills

SELF-EVALUATION WORK SHEET

Respond to the following questions honestly and sincerely. They are meant to assist you in self-assessment.

1. List your three strongest attributes as related to people, data, or things.
   i.e.; Interpersonal skills related to people
   Accuracy related to data
   Mechanical ability related to things
   ______________ related to ______________
   ______________ related to ______________
   ______________ related to ______________
2. List your three weakest attributes as related to people, data, or things.
   ______________ related to ______________
   ______________ related to ______________
   ______________ related to ______________
3. How do you express yourself? excellent, good, fair, poor
   Orally ______________ In Writing ______________
4. Do you work well as a leader of a group or team? Yes ______ No ______
5. Do you prefer to work alone and on your own? Yes ______ No ______
6. Can you work under stress/pressure? Yes ______ No ______
7. Do you enjoy new ideas and situations? Yes ______ No ______
8. Are you comfortable with routines/schedules? Yes ______ No ______
9. Which work setting do you prefer?
   Single-physician setting ______ Multiple-physician setting ______
   Small clinic setting ______ Large clinic setting ______
   Single specialty setting ______ Multi-specialty setting ______
10. Are you willing to relocate? ______ Willing to travel? ______

EVALUATION OF CHAPTER KNOWLEDGE

How has your instructor evaluated the knowledge you have achieved?

Knowledge	**Instructor Evaluation** *Good*	*Average*	*Poor*
Possesses the ability to name the steps of job analysis and research	_____	_____	_____
Describes the function and use of a contact tracker	_____	_____	_____
Differentiates among chronological, functional, and targeted resumes	_____	_____	_____
Implements power words to compose accomplishment statements for resumes	_____	_____	_____
Identifies the purpose and content of a cover letter	_____	_____	_____
Demonstrates effective behavior during interview sessions	_____	_____	_____
Understands the importance of displaying professionalism	_____	_____	_____
Identifies benefits of follow-up letters	_____	_____	_____
Utilizes self-assessment techniques to determine optimal employment goals	_____	_____	_____

Student's Initials: _____ Instructor's Initials: _____

Grade: _______

Study Guide Software Instructions

MINIMUM SYSTEM REQUIREMENTS

486 or better
8 Mb RAM
Windows 3.1 or Windows 95
Graphics adapter sVGA, 640 × 480, 256 colors, small fonts mode

INSTALLING THE CMA PROGRAM

Before you use the *Comprehensive Medical Assisting Software* (CMA), you must install it on your hard disk. The installer decompresses and copies files from the *Comprehensive Medical Assisting* floppy disks onto your hard disk and creates a Comprehensive Medical Assisting program group. Before installing the program, make a back-up copy of the *Comprehensive Medical Assisting* disks. Then install the program using your back-up copies:

1. Insert the *Comprehensive Medical Assisting* Program Disk 1 into your floppy drive.
2. At the Windows Program Manager, choose **Run** from the File menu.
   Note: Although CMA is designed to run on Windows 3.1, it also runs on Windows 95. If you are installing CMA on a Windows 95 system, open the Start menu and choose **Run** to begin the installation.
3. In the Command Line blank, type **a:\install** (where "a:" represents your floppy drive). Click on **OK.**
4. In the Select Installation Drive dialog box, select the hard disk where you want to install the software and click **OK.**
5. On the command line in the Installation Directory dialog box, type the name of the directory where you want to install the software. The default location is **C:\CMA**. After you type a location, click on **OK.** If you specify a new directory (that is, one that does not yet exist), the installer creates the new directory.
6. The installer now copies files onto your hard disk. When all files from Program Disk 1 are copied, the installer prompts you to switch disks. Insert the next program disk into your floppy drive and click on **OK.**

7. A dialog box asks you to select the location for saving your data. Choose one of the following options and click on **OK:**
   - **Save data in CMA directory:** Choose this option if you are going to store your work in the directory where you are installing CMA.
   - **Save data on A:\:** Choose this option if you are going to store your work on a floppy disk.
   - **Save data to other location:** Choose this option if you are going to store you work in a different location. If you choose Other, the next dialog box asks you to specify a location for your data: type the full path to where you want to store your work, then click on **OK.**

   Note: The installer adds the full path to your data location at the end of the Command Line for the CMA program icon. For example, if you specify the **A:** drive for data storage and you view the properties of the CMA program icon, you will see **C:\CMA\CMA.EXE -C A:** in the Command Line (where **C:** is your hard disk and **\CMA** the directory where you installed CMA). The only time you would need to change the Command Line is if you decide, after installing CMA, that you want to store files in a different location.
8. An information dialog box tells you that installation is complete. Click on **OK.** You are now back at the Program Manager, with your new Delmar's CMA program group open on your desktop.

Note: If CMA is installed on a network drive, the system administrator will need to create a program icon at each workstation on the network that will be using the CMA software. Follow the instructions in your Windows User's Manual for creating an icon.

NETWORK INSTALLATION AND OPERATION

Installing *Comprehensive Medical Assisting Software* (CMA) on a network is the same as installing the program on a local hard disk. Follow the procedures outlined in "Installing the CMA Program" specifying a network drive instead of a stand-alone hard drive. To log on and run CMA on a network, the student follows the same procedures outlined in "Starting the Program" and "Working on CMA Exercises."

STARTING THE PROGRAM

1. Start Windows and open the *Delmar's CMA* program group.
2. Double-click on the *Delmar's CMA* icon.
3. The title screen displays. The log-on procedure varies according to whether or not you have logged on previously.

Initial Log-On:

If this is your first time using CMA, you need to register yourself as follows:

a In the Students dialog box, click on **New Student.**

b. In the New Student dialog box, type your first name, last name, class name (optional), and a password (up to 8 characters, with no spaces). Use the mouse or the **Tab** key to move from one field to the next.

c. When your information is complete and correct, click on **OK** or press **Enter.** In the Verify Password dialog box, retype your password and click on **OK** or press **Enter.**

d. The Main Menu displays.
   - Choose a unit by clicking on the unit's name in the list to the left. When you select a unit, its chapters appear in a list to the right.
   - Choose a chapter by clicking on the chapter's name. When you select a chapter, its exercises appear as buttons at the bottom of the screen.
   - Choose an exercise by clicking on its button.

Subsequent Log On

When you return to CMA after your initial log-on:

a. Double-click on your name in the Students dialog box or highlight your name and click on **Select.**

b. Enter your password in the Password dialog box and click on **OK** or press **Enter.**

c. If you have forgotten your password, click on the **Exit** button to close the program and use another variation of your name with a new password *that you won't forget* or inform your instructor so he or she can contact Delmar Customer Support.

If you were working on an exercise that you did not complete when you exited the program previously, a Bookmark dialog box tells you where you left off and allows you to go to the beginning of that exercise, to the particular question you last worked with, or to the Main Menu. If you were not in the middle of an exercise when you exited the program previously, CMA takes you to the Main Menu.

WORKING ON CMA EXERCISES

1. Start CMA and log on.
2. Select an exercise to work on.
   - If you were in the middle of an exercise the last time you logged off CMA, a Bookmark dialog box gives you several options. Click on **Continue where you left off** to resume working where you left off, **Return to beginning of the exercise** to go back to the beginning of the exercise you were working on, or **Cancel** to go to the Main Menu (where you can select a different exercise).
   - If you were not in the middle of an exercise the last time you logged off CMA, the program takes you to the Main Menu. Select a unit and chapter, then select an exercise.
3. Answer the questions for the exercise. Use the buttons at the top and bottom of the screen to move around within the program:
   - To return to the Main Menu (to work on a different exercise), click on the **Menu** button at the top of the screen.
   - To get directions for completing the exercise, click on the **Help** button at the top of the screen.
   - To go to the previous or next screen in a multiple choice or short answer exercise, click on the left arrow or right arrow button in the bottom right corner of the screen. In other exercise types, all of the questions will appear on one screen. If you are reviewing a previously

completed exercise, you can click on the buttons displaying the correct answers to review the feedback information.

Note: You will only be able to go to the next screen in an exercise by clicking on the right arrow button if you are reviewing a previously completed exercise. If you are working on a Matching, Graphical Matching, or Graphical Short Answer exercise, the right arrow button will not display since all of the questions appear on a single screen. In these cases you can review previously answered questions by clicking on the question button.

- To exit the program at any time, click on the **Exit** button at the top of the screen.

4. After you have gone through all questions in the exercise, the program scores your work and returns you to the Main Menu. To view a Report of your work on any CMA exercise, use the Report option on the File menu.

REPORT OPTIONS

1. To view a Summary Report of your work in CMA, select the Report option in the File menu.
2. The Summary Report lists, for each exercise worked on, the work date, chapter number, exercise, score, and whether or not the exercise was completed. The Summary Report stores up to 500 records and can be printed by clicking on the **Print** button.
3. You can view a Detailed Report for any line item in the Summary Report by highlighting a Summary Report entry and clicking the **Details** button. The Detailed Report lists the chapter number, exercise, work date, each question number, and your performance on each question. Each question is scored on a three-level scale. You get full credit for the question if you answer it correctly on the first attempt. You get half credit for the question if you answer it on the second try. If you answer it incorrectly on the second attempt, you do not receive any points for the question.

ON-LINE HELP

Context-sensitive Help is available by clicking on the Help button on any screen or window. Clicking on the Help button in an activity screen displays directions on how to complete the activity. The *General Help* option of the Help menu lists all of the topics for which Help is available. You can also select items from this list to view detailed Help text on a particular topic.